Quantitative PET and SPECT

Quantitative PET and SPECT

Editors

Lioe-Fee de Geus-Oei
Floris H. P. van Velden

MDPI • Basel • Beijing • Wuhan • Barcelona • Belgrade • Manchester • Tokyo • Cluj • Tianjin

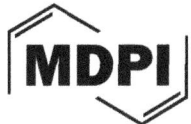

Editors
Lioe-Fee de Geus-Oei
Department of Radiology,
Section of Nuclear Medicine,
Leiden University
Medical Center,
The Netherlands

Floris H. P. van Velden
Department of Radiology,
Section of Medical
Technology, Leiden
University Medical Center,
The Netherlands

Editorial Office
MDPI
St. Alban-Anlage 66
4052 Basel, Switzerland

This is a reprint of articles from the Special Issue published online in the open access journal *Diagnostics* (ISSN 2075-4418) (available at: https://www.mdpi.com/journal/diagnostics/special_issues/Quantitative_PET_SPECT).

For citation purposes, cite each article independently as indicated on the article page online and as indicated below:

LastName, A.A.; LastName, B.B.; LastName, C.C. Article Title. *Journal Name* **Year**, *Volume Number*, Page Range.

ISBN 978-3-0365-5615-4 (Hbk)
ISBN 978-3-0365-5616-1 (PDF)

Cover image courtesy of Sebastiaan ter Burg.

© 2022 by the authors. Articles in this book are Open Access and distributed under the Creative Commons Attribution (CC BY) license, which allows users to download, copy and build upon published articles, as long as the author and publisher are properly credited, which ensures maximum dissemination and a wider impact of our publications.
The book as a whole is distributed by MDPI under the terms and conditions of the Creative Commons license CC BY-NC-ND.

Contents

About the Editors vii

Floris H. P. van Velden and Lioe-Fee de Geus-Oei
Editorial on Special Issue "Quantitative PET and SPECT"
Reprinted from: *Diagnostics* 2022, 12, 1989, doi:10.3390/diagnostics12081989 1

Julian M. M. Rogasch, Frank Hofheinz, Lutz van Heek, Conrad-Amadeus Voltin, Ronald Boellaard and Carsten Kobe
Influences on PET Quantification and Interpretation
Reprinted from: *Diagnostics* 2022, 12, 451, doi:10.3390/diagnostics12020451 5

Sjoerd Rijnsdorp, Mark J. Roef and Albert J. Arends
Impact of the Noise Penalty Factor on Quantification in Bayesian Penalized Likelihood (Q.Clear) Reconstructions of ^{68}Ga-PSMA PET/CT Scans
Reprinted from: *Diagnostics* 2021, 11, 847, doi:10.3390/diagnostics11050847 31

Ching-Ching Yang
Compensating Positron Range Effects of Ga-68 in Preclinical PET Imaging by Using Convolutional Neural Network: A Monte Carlo Simulation Study
Reprinted from: *Diagnostics* 2021, 11, 2275, doi:10.3390/diagnostics11122275 45

Matthew D. Walker, Jonathan I. Gear, Allison J. Craig and Daniel R. McGowan
Effects of Respiratory Motion on Y-90 PET Dosimetry for SIRT
Reprinted from: *Diagnostics* 2022, 12, 194, doi:10.3390/diagnostics12010194 57

Stijn De Schepper, Gopinath Gnanasegaran, John Dickson and Tim Van den Wyngaert
Absolute Quantification in Diagnostic SPECT/CT: The Phantom Premise
Reprinted from: *Diagnostics* 2021, 11, 2333, doi:10.3390/diagnostics11122333 67

Ramsha Iqbal, Lemonitsa H. Mammatas, Tuba Aras, Wouter V. Vogel, Tim van de Brug, Daniela E. Oprea-Lager, Henk M. W. Verheul, Otto S. Hoekstra, Ronald Boellaard and Catharina W. Menke-van der Houven van Oordt
Diagnostic Performance of [^{18}F]FDG PET in Staging Grade 1–2, Estrogen Receptor Positive Breast Cancer
Reprinted from: *Diagnostics* 2021, 11, 1954, doi:10.3390/diagnostics11111954 83

Mark J. Roef, Sjoerd Rijnsdorp, Christel Brouwer, Dirk N. Wyndaele and Albert J. Arends
Evaluation of Quantitative Ga-68 PSMA PET/CT Repeatability of Recurrent Prostate Cancer Lesions Using Both OSEM and Bayesian Penalized Likelihood Reconstruction Algorithms
Reprinted from: *Diagnostics* 2021, 11, 1100, doi:10.3390/diagnostics11061100 97

Yu-Hung Chen, Sung-Chao Chu, Ling-Yi Wang, Tso-Fu Wang, Kun-Han Lue, Chih-Bin Lin, Bee-Song Chang, Dai-Wei Liu, Shu-Hsin Liu and Sheng-Chieh Chan
Prognostic Value of Combing Primary Tumor and Nodal Glycolytic–Volumetric Parameters of ^{18}F-FDG PET in Patients with Non-Small Cell Lung Cancer and Regional Lymph Node Metastasis
Reprinted from: *Diagnostics* 2021, 11, 1065, doi:10.3390/diagnostics11061065 109

Gijsbert M. Kalisvaart, Willem Grootjans, Judith V. M. G. Bovée, Hans Gelderblom, Jos A. van der Hage, Michiel A. J. van de Sande, Floris H. P. van Velden, Johan L. Bloem and Lioe-Fee de Geus-Oei
Prognostic Value of Quantitative [^{18}F]FDG-PET Features in Patients with Metastases from Soft Tissue Sarcoma
Reprinted from: *Diagnostics* 2021, 11, 2271, doi:10.3390/diagnostics11122271 127

Khanyisile N. Hlongwa, Kgomotso M. G. Mokoala, Zvifadzo Matsena-Zingoni, Mariza Vorster and Mike M. Sathekge
The Use of ^{18}F-FDG PET/CT Metabolic Parameters in Predicting Overall Survival in Patients Undergoing Restaging for Malignant Melanoma
Reprinted from: *Diagnostics* 2022, 12, 595, doi:10.3390/diagnostics12030595 139

Wyanne A. Noortman, Dennis Vriens, Charlotte D. Y. Mooij, Cornelis H. Slump, Erik H. Aarntzen, Anouk van Berkel, Henri J. L. M. Timmers, Johan Bussink, Tineke W. H. Meijer, Lioe-Fee de Geus-Oei and Floris H. P. van Velden
The Influence of the Exclusion of Central Necrosis on [^{18}F]FDG PET Radiomic Analysis
Reprinted from: *Diagnostics* 2021, 11, 1296, doi:10.3390/diagnostics11071296 151

Yu-Hua Dean Fang, Jonathan E. McConathy, Talene A. Yacoubian, Yue Zhang, Richard E. Kennedy and David G. Standaert
Image Quantification for TSPO PET with a Novel Image-Derived Input Function Method
Reprinted from: *Diagnostics* 2022, 12, 1161, doi:10.3390/diagnostics12051161 165

Rik Schalbroeck, Lioe-Fee de Geus-Oei, Jean-Paul Selten, Maqsood Yaqub, Anouk Schrantee, Therese van Amelsvoort, Jan Booij and Floris H. P. van Velden
Cerebral [^{18}F]-FDOPA Uptake in Autism Spectrum Disorder and Its Association with Autistic Traits
Reprinted from: *Diagnostics* 2021, 11, 2404, doi:10.3390/diagnostics11122404 181

Christos Sachpekidis, Matthias Türk and Antonia Dimitrakopoulou-Strauss
Quantitative, Dynamic ^{18}F-FDG PET/CT in Monitoring of Smoldering Myeloma: A Case Report
Reprinted from: *Diagnostics* 2021, 11, 649, doi:10.3390/diagnostics11040649 191

Sjoerd Rijnsdorp, Mark J. Roef and Albert J. Arends
Correction: Rijnsdorp et al. Impact of the Noise Penalty Factor on Quantification in Bayesian Penalized Likelihood (Q.Clear) Reconstructions of ^{68}Ga-PSMA PET/CT Scans. *Diagnostics* 2021, 11, 847
Reprinted from: *Diagnostics* 2021, 11, 1371, doi:10.3390/diagnostics11081371 201

About the Editors

Lioe-Fee de Geus-Oei

Lioe-Fee de Geus-Oei (MD, PhD) is a Professor of Radiology, particularly Nuclear Medicine, at the Leiden University Medical Center (LUMC), where she is Head of the Nuclear Medicine Research Group, chairwoman of the Education Management Team, and a member of the Radiology Management Team. In addition, she is a part-time clinical Professor of Molecular Imaging, Innovation and Translation at the University of Twente and Medical Delta Professor at the LUMC and Delft University of Technology. She is also on the Executive Board of the European Organisation for Research and Treatment of Cancer (EORTC) Imaging Group in Brussels and on the Oncology and Theranostics Committee of the European Association of Nuclear Medicine (EANM) in Vienna.

Floris H. P. van Velden

Floris H. P. van Velden (PhD) is a Medical Physics Expert in Nuclear Medicine at the Radiology department of the LUMC, where he is the Head of the Medical Technology unit. He is a member of the Radiomics and Big Data Subcommittee of the EORTC Imaging Group in Brussels and a member of the Imaging Committee of the Haemato Oncology Foundation for Adults in the Netherlands (HOVON) in Amsterdam. His research currently focuses on quantification in PET/CT and SPECT/CT, and predominantly on radiomics and image reconstruction.

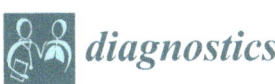

Editorial

Editorial on Special Issue "Quantitative PET and SPECT"

Floris H. P. van Velden [1,*] and Lioe-Fee de Geus-Oei [1,2]

1. Section of Nuclear Medicine, Department of Radiology, Leiden University Medical Center, 2333 ZA Leiden, The Netherlands
2. Biomedical Photonic Imaging Group, University of Twente, 7522 NB Enschede, The Netherlands
* Correspondence: f.h.p.van_velden@lumc.nl

Since the introduction of personalized (or precision) medicine, where individually tailored treatments are designed to deliver the right treatment to the right patient at the right time, the primary focus of imaging has moved from detection and diagnosis to tissue characterization, determination of prognosis, prediction of treatment efficacy, and measurement of treatment response [1]. Precision (personalized) imaging relies heavily on the use of hybrid imaging technologies and a variety of quantitative imaging biomarkers. The growing number of promising theragnostics, treatment strategies that combine radiolabeled therapeutics with diagnostics, require accurate quantification for pre- and post-treatment dosimetry. Furthermore, quantification is essential in the pharmacokinetic analysis of promising new radiotracers and drugs, and in the assessment of drug resistance. This Special Issue highlights trending research topics of two quantitative imaging tools used in nuclear medicine, positron emission tomography (PET) and single photon emission computed tomography (SPECT).

PET is by nature a quantitative imaging tool, relating the time–activity concentration in tissues and the basic functional parameters governing the biological processes being studied. The quantitative accuracy and interpretation of PET images are influenced by many factors, which are summarized in the review of Rogasch and colleagues, emphasizing the need to implement quality control and standardized imaging protocols [2]. In this Special Issue, three research articles address factors influencing quantitative accuracy and/or interpretation of PET images, such as image reconstruction. Based on the evaluation of multiple Bayesian penalized likelihood (BPL) reconstructions of phantom scans, Rijnsdorp et al. identified the optimal noise penalty factor for BPL reconstruction of clinical ^{68}Ga-PSMA PET/CT scans in terms of detectability and reproducibility [3]. A second factor impacting the quantitative accuracy of PET is the spatial resolution, which is influenced by, amongst others, the positron range of the imaged isotope. In this Special Issue, Yang developed a convolutional neural network, originally designed to convert magnetic resonance imaging (MRI) into pseudo computed tomography (CT) scans, to correct for the positron range in preclinical ^{68}Ga-PET imaging [4]. Third, respiratory motion degrades the quantification accuracy of PET imaging [5] and, when left uncorrected, could thereby impact the evaluation of selective internal radiation therapy (SIRT) dosimetry. Walker and colleagues showed that post-therapy ^{90}Y SIRT PET/CT imaging, in terms of tumor quantification and dosimetric measures, is improved by quiescent period respiratory motion correction [6].

Recent innovations in SPECT reconstruction techniques have allowed SPECT to move from relative/semi-quantitative measures to absolute quantification [7]. So far, absolute SPECT is only limitedly translated to diagnostic nuclear medicine, requiring proper validations with a ground truth, such as imaging phantoms. The review by De Schepper and colleagues showed that these validations are currently feasible with the use of application-specific phantoms produced by the current state-of-the-art in additive manufacturing or 3D printing [8].

The strength of PET and SPECT is that they permit whole-body molecular imaging in a noninvasive way, evaluating multiple disease sites. In this Special Issue, Iqbal et al.

investigated the diagnostic accuracy of ^{18}F-FDG PET for staging of patients with grade 1–2 estrogen receptor positive (ER+) breast cancer and showed that ^{18}F-FDG PET inadequately staged almost 30% of these patients, illustrating the urgent need for new radiotracers to improve the current imaging staging procedures for these patients [9].

Serial scanning allows the measurement of functional changes over time during therapeutic interventions. In this Special Issue, Roef and colleagues determined the repeatability of ^{68}Ga-PSMA lesion uptake in both relapsing and metastatic tumors and showed that a minimum response of 50% seems appropriate in this clinical situation [10], which is higher than 30% recommended by the PET Response Criteria in Solid Tumors [11]. In this Special Issue, three articles investigated the prognostic value of ^{18}F-FDG PET imaging. Chen et al. investigated whether the combination of primary tumor and nodal PET parameters can predict survival outcomes in patients with nodal metastatic non-small cell lung cancer without distant metastasis and demonstrated that by using this combination of PET features (in specific a combination of total lesion glycolysis values; TLG) with clinical factors risk stratification can be refined, facilitating tailored therapeutic strategies for these patients [12]. In addition, Kalisvaart and colleagues determined the added prognostic value of PET features in patients with metastases from soft tissue sarcoma, identifying the maximum and peak standardized uptake values as independent prognostic factors for overall survival in these patients [13]. Finally, Hlongwa et al. demonstrated that high whole-body TLG, and metabolic tumor volumes and TLG of the primary tumor were prognostic factors for overall survival in patients with malignant melanoma [14].

Images can no longer be treated strictly as pictures but instead must use innovative approaches based on numerical analysis. Medical images contain much more information hidden in the millions of voxels that cannot be assessed by the human eye. Recent developments in computer science have introduced computational methods that can capture this concealed information, which is studied in the field of radiomics that includes (a variety of) quantitative imaging biomarkers. Radiomics have the potential to improve knowledge of tumor biology and, combined with clinical data and other biomarkers, guide clinical management decisions, thereby contributing to precision medicine [15]. Currently, there is no consensus regarding the inclusion of regions of central necrosis during tumor delineation for radiomic analysis. In this Special Issue, Noortman and colleagues showed that central necrosis of tumors on ^{18}F-FDG PET significantly impacts radiomic feature values but did not seem to impact the predictive performance of the radiomics model [16].

Only with a dynamic scan is it possible to follow the kinetics (uptake, retention, clearance) of the radiotracer quantitatively [17]. However, the pharmacokinetic analysis often requires an arterial input function (AIF) that is acquired by an invasive arterial blood sampling procedure. As a noninvasive surrogate to the AIF, Fang et al. developed an image-derived input function using a model-based matrix factorization to measure the volume of distribution that quantifies the 18-kDa translocator protein (TSPO) of ^{18}F-DPA-714 PET in the human brain [18]. In another, more exploratory and noninvasive dynamic PET study to assess the presynaptic dopamine synthesis capacity using ^{18}F-FDOPA in the human brain, Schalbroeck et al. revealed that, among autistic adults, specific autistic traits can be associated with reduced striatal dopamine synthesis capacity [19]. Last but not least, this Special Issue also identifies a potential role for dynamic PET to monitor treatment response in smoldering myeloma using ^{18}F-FDG, as illustrated by a case report by Sachpekidis et al. [20].

In conclusion, the manuscripts published in this Special Issue highlight hot topics on quantitative PET and SPECT, discussing developments in the field of radiomics, the rise of artificial intelligence techniques, and the problems that have to be solved to be able to move towards validated and clinically accepted quantitative imaging biomarkers for precision medicine. We would like to sincerely thank all authors for their contributions and hope that the readers will enjoy reading this Special Issue.

Author Contributions: Writing—original draft preparation, F.H.P.v.V. and L.-F.d.G.-O.; writing—review and editing, F.H.P.v.V. and L.-F.d.G.-O. All authors have read and agreed to the published version of the manuscript.

Funding: This research received no external funding.

Conflicts of Interest: The authors declare no conflict of interest.

References

1. European Society of Radiology. Medical imaging in personalised medicine: A white paper of the research committee of the European Society of Radiology (ESR). *Insights Imaging* **2015**, *6*, 141–155. [CrossRef] [PubMed]
2. Rogasch, J.M.M.; Hofheinz, F.; van Heek, L.; Voltin, C.-A.; Boellaard, R.; Kobe, C. Influences on PET Quantification and Interpretation. *Diagnostics* **2022**, *12*, 451. [CrossRef] [PubMed]
3. Rijnsdorp, S.; Roef, M.J.; Arends, A.J. Impact of the Noise Penalty Factor on Quantification in Bayesian Penalized Likelihood (Q.Clear) Reconstructions of ^{68}Ga-PSMA PET/CT Scans. *Diagnostics* **2021**, *11*, 847. [CrossRef] [PubMed]
4. Yang, C.-C. Compensating Positron Range Effects of Ga-68 in Preclinical PET Imaging by Using Convolutional Neural Network: A Monte Carlo Simulation Study. *Diagnostics* **2021**, *11*, 2275. [CrossRef] [PubMed]
5. Grootjans, W.; Rietbergen, D.D.; van Velden, F.H. Added Value of Respiratory Gating in Positron Emission Tomography for the Clinical Management of Lung Cancer Patients. *Semin Nucl. Med.* **2022**, in press. [CrossRef] [PubMed]
6. Walker, M.D.; Gear, J.I.; Craig, A.J.; McGowan, D.R. Effects of Respiratory Motion on Y-90 PET Dosimetry for SIRT. *Diagnostics* **2022**, *12*, 194. [CrossRef] [PubMed]
7. Collarino, A.; Pereira Arias-Bouda, L.M.; Valdes Olmos, R.A.; van der Tol, P.; Dibbets-Schneider, P.; de Geus-Oei, L.F.; van Velden, F.H.P. Experimental validation of absolute SPECT/CT quantification for response monitoring in breast cancer. *Med. Phys.* **2018**, *45*, 2143–2153. [CrossRef] [PubMed]
8. De Schepper, S.; Gnanasegaran, G.; Dickson, J.C.; Van den Wyngaert, T. Absolute Quantification in Diagnostic SPECT/CT: The Phantom Premise. *Diagnostics* **2021**, *11*, 2333. [CrossRef] [PubMed]
9. Iqbal, R.; Mammatas, L.H.; Aras, T.; Vogel, W.V.; van de Brug, T.; Oprea-Lager, D.E.; Verheul, H.M.W.; Hoekstra, O.S.; Boellaard, R.; Menke-van der Houven van Oordt, C.W. Diagnostic Performance of [^{18}F]FDG PET in Staging Grade 1–2, Estrogen Receptor Positive Breast Cancer. *Diagnostics* **2021**, *11*, 1954. [CrossRef] [PubMed]
10. Roef, M.J.; Rijnsdorp, S.; Brouwer, C.; Wyndaele, D.N.; Arends, A.J. Evaluation of Quantitative Ga-68 PSMA PET/CT Repeatability of Recurrent Prostate Cancer Lesions Using Both OSEM and Bayesian Penalized Likelihood Reconstruction Algorithms. *Diagnostics* **2021**, *11*, 1100. [CrossRef] [PubMed]
11. Wahl, R.L.; Jacene, H.; Kasamon, Y.; Lodge, M.A. From RECIST to PERCIST: Evolving Considerations for PET response criteria in solid tumors. *J. Nucl. Med.* **2009**, *50* (Suppl. S1), 122S–150S. [CrossRef] [PubMed]
12. Chen, Y.-H.; Chu, S.-C.; Wang, L.-Y.; Wang, T.-F.; Lue, K.-H.; Lin, C.-B.; Chang, B.-S.; Liu, D.-W.; Liu, S.-H.; Chan, S.-C. Prognostic Value of Combing Primary Tumor and Nodal Glycolytic–Volumetric Parameters of ^{18}F-FDG PET in Patients with Non-Small Cell Lung Cancer and Regional Lymph Node Metastasis. *Diagnostics* **2021**, *11*, 1065. [CrossRef] [PubMed]
13. Kalisvaart, G.M.; Grootjans, W.; Bovée, J.V.M.G.; Gelderblom, H.; van der Hage, J.A.; van de Sande, M.A.J.; van Velden, F.H.P.; Bloem, J.L.; de Geus-Oei, L.-F. Prognostic Value of Quantitative [^{18}F]FDG-PET Features in Patients with Metastases from Soft Tissue Sarcoma. *Diagnostics* **2021**, *11*, 2271. [CrossRef] [PubMed]
14. Hlongwa, K.N.; Mokoala, K.M.G.; Matsena-Zingoni, Z.; Vorster, M.; Sathekge, M.M. The Use of ^{18}F-FDG PET/CT Metabolic Parameters in Predicting Overall Survival in Patients Undergoing Restaging for Malignant Melanoma. *Diagnostics* **2022**, *12*, 595. [CrossRef] [PubMed]
15. Noortman, W.A.; Vriens, D.; Grootjans, W.; Tao, Q.; de Geus-Oei, L.F.; Van Velden, F.H. Nuclear medicine radiomics in precision medicine: Why we can't do without artificial intelligence. *Q. J. Nucl. Med. Mol. Imaging* **2020**, *64*, 278–290. [CrossRef] [PubMed]
16. Noortman, W.A.; Vriens, D.; Mooij, C.D.Y.; Slump, C.H.; Aarntzen, E.H.; van Berkel, A.; Timmers, H.J.L.M.; Bussink, J.; Meijer, T.W.H.; de Geus-Oei, L.-F.; et al. The Influence of the Exclusion of Central Necrosis on [^{18}F]FDG PET Radiomic Analysis. *Diagnostics* **2021**, *11*, 1296. [CrossRef] [PubMed]
17. Lammertsma, A.A. Forward to the Past: The Case for Quantitative PET Imaging. *J. Nucl. Med.* **2017**, *58*, 1019–1024. [CrossRef] [PubMed]
18. Fang, Y.-H.D.; McConathy, J.E.; Yacoubian, T.A.; Zhang, Y.; Kennedy, R.E.; Standaert, D.G. Image Quantification for TSPO PET with a Novel Image-Derived Input Function Method. *Diagnostics* **2022**, *12*, 1161. [CrossRef] [PubMed]
19. Schalbroeck, R.; de Geus-Oei, L.-F.; Selten, J.-P.; Yaqub, M.; Schrantee, A.; van Amelsvoort, T.; Booij, J.; van Velden, F.H.P. Cerebral [^{18}F]-FDOPA Uptake in Autism Spectrum Disorder and Its Association with Autistic Traits. *Diagnostics* **2021**, *11*, 2404. [CrossRef] [PubMed]
20. Sachpekidis, C.; Türk, M.; Dimitrakopoulou-Strauss, A. Quantitative, Dynamic ^{18}F-FDG PET/CT in Monitoring of Smoldering Myeloma: A Case Report. *Diagnostics* **2021**, *11*, 649. [CrossRef] [PubMed]

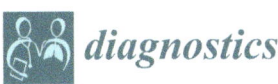

Review

Influences on PET Quantification and Interpretation

Julian M. M. Rogasch [1,2], **Frank Hofheinz** [3], **Lutz van Heek** [4], **Conrad-Amadeus Voltin** [4], **Ronald Boellaard** [5] and **Carsten Kobe** [4,*]

[1] Department of Nuclear Medicine, Charité—Universitätsmedizin Berlin, Corporate Member of Freie Universität Berlin and Humboldt-Universität zu Berlin, 13353 Berlin, Germany; julian.rogasch@charite.de
[2] Berlin Institute of Health at Charité, Universitätsmedizin Berlin, 10178 Berlin, Germany
[3] Institute of Radiopharmaceutical Cancer Research, Helmholtz Center Dresden-Rossendorf, 01328 Dresden, Germany; hofheinz@hzdr.de
[4] Department of Nuclear Medicine, Faculty of Medicine and University Hospital Cologne, University of Cologne, 50937 Cologne, Germany; lutz.van-heek@uk-koeln.de (L.v.H.); conrad-amadeus.voltin@uk-koeln.de (C.-A.V.)
[5] Department of Radiology and Nuclear Medicine, Cancer Center Amsterdam (CCA), Amsterdam University Medical Center, Free University Amsterdam, 1081 HV Amsterdam, The Netherlands; r.boellaard@amsterdamumc.nl
* Correspondence: carsten.kobe@uk-koeln.de; Tel.: +49-221-478-7534

Abstract: Various factors have been identified that influence quantitative accuracy and image interpretation in positron emission tomography (PET). Through the continuous introduction of new PET technology—both imaging hardware and reconstruction software—into clinical care, we now find ourselves in a transition period in which traditional and new technologies coexist. The effects on the clinical value of PET imaging and its interpretation in routine clinical practice require careful reevaluation. In this review, we provide a comprehensive summary of important factors influencing quantification and interpretation with a focus on recent developments in PET technology. Finally, we discuss the relationship between quantitative accuracy and subjective image interpretation.

Keywords: positron emission tomography; quantitative accuracy; contrast recovery; signal-to-noise ratio; image interpretation; image quality

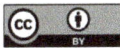

1. Introduction

The purpose of this review is to provide a state-of-the-art overview of factors influencing common quantitative image parameters in positron emission tomography (PET) as well as image interpretation, which is usually not quantitative. To address this dichotomy, the chapter on "quantification" relates to factors with a bearing on quantitative accuracy, while the second chapter "interpretation" focusses on variables that affect the subjective, reader-dependent, mostly visual interpretation of images and their effects on diagnostic accuracy and response assessment. Some sections of the article put special emphasis on [18F]fluorodeoxyglucose (FDG), owing both to the unique clinical importance of [18F]FDG and its vast literature as well as the issue of dietary preparation and influences of blood glucose levels on quantification in [18F]FDG-PET.

PET quantification, as defined in this review article, comprises primarily those methodological factors that determine how accurately the radiopharmaceutical with its biodistribution in an individual patient is depicted. It focusses on those aspects that are potentially relevant for daily routine clinical care (Figure 1).

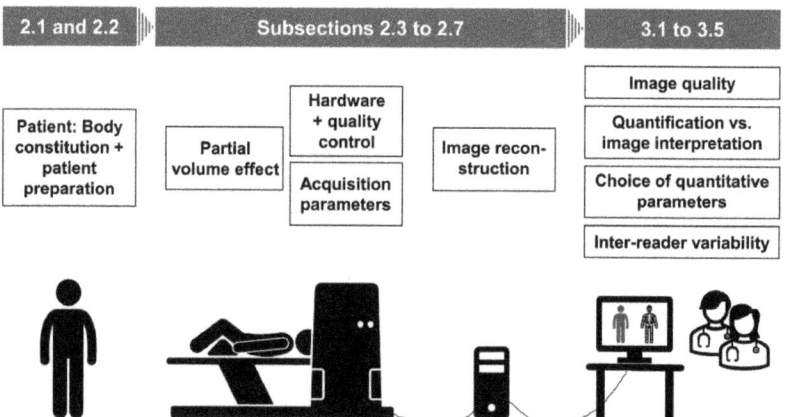

Figure 1. Article structure: From patient preparation to image interpretation. Every step of preparing the patient, acquiring and processing PET images, and choosing criteria to quantify and interpret the data potentially affects quantitative and diagnostic accuracy. Each of these steps is addressed by successive subsections of this article.

2. Factors Affecting PET Quantification

The essence of PET quantification is lesion contrast recovery (CR), which describes the relative recovery of the true focal activity concentration. Figure 2 illustrates the most relevant factors influencing lesion CR in PET.

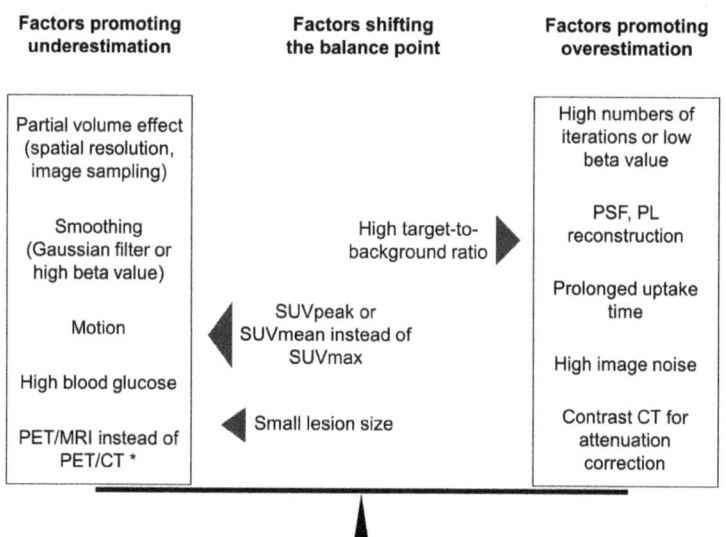

Figure 2. The thin line of quantitative accuracy in PET. Quantitative accuracy of PET in lesions (i.e., recovery of the true activity concentration) can be imagined as a pair of balances between factors that promote either under- or overestimation of the true activity. Additionally, the point at which the combination of these contrasting factors achieves quantitative accuracy is influenced by lesion-specific and methodological factors (e.g., the choice of standardized uptake value (SUV) parameter). * Reported lesion SUVs in PET/MRI are lower than those in PET/CT; however, this may not be true for every lesion in every tissue. PSF, point spread function; PL, penalized likelihood.

2.1. Patient

The patient's physiology and constitution influence the biodistribution of radiopharmaceuticals, especially of [^{18}F]FDG, although they mainly affect standardized uptake values (SUV) in normal organs, such as the liver, brain, lung, skeletal muscles, and blood pool [1]. In a number of normal organs, the SUV corrected for body mass is positively correlated with the body mass index (BMI) [1–3]. This correlation can be partly explained mathematically by the incorrect estimation of the distribution volume in obese patients if total body mass is used instead of lean body mass (due to the relatively low [^{18}F]FDG accumulation in fat tissue [4]) [5]. However, when compared to SUV in prostate-specific membrane antigen (PSMA)-PET, those in [^{18}F]FDG-PET are more closely correlated with BMI [5]. This suggests effects on SUV in obese patients that are specific for [^{18}F]FDG, possibly stemming from the positive correlation between BMI and blood glucose [3,6].

Mildly to moderately reduced kidney function (estimated glomerular filtration rate <60 ml/min) may not influence either normal organ SUV or blood pool clearance [6,7], unless kidney function is so far reduced that the patient requires hemodialysis [8]. Normal brain [^{18}F]FDG uptake varies with age, sex, and the presence or absence of diabetes mellitus [1,6,9,10]. In women, [^{18}F]FDG uptake in the ovaries and breast tissue varies with progesterone levels and age [11,12].

Notably, tumor SUVmax and SUVmean were not shown to vary systematically with the above-named physiological factors in a large meta-analysis of >20.000 individuals [1]. However, if tumor SUV is related to normal tissue SUV, these factors may have an indirect effect.

2.2. Patient Preparation

[^{18}F]FDG uptake in tumors, inflammatory cells and brain tissue is mainly brought about by insulin-independent glucose transporters (GLUT) 1 or 3 [13–19]. Their metabolic rate (i.e., the absolute glucose uptake per time) is mostly constant at varying blood glucose levels, resulting in a lowering of absolute [^{18}F]FDG uptake (i.e., SUV) by up to 50% if glucose levels are highly elevated. This is due to the competition of glucose and [^{18}F]FDG for transporter molecules [6,20,21]. Conversely, raising blood glucose and/or insulin levels increases [^{18}F]FDG uptake in the liver, skeletal muscles, and myocardium mainly via GLUT2 and 4 [1,6,22]. Physical exercise increases skeletal muscle [^{18}F]FDG uptake via GLUT4 [23]. Therefore, to achieve optimal results for lesion-to-background ratios in [^{18}F]FDG-PET, a low blood glucose level and insulin level should be ensured at the time of injection, and recommendations regarding physical activity should be observed [24].

Some drugs affect [^{18}F]FDG uptake in normal organs. Examples of this are the variations in brain and cardiac uptake caused by sedatives [25,26] or elevated bone marrow uptake following administration of hematopoietic cytokines [27].

Regarding other tracers, specific recommendations to pause potentially interfering substances may also be important. The influence of somatostatin analogues on the uptake of neuroendocrine tumors in somatostatin receptor-specific PET [28] and of antihormonal treatment on PSMA uptake in prostate cancer cells [29,30] are currently under investigation. Further determinants of the biodistribution of various other radiopharmaceuticals are also beyond the scope of this article but have been addressed by previous reviews. These include physiological and pharmacological factors [31], the in vivo degradation of peptide-based PET radiopharmaceuticals [32], and interactions between the lesion microenvironment and radiopharmaceuticals [33–36].

Likewise, advances in kinetic modeling and parametric PET imaging [37] for the prediction and validation of pharmacokinetic models, e.g., in radioligand therapy [38] or in neurology [39,40], have been discussed elsewhere.

2.3. Partial Volume Effect

A general problem in the quantitative evaluation of PET data is the rather low spatial resolution. Even though improved scanner technology and reconstruction algorithms lead to a noticeably improved reconstructed spatial resolution compared to older systems (about

4 mm vs. 6 mm) [41], it is still much worse than the resolution of computed tomography (CT) or magnetic resonance imaging (MRI). The low resolution causes unavoidable partial volume effects, which can lead to a severe underestimation of tracer uptake, depending on the lesion size. Assuming a spherical lesion with homogeneous tracer accumulation and a spatial resolution approximated by a Gaussian point spread function (PSF) with 4 mm full width at half maximum (FWHM), the effect becomes relevant at a lesion diameter of about 10 mm. Here, the recovery of the maximum activity is still 97%, but it drops sharply with decreasing diameter, e.g., to 86% for an 8 mm diameter or 63% for a diameter of 6 mm (Figure 3) [42].

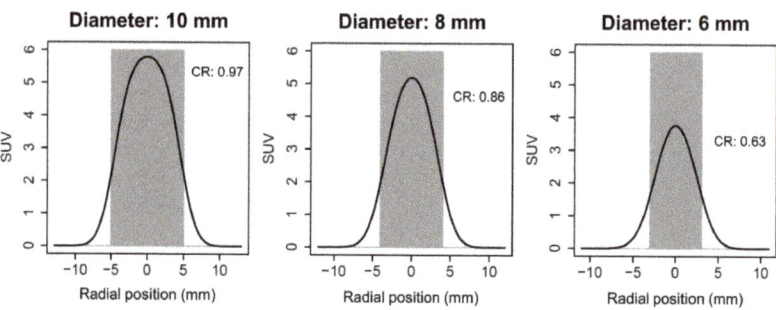

Figure 3. Reconstructed spatial resolution. The effect of limited reconstructed spatial resolution on lesion contrast recovery (CR) at different lesion diameters is demonstrated here, while the additional effect of image spacing is disregarded. In this example, spatial resolution is always 4 mm full width at half maximum (FWHM). The true lesion activity is shown in light grey, and the displayed activity is shown by the black line. In a 10-mm lesion (left), CR is 0.97, which is close to the optimum of 1.0 but decreases considerably with decreasing lesion diameter despite equal true activity. Please note that these values are calculated for lesions with absent background activity. If background activity is present, relative CR increases systematically.

While these figures can easily be computed using the convolution of PSF and object geometry, they are of limited value in routine clinical practice since they apply only to the idealized situation described above. The recovery for lesions of a different shape and inhomogeneous tracer accumulation can differ widely from the figures presented [43], and it is therefore not possible to achieve reliable partial volume correction using these results.

Another factor besides spatial resolution that contributes to the partial volume effect is image sampling, meaning, in the context of PET, the distribution of a natural, irregular volume into cuboid voxels of a fixed size. Each voxel value then reflects the average activity in this voxel volume. In the case of lesion borders, some of the marginal activity is projected into the vicinity of the lesion (so-called spill-out; Figure 4A) while, conversely, activity at the lesion surface is diluted by background activity (spill-in). Furthermore, the activity within lesions is usually heterogenous due to numerous cell clusters of different tracer avidity. The projection of such clusters into comparably large voxel volumes with fixed size inevitably leads to attenuation of the true magnitude of heterogeneity and to a loss of spatial resolution of small heterogenous areas (Figure 4B). Consequently, PET systematically underestimates intralesional heterogeneity. The larger the voxel size, the higher the likelihood of underestimating both the true maximum activity within the lesion and the variety and heterogeneity of activities [42].

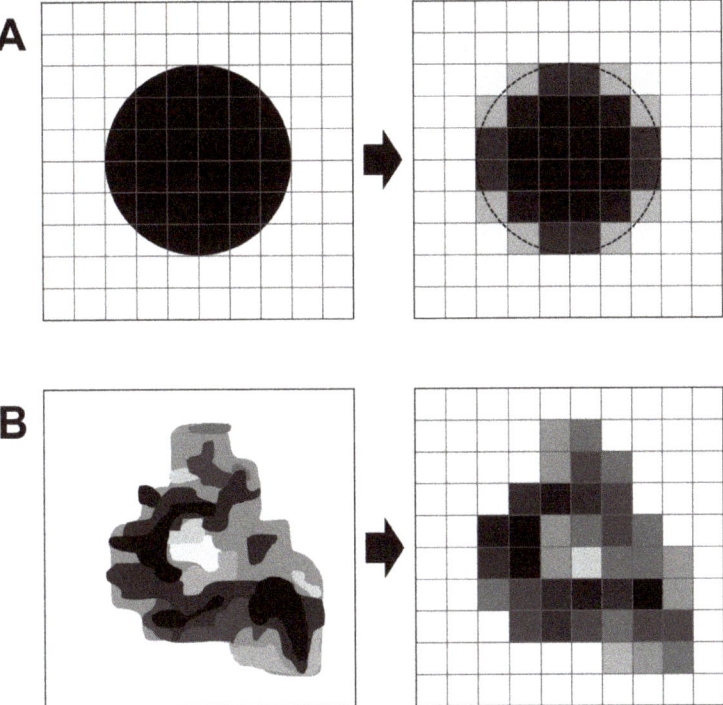

Figure 4. Image spacing. The effect of image spacing is illustrated in two dimensions (but would have to be extrapolated to three dimensions for PET data). (**A**) An idealized homogenous, spherical lesion is displayed on the left side with the superimposed voxel grid. The depiction of this lesion is shown on the right. At the lesion border (surface), image spacing results in a dilution of lesion activity by background activity (spill-in). In the usual case of a hot lesion, this spill-in leads to underestimation of the average lesion activity. Conversely, some of the marginal lesion activity may be visualized outside of the true lesion border (spill-out), and the lesion may appear larger than it truly is (dotted line). (**B**) In a lesion with heterogeneous activity (illustrated by different grey values), image spacing leads to an underestimation of intralesional heterogeneity because each voxel only represents an average activity, and both maximum and minimum intensities are attenuated. The minimum spatial resolution is determined by the voxel size. In (**B**), the effects of spill-in and spill-out at the lesion border are disregarded for simplification.

Both factors must be kept in mind when interpreting the SUV, especially SUVmax, of small lesions.

2.4. Hardware

2.4.1. Silicon Photomultiplier (SiPM) Technology

The photomultiplier converts the photon emitted from the scintillation crystal into an electronic signal. Compared to conventional photomultiplier tubes (PMT), silicon photomultipliers (SiPM) in recently developed PET/CT scanners are smaller, provide up to 100% coverage of the scintillation crystal surface and offer high photon sensitivity, low noise, and fast timing resolution [44]. The chief advantages of SiPM are higher effective sensitivity and improved signal-to-noise ratios (SNR).

To estimate the independent added value of SiPM technology, performance metrics can be compared with otherwise similar PMT-based scanner models. Most importantly, these scanners should feature a similar length of the axial field of view (FOV) because the system sensitivity (cps/kBq), a main determinant of the SNR, increases quadratically with an increase in axial FOV (e.g., system sensitivity gain of approx. 80% for an axial FOV increase of 33%) [45]. The potential gain associated with SiPM is dependent on the relative coverage of the detector area with SiPM elements and their specific timing resolution relative to the PMT comparator. If, for example, a SiPM system with low relative coverage of <60% and a modest timing resolution of 382 ps [44,45] is compared to a bismuth germanate (BGO) PMT scanner with similar axial FOV length [46], the SiPM system's sensitivity can be similar or even slightly inferior (20.8 vs. 23.3 cps/kBq) [45]. In contrast, a SiPM system with 100% detector coverage and 214 ps timing resolution [47] can offer increased system sensitivity over a comparable PMT system with lutetium oxyorthosilicate (LSO) crystals [48] that exceeds the expected difference based on the slightly larger axial FOV (16.4 vs. 9.6 cps/kBq with a 25.6 vs. 22.1 cm FOV) [47]. If further improvements in timing resolution are achieved with future generations of SiPM [44], this could bring with it a proportional increase in effective sensitivity (noise equivalent counts; NEC) [49,50]. Such a gain in counts could translate into an SNR gain that is equivalent to the square root of the relative improvement in timing resolution [49,51].

Additionally, the development of small SiPM elements has enabled small voxel sizes down to $1 \times 1 \times 1$ mm^3 [52] with potential superiority over PMT-based systems in reconstructed spatial resolution and quantitative accuracy in the case of small lesions [53–56].

2.4.2. PET/CT vs. PET/MRI

CT-based attenuation correction (CT-AC) for PET has the advantage of directly and reliably translating tissue densities from CT Hounsfield units (e.g, acquired with 120 keV) into linear attenuation correction factors for 511 keV photons [57]. In contrast, MR-based attenuation correction (MR-AC) in PET/MRI relies on different, vendor-dependent MR sequences that are used to automatically segment the body into three or four compartments (air, bone, soft tissue, and fat) [58]. These compartments are assigned specific linear attenuation correction factors for 511 keV photons. However, several sources of error exist, including extracorporeal components such as headphones, dense hair or MR coils [59], incorrect attenuation correction factors for bone and lung tissue [60], incorrect segmentation of such compartments, and MR image truncation [61]. Systematic underestimation of SUV in bone tissue or lesions close to the bone of >10% compared to PET/CT has been described [60,62], whereas SUV differences were <5% in other normal tissues [60]. It should also be noted that cross-calibration of PET/MRI scanners is generally hampered by water-filled phantoms, which are commonly used for SUV calibration in PET/CT and can produce substantial artifacts in the MR-AC sequence with corresponding SUV errors [63,64]. In such phantoms, inter-vendor differences in MR-AC maps [61] can lead to SUV differences in phantom spheres of 10–20% [58].

Studies that have investigated normal organ and lesion SUV in patients undergoing both PET/CT and PET/MRI after a single injection of [^{18}F]FDG were mostly biased by a non-randomized scan order. Lesion SUV were usually lower on the first examination, which can partly be explained by the increasing [^{18}F]FDG accumulation in most (malignant) lesions beyond 60 min after tracer administration. However, systematically different normal organ SUVs have been reported for [^{18}F]FDG as well, which most likely result from MR-AC inaccuracies [60,65,66]. Furthermore, as such studies can only compare one single PET/CT scanner with one PET/MRI scanner and have usually only investigated one specific set of reconstruction parameters, it is difficult to draw a generalized conclusion regarding the comparability of SUV in clinical PET/CT and PET/MRI.

2.5. Quality Control

High image quality is of general importance, but special requirements are necessary in the case of SUV quantification. Three quantities are needed for the computation of SUV: the injected activity, the activity concentration in the lesion as determined in the image data, and the distribution volume of the radiopharmaceutical (usually approximated by the body mass of the patient). Errors in these quantities lead directly to errors in the SUV of the same magnitude; e.g., a 10% error in the patient body mass leads to a 10% error in SUV. An accurate determination of the patient's body mass is therefore indispensable for quantitative purposes and of special importance if follow-up studies are to be compared.

The accuracy of the measured target activity concentration depends on accurate cross-calibration of the scanner with the dose calibrator that is used to measure injected activities. Frequent verification is therefore mandatory, and the European Association of Nuclear Medicine (EANM) recommends quarterly cross-calibrations [24]. To determine the injected net activity, the activity in the syringe has to be measured before and after injection. Furthermore, since the activity concentration in the lesion and the injected activity are measured with different devices, correct decay correction requires the two devices to have synchronized clocks. The optimal way to achieve this is by connecting both devices to the same time server. If this is not possible, regular verification of a synchronized time is necessary. Although all these errors are potentially severe, it should be noted that they can easily be avoided by following existing guidelines published by the EANM [24] or the EANM Research Ltd. (EARL) initiative [67].

2.6. Acquisition Parameters

2.6.1. Uptake Time after Tracer Administration

Lesional uptake of [^{18}F]FDG is more or less irreversible in neoplastic cells [68,69] due to intracellular trapping of the phosphorylated molecule, although reversible uptake has been demonstrated in inflammatory tissue [18]. The SUV of tumor lesions, therefore, increases steadily over time after [^{18}F]FDG injection [70,71]. Normal organ SUV may either decline over time (blood pool, bowel, and fat tissue), remain relatively stable (liver and lung) or increase (cerebellum, spleen, bone marrow, and muscles) [72,73]. Therefore, to ensure the repeatability of SUV measurements, a similar uptake time should be observed [24]. It should be noted that tumor uptakes of [^{68}Ga]Ga-PSMA-11 [74] and the somatostatin receptor-specific agents [^{68}Ga]Ga-DOTATOC and -DOTATATE [75] have recently also been described as irreversible.

2.6.2. Acquisition Duration per Bed Position

SUV are corrected for injected activity and acquisition time per bed position. Due to this correction, they are less directly affected by changes in these variables than image noise (Section 3.2.1). This is especially true for SUVmean and, to a lesser degree, for SUVpeak, which are both relatively stable even after reduction of acquisition time to 50% or less [76–80]. In contrast, SUVmax can vary substantially because this is, by definition, the outlier, which is most affected by increasing relative errors with declining count statistics [76,80]. However, systematic SUVmax increases of >5–10% have not typically been observed at acquisition times per bed position of >30–60s, at least during investigations of SiPM-equipped systems and/or patients with BMI <25 kg/m^2 [79,81,82].

2.6.3. Respiratory Motion Correction

As static PET images require considerable acquisition time for each bed position, a bed position covers several breathing cycles, and the final image represents the average of detected activity in each location. The true signal in organs and lesions that are subject to respiratory motion is thereby distorted and blurred along the vector of motion. This results in lower maximum activity but higher apparent lesion volume of the target lesion at an equal relative SUV threshold. This has been reported, e.g., for pulmonary lesions (especially in the lower and middle parts of the lung), liver lesions, and pancreatic lesions [83–88]. Several techniques for respiratory motion correction have been proposed [89].

In cardiac PET imaging, contraction of the myocardium further contributes to the quantitative inaccuracy of uncorrected static PET protocols [90,91].

2.7. Image Reconstruction

The effect of image reconstruction algorithms on quantitative accuracy in PET has been studied extensively, and three recent reviews cover current knowledge and views on time of flight (TOF) integration [44] as well as PSF modelling and Bayesian penalized likelihood (PL) reconstruction [92,93].

Briefly, TOF increases the lesion's CR and SUV compared to non-TOF PET at a comparable level of image noise [94–96]. This effect is especially prominent in low-contrast lesions [95].

PSF reconstruction, or resolution modelling, refers to compensation for the scanner's specific PSF throughout the transaxial FOV as part of the reconstruction process. This improves reconstructed spatial resolution [97,98] and increases lesion SUV [99,100] but can lead to overestimation of the true activity due to so-called Gibbs' artifacts [92,93]. Compared with non-PSF reconstructed images, this can increase lesion SUVmax, SUVmean and SUVpeak by up to 30% on average [100–102]. To correct for these increases, an additional Gaussian filter can be applied during image reconstruction or to the final images [100,102]. With appropriate filter width (FWHM) based on sphere CR from standardized phantom measurements, PSF-induced SUV increases can be negated, resulting in comparable lesion SUVs to those in non-PSF data. Kaalep et al. showed that by filtering PSF-reconstructed data that were compliant with the updated EARL2 standard, SUV and metabolic tumor volumes (MTV) in lung cancer and lymphoma lesions could be achieved that were similar to non-PSF data (EARL1-compliant) [102]. Houdu et al. demonstrated that prognostically relevant SUVmax thresholds in patients with lung cancer are only valid in data reconstructed in compliance with the same standard as the dataset that defined this prognostic threshold [103]. A harmonization of PET data is therefore recommended when quantitative data are to be analyzed from different PET systems.

Bayesian PL reconstruction is an iterative method that employs the Bayesian principle of integrating estimates about the physical properties of the unknown image as a prior probability with the aim of improving its prediction [104]. Furthermore, a penalization/regularization term *beta* is included that penalizes large intensity differences between neighboring voxels and thereby aims at controlling the noise and Gibbs' artifacts. The beta factor, which is user-defined, determines the weight (importance) of this penalty [105,106]. Using a commercially available PL reconstruction (General Electric [GE] Q.Clear), several phantom studies have shown that PL reconstruction can increase the CR of standardized sphere inserts compared to conventional TOF and PSF reconstruction [41,46,101,107,108]. Although this effect can lead to overestimation of the true activity in larger lesions if the SUVmax is used [101], the increase in CR may be especially prominent in microspheres with diameters <10 mm, in which conventional algorithms usually underestimate the true activity substantially [109]. This has been confirmed by increasing lesion SUVmax compared with TOF and PSF reconstruction, particularly in small pulmonary lesions [110,111]. However, this difference is directly dependent on the user-defined penalization factor beta during PL reconstruction, and at beta values of 300 to 600, which have been rated as optimal for visual reading of [^{18}F]FDG-PET images by human readers [107,112,113], inter-method SUV differences may no longer be significant [41,108,111].

Besides these clinically established algorithms, several reconstruction algorithms based on artificial intelligence, namely deep learning techniques, have recently been proposed [114].

Any current PET image reconstruction algorithm includes correction for scatter, randoms, dead time, and attenuation. Regarding CT-AC, the presence of an intravenous contrast agent in the target tissue results in overestimation of attenuation and, therefore, higher SUV. In tumor lesions, such increases are usually <10% [115–117] and have been deemed irrelevant for visual assessment in previous studies [118,119]. However, in organs with a particularly high concentration of the contrast agent (e.g., the liver, kidney, or blood vessels), these deviations can be higher [116,120,121]. Thus, using a non-contrast-enhanced CT for attenuation correction is recommended when quantification by SUV is planned [24].

3. Factors Affecting PET Interpretation

Interpretation of PET images aims at classifying lesions or tissues according to their differential diagnosis at a single time point or at evaluating changes in lesion or tissue biology over time. Both may contain prognostic or predictive information.

Figure 5 presents the most relevant factors influencing PET interpretation. Selected factors are discussed in the following respective sections.

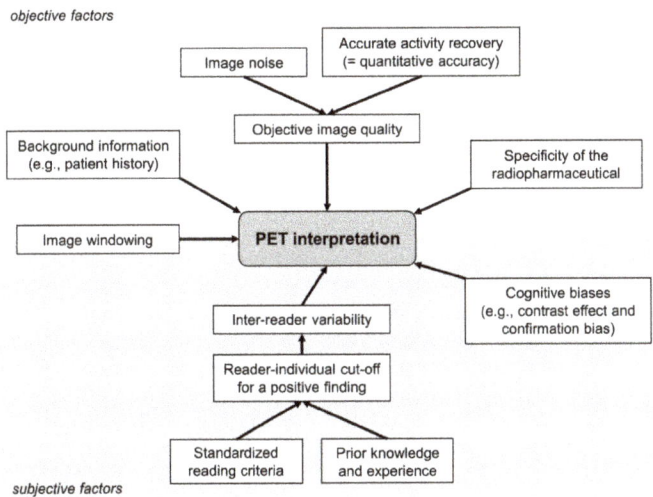

Figure 5. Factors affecting PET interpretation.

3.1. Specificity of the Radiopharmaceutical

In any thorough examination of the factors confounding quantitative accuracy, it should be kept in mind that the appropriateness of the radiopharmaceutical to assess the tissue or lesion characteristics of interest may be of utmost importance to the reader's certainty and correctness in interpreting PET images. If the radiopharmaceutical does not allow the classification of a lesion on a biochemical basis, e.g., the differentiation of a malignant or benign cause, the achievement of quantitative accuracy will not be helpful or relevant.

This becomes most evident with [^{18}F]FDG, which is specific neither to malignant lesions nor to discrete tumor entities. In oncology, this hampers the differentiation between inflammatory changes and neoplastic tissue [15,18] or benign lesions and well-differentiated malignant lesions with low [^{18}F]FDG avidity [122–125]. Various radiopharmaceuticals with higher tumor specificity have therefore been developed to increase diagnostic accuracy for certain tumor entities, e.g., [^{68}Ga]Ga-PSMA-11 or [^{18}F]F-PSMA-1007 in prostate cancer [126,127], somatostatin receptor-specific tracers for neuroendocrine tumors [128], radiolabeled peptides in brain tumors [129] or [^{18}F]fibroblast activation protein inhibitor (FAPI) for different carcinoma types [130]. However, sources of false positive or negative findings still remain with these tracers [131–134] and must be considered during image interpretation.

In cardiovascular imaging with [^{18}F]FDG-PET, insufficiently suppressed physiologic [^{18}F]FDG uptake by the myocardium can complicate the differentiation from inflammatory changes [135], while postoperative changes or sterile inflammation can be difficult to differentiate from active infection [136–138]. Alternative tracers that are more specific for inflammation [139,140] or bacterial infection [141] might facilitate interpretation.

3.2. Image Quality and Lesion Detection

In the visual assessment of PET images in routine clinical practice, quantitative accuracy cannot usually be directly assessed because the ground truth is unknown. However, the subjective, perceived image quality can be rated, and quantitative measures can be used to derive an objectified surrogate for image quality. In this sense, a maximized contrast-to-noise ratio (CNR) reflects high image quality [142], because high lesion CR and low background noise are both key to achieving high diagnostic accuracy (i.e., to minimize false-negative and false-positive results). Therefore, all previously discussed factors on CR and image noise have a direct influence on image quality.

3.2.1. Injected Activity and Acquisition Time

Subjective image quality is affected by the relationship between injected activity per kilogram body mass and acquisition time per bed position. A low product of the two factors results in excessive image noise and possibly increased rates of false-positive results and decreased reader confidence [76,143,144]. The EANM, therefore, recommends a minimum of 7 MBq/kg*min for [^{18}F]FDG-PET using a contemporary PET system with >30% overlap between bed positions [24]. Alternatively, a formula that includes the quadratic weight can be used, which could better compensate for loss in image quality in patients >75 kg [24]. Moreover, EARL also provides a procedure that can be followed to determine a lower activity prescription for systems with very high sensitivity or improved timing resolution (e.g., <300 ps) [145].

The anticipated benefits of PET hardware and software improvements over the last decade are perhaps reflected in figures for the lower minimum of injected activities required for state-of-the-art PET systems. Using an older non-TOF PET scanner with BGO crystals and 15.7 cm axial FOV [146], Geismar et al. recommended 10 MBq/kg*min for [^{18}F]FDG-PET in patients with a BMI >22 kg/m^2, while 8 MBq/kg*min was recommended only in patients with BMI <22 kg/m^2 [144]. Using a modern SiPM-equipped PET scanner with 20 cm axial FOV and PL reconstruction [54], Trägårdh et al. proposed 6 MBq/kg*min for [^{18}F]FDG-PET to achieve acceptable image quality and lesion visibility [76]. Moreover, the authors recommended 8 MBq/kg*min for [^{18}F]F-PSMA-1007 based on the same scanner and PL reconstruction [143].

Wickham et al. [147] investigated the relationship between subjective and quantified measures of image quality in 111 clinical [^{18}F]FDG-PET/CT scans (oncology, hematology, and infection) using a PMT-based PET scanner with a 22.1 cm axial FOV [148]. The optimal formula to predict high image quality included sex (higher activity in women), body mass and height. Neither patient age nor normalized body metrics or different, more sophisticated measures of body tissue composition provided added value in predicting image quality [147].

However, although a standardized measure of image quality is used, the studies cited here are still not directly comparable, as the axial FOV length differed substantially. To address this problem, the FOV length or–more accurately–the system's sensitivity in cps/kBq would have to be included in the formula to calculate the required injected activity. This becomes especially evident with recent PET systems with extra-large axial FOV of >25 cm and their potential to substantially reduce required acquisition times [47,149,150].

Furthermore, some publications have relativized the general assumption that injected activity and acquisition time are linearly interchangeable when aiming at constant image noise. These studies have demonstrated that image quality (namely image noise) in overweight patients >80–90 kg benefits especially from increased acquisition time per bed position [77,151,152].

3.2.2. SiPM Technology

The increase in effective sensitivity enabled by modern SiPM could be translated into an equivalent reduction in injected activity or acquisition time while retaining equal image quality as PMT [49,51]. Intraindividual comparisons of clinical PET data between scanners equipped with either SiPM or PMT are scarce because this requires a second scan in a randomized protocol to prevent bias from systematically different uptake times between the scans. Sekine et al. used a randomized protocol to investigate the potential to reduce injected [^{18}F]FDG activity required (or acquisition time) through the use of an SiPM TOF PET/MRI instead of a PMT TOF PET/CT in 74 patients with different types of malignant tumors. Image quality (artifacts, noise, and sharpness) was rated as acceptable at up to 40% reduction in simulated acquisition time with the SiPM PET/MRI. However, the potential to reduce acquisition time with the PMT PET/CT was not specifically investigated. Moreover, the SiPM PET/MRI had a 25 cm axial FOV compared to the 15.7 cm FOV of the PET/CT system, which partly explains differences in image quality (especially image noise) independent of the photomultiplier technology [153].

López-Mora et al. reported higher lesion detection rates with a SiPM PET/CT compared to a PMT PET/CT in 22 of 100 patients using [^{18}F]FDG or [^{18}F]fluorocholine (58 patients underwent SiPM PET first; axial FOV were similar). This resulted in a modified disease stage in 7 of these 22 patients based on SiPM PET/CT [154]. Similarly, Baratto et al. found higher lesion detection rates in 13 of 94 patients with [^{68}Ga]Ga-DOTATATE using SiPM vs. PMT PET/CT in randomized order (SiPM, 20 cm axial FOV; PMT, 15.7 cm) [155].

Consequently, SiPM technology may well produce improvements in image quality and lesion detection rates. However, the magnitude of improvement that can be achieved in clinical scans is likely to vary with different SiPM designs.

3.2.3. Image Reconstruction

Among the technical factors that affect PET interpretation, image reconstruction is especially influential because it directly affects both image noise and lesion CR to a potentially high degree (Figure 6).

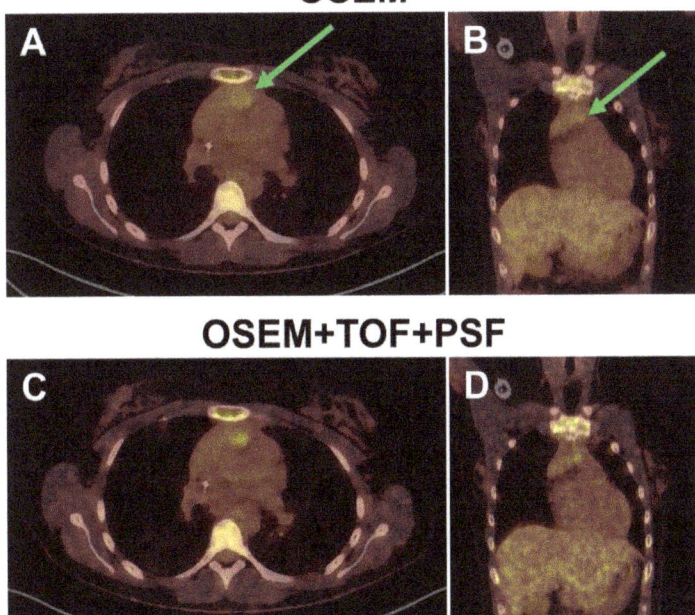

Figure 6. Fused transaxial as well as coronal PET/CT slices through residual mediastinal lymphoma tissue of a 23-year-old female patient reconstructed with the OSEM algorithm (**A**,**B**) and with OSEM combined with TOF and PSF (**C**,**D**). While the lesional [^{18}F]FDG uptake was defined as Deauville score 3 based on OSEM reconstruction, it would exceed the liver uptake when assessed based on images reconstructed with TOF and PSF (=Deauville score 4). This could alter the assessment from "adequate" to "inadequate" metabolic response.

Compared to standard ordered subset expectation maximization (OSEM) reconstruction, OSEM with TOF shows improved noise characteristics [49,94,156–158]. Surti et al. showed that TOF reconstruction improves detection rates of simulated liver and lung lesions by human readers. This improvement was pronounced in heavy patients with BMI $\geq$ 26 kg/m^2 [159]. The same group further demonstrated that TOF improved lesion detection, especially in low-contrast lesions [160].

PSF compensation can also increase the SNR [157,158] and thereby the subjectively rated image quality [157,161,162]. Investigations with an anthropomorphic phantom or with simulated liver and lung lesions have shown that TOF and PSF can have a supplementary effect on increasing lesion detection rates [161,163]. Conflicting results were reported by other authors who did not find higher lesion conspicuity or detection rates with PSF in small patient samples [162,164,165]. These discrepancies may stem from the fact that the ability of PSF to increase lesion CR is most prominent at the periphery of the transaxial FOV [98,166,167] and in small, high-contrast lesions [95], such as pulmonary nodules. This is illustrated by the observation of Schaefferkoetter et al. of an improvement in lesion detection rates with PSF limited mainly to the lung, while the detection rates achieved with TOF extended to the liver and lung [161].

Based on the potential of PL reconstruction to systematically improve SNR compared to OSEM-based algorithms [108,113,168], several authors have reported improved SNR and image quality with different radiopharmaceuticals, such as [^{18}F]FDG [107,112,113], [^{18}F]F-PSMA-1007 [143], [^{68}Ga]Ga-PSMA-11 [169,170], [^{68}Ga]Ga-DOTATATE [171] or ^{89}Zr-labelled tracers [172]. PL reconstruction has repeatedly been shown to increase conspicuity and detection rates of pulmonary lesions, even compared to OSEM with PSF and/or TOF [112,113,164,173,174]. Figure 7 shows a case example.

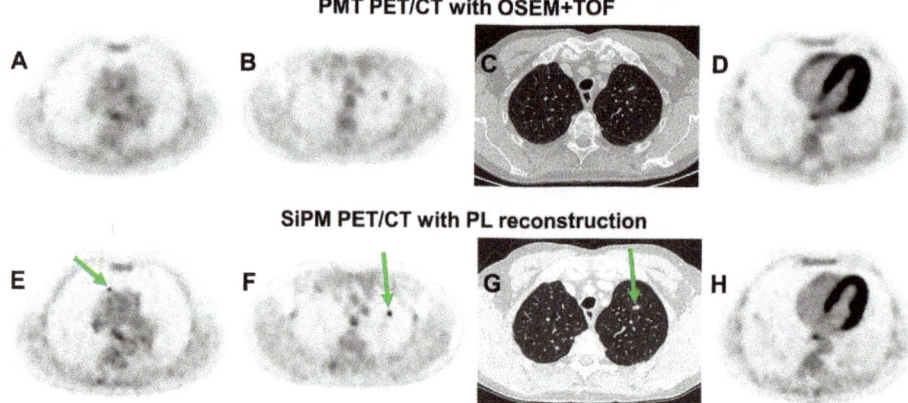

Figure 7. Images of two [^{18}F]FDG-PET/CT examinations in a 63-year-old man with hepatic and pulmonary aspergillosis. The earlier examination was performed with a scanner equipped with conventional photomultiplier tubes (PMT) and reconstructed with OSEM and TOF (**A–D**). The second examination after 5 months used a SiPM-equipped PET scanner and PL reconstruction with a penalization factor beta of 450 (**E–H**). Two pulmonary lesions that showed only moderate [^{18}F]FDG uptake during the earlier examination (**A,B**) appeared substantially more intense on the second scan (**E,F**). However, uptake in hepatic lesions declined (not shown), and both pulmonary lesions were unaltered in the CT scan (**C,G**), which suggested that the higher conspicuity of the pulmonary lesions was a result of improved reconstructed spatial resolution and lesion contrast recovery (CR) with the SiPM scanner and PL reconstruction. Based on phantom measurements, reconstructed spatial resolution was estimated at 7.8 mm full width at half maximum (FWHM) with the PMT scanner and 4.7 mm with the SiPM scanner. The improvement in image sharpness can also be seen in the myocardium (**D,H**).

In contrast, in a small sample of 13 patients undergoing [^{18}F]fluorocholine PET/CT for prostate cancer staging, PL with different beta values showed a comparable number of positive lymph nodes to that revealed by OSEM with PSF and TOF [175].

When estimating diagnostic accuracy from reported lesion detection rates, it is important to recognize that there is usually no gold standard available with which to assess the correctness of detected lesions and that such analyses are therefore unable to evaluate specificity. As an exception, Teoh et al. retrospectively investigated the diagnostic accuracy of OSEM + TOF and PL reconstruction using SUVmax and visual reading in 121 pulmonary nodules. Here, histological verification was available. Diagnostic sensitivity and accuracy were similar with both algorithms, while specificity tended to be lower with PL than with OSEM + TOF, especially in lesions >10 mm diameter [173].

Furthermore, no blanket conclusion on differences in image noise or lesion detection between reconstruction algorithms should be drawn from isolated results comparing two algorithms with only one set of parameters each (e.g., number of iterations or type of in-plane filter). Such parameters, namely the in-plane filter width or, in the case of PL reconstruction, the beta value, can have drastic effects on image noise and lesion CR (Figure 2). A higher filter width or beta value systematically decreases both image noise and CR. Reconstruction algorithms should therefore be compared with multiple sets of parameters to investigate real systematic differences between the methods [108]. It may otherwise be observed that such differences can only be detected under specific conditions [41,175].

In a study on 52 patients with lymphoma, 5 patients undergoing [^{18}F]FDG-PET for restaging were divergently classified as non-responders (Deauville score 4–5) with PL reconstruction but as responders (Deauville 1–3) with OSEM (without TOF or PSF; compliant with the EARL1 standard) [176].

3.3. Relationship between Objective and Subjective Image Quality

Although CNR, SNR and NEC are surrogates for image quality, none of these single parameters sufficiently reflects subjective image quality as a whole [147,177]. However, adequately defined quantitative assessments may each measure specific aspects of subjective image quality, such as image sharpness, lesion contrast or image noise [178].

Several studies on subjective image quality in whole-body [^{18}F]FDG-PET with PL reconstruction found that image quality was highest at beta values of 450 (to 600) despite lower lesion CR or "image sharpness" at these beta values compared to lower values [41,108,112,175,179]. This confirms that subjective image quality is a combination of lesion contrasts and image noise and that readers may demand adequately low noise levels even if this comes at the expense of lesion CR (i.e., quantitative accuracy). In low-count conditions, this tendency to prefer smooth, low-noise images with beta values >600 over "sharper" images could become even more evident [112,170]. Thus, images that are rated best regarding subjective image quality are not necessarily those with the highest quantitative accuracy. Conversely, Zhang et al. reported that lesion SUVmax and detection rates in [^{18}F]FDG-PET remained significantly unchanged despite decreasing acquisition time per bed position from 900 s to 60 s and steadily decreasing subjective image quality [180]. Quantitative accuracy may therefore not necessarily require optimal (subjective) image quality. As these criteria may not be equally fulfilled by a single reconstructed dataset, a reconstruction of separate datasets has been proposed for visual reading or optimized quantification in routine clinical practice [24,181,182].

3.4. Relationship between PET Quantification and Image Interpretation

3.4.1. Quantitative or Visual Interpretation Criteria?

Interpretation of PET images in routine clinical practice primarily follows visual criteria, i.e., the assessment of generalized or focal pathologies in tracer accumulation, while quantitative parameters, including SUV, provide orientation or additional information at most [24]. As the use of SUV to quantify tracer uptake increased, it was anticipated that this would represent a standardized, reliable criterion to classify lesions with their biological properties and prognostic implications. Consequently, diagnostic SUV thresholds have been proposed for pulmonary nodules [183], lymph node staging in lung cancer [184], adrenal lesions [185], musculoskeletal tumors [186], tumor delineation in gliomas [187], and response assessment in lymphoma [188] among other things. Thus, it is reasonable to assume that the achievement of quantitative accuracy will bring certainty and correctness to lesion interpretation.

However, lesion SUVs in [^{18}F]FDG-PET show a test-retest variability in the same patient with the same PET scanner of up to 20% [189] and are usually even less comparable between different scanners and centers or under routine clinical conditions [190]. This has undermined any attempts to establish widely adoptable SUV thresholds unless rigorous harmonization measures are followed [101,103,181]. Given the inability to derive generalizable SUV thresholds, it has not yet been possible to prove that SUV or any other quantitative measures used in clinical practice provide additional value over visual assessment alone for routine clinical diagnostics [24].

3.4.2. SUV: Which Parameter?

If SUV measurements are taken to support the visual assessment of PET images in routine clinical practice, this probably occurs most often in assessments of the response to therapy. However, as stated above, the validity of these measures is determined by the test-retest variability. Despite the common use of SUVmax in clinical practice, arising from its convenience, SUVpeak and SUVmean have been shown to be slightly less variable under test-retest conditions [189,191]. However, SUVmean and SUVpeak are affected by the reproducibility of the size and placement of the volume of interest (VOI) [192], which requires appropriate standardization or automation. Consequently, the choice of SUV parameter can fundamentally change the assessment of disease progression or response to treatment in the majority of cases [193]. A consensus was therefore needed, and Wahl et al. proposed the PET Response Criteria In Solid Tumors (PERCIST 1.0) in 2009 with the aim of standardizing the SUV parameters (SULpeak = SUVpeak corrected for lean body mass), the VOI size, the definition and number of appropriate target lesions and thresholds for response categories [194]. Still, the repeatability of the liver SULmean under clinical conditions in the same patient during treatment has been shown to be only fair (intraclass correlation coefficient <0.6) [195]. Consequently, the use of SUV to support valid clinical response assessment outside of study conditions remains highly challenging.

3.4.3. MTV: Which Delineation Method?

Treatment decisions based on clinical risk stratification might be further improved by including the initial tumor volume in [^{18}F]FDG-PET, as this factor has been shown to be an independent prognostic value for patient survival in conditions such as non-small cell lung cancer [196,197], different gynecological malignancies [198–201], and head and neck cancer [202,203]. Initial results also show a prognostic value of PSMA-PET tumor volume in prostate cancer prior to radioligand therapy with [^{177}Lu]Lu-PSMA-617 [204].

However, measurement of tumor volume is not yet a standardized procedure because numerous methods have been described to delineate the tumor volume, and considerable differences have been reported between those methods [205,206]. The most convenient and common approaches range from the use of fixed absolute or relative activity thresholds to adaptive methods based on the local signal-to-background ratio. Consequently, optimal volume thresholds to separate prognostic groups may differ systematically and foster discordant assessments, although with optimized thresholds, each method on its own may retain its prognostic value [207–209]. Therefore, for both scientific and clinical use, tumor volume should be calculated by parameters that are readily available and promise high reproducibility between different readers and institutions.

3.5. Inter-Reader Variability

Inter-reader or -rater variability can limit the reliability of PET imaging (Figure 5). Numerous studies have analyzed the inter-reader agreement of visual PET assessments, particularly in [^{18}F]FDG-PET for lymphoma and PSMA-PET for prostate cancer. In lymphoma patients, several studies have reported high inter-rater agreement using the standardized Deauville criteria [210,211], although conflicting results have also been reported [188,212]. It has been shown that reader training and discussions over divergent assessments increase agreement even among "expert" readers [213]. It has been suggested that SUV-based criteria in lymphoma might improve inter-reader agreement because they are unaffected by visual contrast effects [188]. However, both SUV measurements and visual Deauville criteria may be affected by image reconstruction, such as PL reconstruction [176]. Furthermore, besides the reader's subjective assessment of a certain lesion, in a setting in which several lesions of interest are present (e.g., in restaging in lymphoma or metastatic tumors), additional inter-reader variability can result from a divergent choice of the decisive target lesion [213].

A systematic comparison of inter-reader agreement based on quantitative measures and based on visual reading has rarely been performed, and there is still little evidence of any additional value of the quantitative approach. Furthermore, any quantitative criteria and diagnostic thresholds are a result of certain methodological and technical conditions, which may change over time and require adaptation. However, it has been demonstrated that inter-rater agreement in response assessment with [^{18}F]FDG-PET in non-small cell lung cancer or metastatic breast cancer can be considerably improved through the use of the target lesion SULpeak (PERCIST 1.0 criteria) in comparison with a subjective assessment [194,214,215].

Regarding PSMA-PET for prostate cancer, several standardized evaluation criteria have recently been proposed [216–219] with the aim of improving inter-reader agreement [219] and to aid inexperienced readers [220]. However, inter-reader concordance remains higher between experienced readers [221] and, depending on the specific diagnostic task, substantial to almost perfect agreement has usually been reported [220–223]. Similar degrees of inter-reader agreement were achieved with different reporting criteria [224]. However, standardized reading criteria do not negate the dissimilarities in the images obtained using different types of PET hardware and methods of image reconstruction, and both SiPM technology [79] and PSF reconstruction [225] have been found to result in systematically higher lesion conspicuity despite standardized reporting criteria (PSMA-RADS) [216].

4. Conclusions and Perspectives

As we have demonstrated here, a variety of factors influence PET quantification and interpretation. All variables should be considered potential sources of error when interpreting clinical PET images. Although the added value of quantitative uptake parameters for clinical decisions is still not well-defined, it should be kept in mind that even simple quantitative measures such as the SUV are highly variable. The emergence of new PET technologies such as SiPM and advanced image reconstruction algorithms further contributes to the complex issue of image quality and quantitative accuracy. Stringent measures of quality control and standardized imaging protocols should therefore be implemented to ensure robust and valid imaging results in routine clinical care. This will also be crucial to explore and validate the clinical utility of machine learning-based image biomarkers. To ensure comparability, we recommend adhering to the procedure guidelines by the EANM. Furthermore, the EARL initiative has proposed standards for a systematic standardization between imaging centers. This may include the reconstruction of different data sets for image interpretation: (1) a data set for optimal visual lesion detection and (2) a data set for standardized and quantitative image interpretation.

Author Contributions: Conceptualization, J.M.M.R. and C.K.; methodology, J.M.M.R., L.v.H. and C.-A.V.; writing—original draft preparation, J.M.M.R., F.H. and C.K.; writing—review and editing, L.v.H., C.-A.V. and R.B.; visualization, J.M.M.R.; supervision, C.K., F.H. and R.B.; project administration, C.K. All authors have read and agreed to the published version of the manuscript.

Funding: This research received no external funding.

Institutional Review Board Statement: Not applicable.

Informed Consent Statement: Written informed consent has been obtained from the patients to publish this paper.

Acknowledgments: J.M.M.R. is a participant in the BIH-Charité Digital Clinician Scientist Program funded by the Charité–Universitätsmedizin Berlin, the Berlin Institute of Health, and the German Research Foundation (DFG).

Conflicts of Interest: The authors declare no conflict of interest.

References

1. Eskian, M.; Alavi, A.; Khorasanizadeh, M.; Viglianti, B.L.; Jacobsson, H.; Barwick, T.D.; Meysamie, A.; Yi, S.K.; Iwano, S.; Bybel, B.; et al. Effect of blood glucose level on standardized uptake value (SUV) in ^{18}F-FDG PET-scan: A systematic review and meta-analysis of 20,807 individual SUV measurements. *Eur. J. Nucl. Med. Mol. Imaging* **2019**, *46*, 224–237. [CrossRef] [PubMed]
2. Keramida, G.; Peters, A.M. FDG PET/CT of the non-malignant liver in an increasingly obese world population. *Clin. Physiol. Funct. Imaging* **2020**, *40*, 304–319. [CrossRef] [PubMed]
3. Sprinz, C.; Zanon, M.; Altmayer, S.; Watte, G.; Irion, K.; Marchiori, E.; Hochhegger, B. Effects of blood glucose level on ^{18}F fluorodeoxyglucose (^{18}F-FDG) uptake for PET/CT in normal organs: An analysis on 5623 patients. *Sci. Rep.* **2018**, *8*, 2126. [CrossRef]
4. Christen, T.; Sheikine, Y.; Rocha, V.Z.; Hurwitz, S.; Goldfine, A.B.; Di Carli, M.; Libby, P. Increased glucose uptake in visceral versus subcutaneous adipose tissue revealed by PET imaging. *JACC Cardiovasc. Imaging* **2010**, *3*, 843–851. [CrossRef] [PubMed]
5. Zhao, J.; Xue, Q.; Chen, X.; You, Z.; Wang, Z.; Yuan, J.; Liu, H.; Hu, L. Evaluation of SUVlean consistency in FDG and PSMA PET/MR with Dixon-, James-, and Janma-based lean body mass correction. *EJNMMI Phys.* **2021**, *8*, 17. [CrossRef]
6. Büsing, K.A.; Schönberg, S.O.; Brade, J.; Wasser, K. Impact of blood glucose, diabetes, insulin, and obesity on standardized uptake values in tumors and healthy organs on ^{18}F-FDG PET/CT. *Nucl. Med. Biol.* **2013**, *40*, 206–213. [CrossRef]
7. Akers, S.R.; Werner, T.J.; Rubello, D.; Alavi, A.; Cheng, G. ^{18}F-FDG uptake and clearance in patients with compromised renal function. *Nucl. Med. Commun.* **2016**, *37*, 825–832. [CrossRef]
8. Toriihara, A.; Kitazume, Y.; Nishida, H.; Kubota, K.; Nakadate, M.; Tateishi, U. Comparison of FDG-PET/CT images between chronic renal failure patients on hemodialysis and controls. *Am. J. Nucl. Med. Mol. Imaging* **2015**, *5*, 204–211.
9. Yoshizawa, H.; Gazes, Y.; Stern, Y.; Miyata, Y.; Uchiyama, S. Characterizing the normative profile of ^{18}F-FDG PET brain imaging: Sex difference, aging effect, and cognitive reserve. *Psychiatry Res.* **2014**, *221*, 78–85. [CrossRef]
10. Turpin, S.; Martineau, P.; Levasseur, M.A.; Lambert, R. Modeling the Effects of Age and Sex on Normal Pediatric Brain Metabolism Using ^{18}F-FDG PET/CT. *J. Nucl. Med.* **2018**, *59*, 1118–1124. [CrossRef]
11. Jung, Y.; Kim, T.H.; Kim, J.Y.; Han, S.; An, Y.S. The effect of sex hormones on normal breast tissue metabolism: Evaluation by FDG PET/CT. *Medicine* **2019**, *98*, e16306. [CrossRef] [PubMed]
12. Kim, T.H.; Kim, M.R.; Jung, Y.; An, Y.S. Relationship between sex hormones levels and ^{18}F-FDG uptake by the ovaries in premenopausal woman. *Radiol. Oncol.* **2019**, *53*, 293–299. [CrossRef] [PubMed]
13. Brown, R.S.; Wahl, R.L. Overexpression of Glut-1 glucose transporter in human breast cancer. An immunohistochemical study. *Cancer* **1993**, *72*, 2979–2985. [CrossRef]
14. Higashi, K.; Ueda, Y.; Sakurai, A.; Mingwang, X.; Xu, L.; Murakami, M.; Seki, H.; Oguchi, M.; Taki, S.; Nambu, Y.; et al. Correlation of Glut-1 glucose transporter expression with [^{18}F]FDG uptake in non-small cell lung cancer. *Eur. J. Nucl. Med.* **2000**, *27*, 1778–1785. [CrossRef] [PubMed]
15. Kubota, R.; Yamada, S.; Kubota, K.; Ishiwata, K.; Tamahashi, N.; Ido, T. Intratumoral distribution of fluorine-18-fluorodeoxyglucose in vivo: High accumulation in macrophages and granulation tissues studied by microautoradiography. *J. Nucl. Med.* **1992**, *33*, 1972–1980.
16. Park, S.G.; Lee, J.H.; Lee, W.A.; Han, K.M. Biologic correlation between glucose transporters, hexokinase-II, Ki-67 and FDG uptake in malignant melanoma. *Nucl. Med. Biol.* **2012**, *39*, 1167–1172. [CrossRef]
17. Paul, R.; Johansson, R.; Kellokumpu-Lehtinen, P.L.; Söderström, K.O.; Kangas, L. Tumor localization with ^{18}F-2-fluoro-2-deoxy-D-glucose: Comparative autoradiography, glucose 6-phosphatase histochemistry, and histology of renally implanted sarcoma of the rat. *Res. Exp. Med.* **1985**, *185*, 87–94. [CrossRef]
18. Yamada, S.; Kubota, K.; Kubota, R.; Ido, T.; Tamahashi, N. High accumulation of fluorine-18-fluorodeoxyglucose in turpentine-induced inflammatory tissue. *J. Nucl. Med.* **1995**, *36*, 1301–1306.

19. Simpson, I.A.; Dwyer, D.; Malide, D.; Moley, K.H.; Travis, A.; Vannucci, S.J. The facilitative glucose transporter GLUT3: 20 years of distinction. *Am. J. Physiol. Endocrinol. Metab.* **2008**, *295*, E242–E253. [CrossRef]
20. Langen, K.J.; Braun, U.; Rota Kops, E.; Herzog, H.; Kuwert, T.; Nebeling, B.; Feinendegen, L.E. The influence of plasma glucose levels on fluorine-18-fluorodeoxyglucose uptake in bronchial carcinomas. *J. Nucl. Med.* **1993**, *34*, 355–359.
21. Lindholm, P.; Minn, H.; Leskinen-Kallio, S.; Bergman, J.; Ruotsalainen, U.; Joensuu, H. Influence of the blood glucose concentration on FDG uptake in cancer—A PET study. *J. Nucl. Med.* **1993**, *34*, 1–6. [PubMed]
22. Namba, H.; Nakagawa, K.; Iyo, M.; Fukushi, K.; Irie, T. A simple method for measuring glucose utilization of insulin-sensitive tissues by using the brain as a reference. *Eur. J. Nucl. Med.* **1994**, *21*, 228–231. [CrossRef]
23. Jensen, T.E.; Sylow, L.; Rose, A.J.; Madsen, A.B.; Angin, Y.; Maarbjerg, S.J.; Richter, E.A. Contraction-stimulated glucose transport in muscle is controlled by AMPK and mechanical stress but not sarcoplasmatic reticulum Ca(2+) release. *Mol. Metab.* **2014**, *3*, 742–753. [CrossRef] [PubMed]
24. Boellaard, R.; Delgado-Bolton, R.; Oyen, W.J.; Giammarile, F.; Tatsch, K.; Eschner, W.; Verzijlbergen, F.J.; Barrington, S.F.; Pike, L.C.; Weber, W.A.; et al. FDG PET/CT: EANM procedure guidelines for tumour imaging: Version 2.0. *Eur. J. Nucl. Med. Mol. Imaging* **2015**, *42*, 328–354. [CrossRef]
25. Lee, Y.A.; Kim, J.I.; Lee, J.W.; Cho, Y.J.; Lee, B.H.; Chung, H.W.; Park, K.K.; Han, J.S. Effects of various anesthetic protocols on ^{18}F-flurodeoxyglucose uptake into the brains and hearts of normal miniature pigs (*Sus scrofa domestica*). *J. Am. Assoc. Lab. Anim. Sci.* **2012**, *51*, 246–252. [PubMed]
26. Israel, O.; Weiler-Sagie, M.; Rispler, S.; Bar-Shalom, R.; Frenkel, A.; Keidar, Z.; Bar-Shalev, A.; Strauss, H.W. PET/CT quantitation of the effect of patient-related factors on cardiac ^{18}F-FDG uptake. *J. Nucl. Med.* **2007**, *48*, 234–239. [PubMed]
27. Yao, W.J.; Hoh, C.K.; Hawkins, R.A.; Glaspy, J.A.; Weil, J.A.; Lee, S.J.; Maddahi, J.; Phelps, M.E. Quantitative PET imaging of bone marrow glucose metabolic response to hematopoietic cytokines. *J. Nucl. Med.* **1995**, *36*, 794–799.
28. Aalbersberg, E.A.; de Wit-van der Veen, B.J.; Versleijen, M.W.J.; Saveur, L.J.; Valk, G.D.; Tesselaar, M.E.T.; Stokkel, M.P.M. Influence of lanreotide on uptake of ^{68}Ga-DOTATATE in patients with neuroendocrine tumours: A prospective intra-patient evaluation. *Eur. J. Nucl. Med. Mol. Imaging* **2019**, *46*, 696–703. [CrossRef]
29. Mathy, C.S.; Mayr, T.; Kürpig, S.; Meisenheimer, M.; Dolscheid-Pommerich, R.C.; Stoffel-Wagner, B.; Kristiansen, G.; Essler, M.; Muders, M.H.; Bundschuh, R.A. Antihormone treatment differentially regulates PSA secretion, PSMA expression and ^{68}Ga-PSMA uptake in LNCaP cells. *J. Cancer Res. Clin. Oncol.* **2021**, *147*, 1733–1743. [CrossRef]
30. Brumberg, J.; Beckl, M.; Dierks, A.; Schirbel, A.; Krebs, M.; Buck, A.; Kübler, H.; Lapa, C.; Seitz, A.K. Detection Rate of ^{68}Ga-PSMA Ligand PET/CT in Patients with Recurrent Prostate Cancer and Androgen Deprivation Therapy. *Biomedicines* **2020**, *8*, 511. [CrossRef]
31. Vallabhajosula, S.; Killeen, R.P.; Osborne, J.R. Altered biodistribution of radiopharmaceuticals: Role of radiochemical/pharmaceutical purity, physiological, and pharmacologic factors. *Semin. Nucl. Med.* **2010**, *40*, 220–241. [CrossRef]
32. Evans, B.J.; King, A.T.; Katsifis, A.; Matesic, L.; Jamie, J.F. Methods to Enhance the Metabolic Stability of Peptide-Based PET Radiopharmaceuticals. *Molecules* **2020**, *25*, 2314. [CrossRef] [PubMed]
33. Lilburn, D.M.L.; Groves, A.M. The role of PET in imaging of the tumour microenvironment and response to immunotherapy. *Clin. Radiol.* **2021**, *76*, 784.e1–784.e15. [CrossRef]
34. Chaturvedi, S.; Hazari, P.P.; Kaul, A.; Anju; Mishra, A.K. Microenvironment Stimulated Bioresponsive Small Molecule Carriers for Radiopharmaceuticals. *ACS Omega* **2020**, *5*, 26297–26306. [CrossRef] [PubMed]
35. Parker, C.C.; Lapi, S.E. Positron Emission Tomography Imaging of Macrophages in Cancer. *Cancers* **2021**, *13*, 1921. [CrossRef]
36. Iravani, A.; Hicks, R.J. Imaging the Cancer Immune Environment and Its Response to Pharmacologic Intervention, Part 1: The Role of ^{18}F-FDG PET/CT. *J. Nucl. Med.* **2020**, *61*, 943–950. [CrossRef] [PubMed]
37. Dimitrakopoulou-Strauss, A.; Pan, L.; Sachpekidis, C. Kinetic modeling and parametric imaging with dynamic PET for oncological applications: General considerations, current clinical applications, and future perspectives. *Eur. J. Nucl. Med. Mol. Imaging* **2021**, *48*, 21–39. [CrossRef]
38. Kletting, P.; Thieme, A.; Eberhardt, N.; Rinscheid, A.; D'Alessandria, C.; Allmann, J.; Wester, H.J.; Tauber, R.; Beer, A.J.; Glatting, G.; et al. Modeling and Predicting Tumor Response in Radioligand Therapy. *J. Nucl. Med.* **2019**, *60*, 65–70. [CrossRef]
39. Wimberley, C.; Lavisse, S.; Hillmer, A.; Hinz, R.; Turkheimer, F.; Zanotti-Fregonara, P. Kinetic modeling and parameter estimation of TSPO PET imaging in the human brain. *Eur. J. Nucl. Med. Mol. Imaging* **2021**, *49*, 246–256. [CrossRef]
40. Lammertsma, A.A. Radioligand studies: Imaging and quantitative analysis. *Eur. Neuropsychopharmacol. J. Eur. Coll. Neuropsychopharmacol.* **2002**, *12*, 513–516. [CrossRef]
41. Rogasch, J.M.; Suleiman, S.; Hofheinz, F.; Bluemel, S.; Lukas, M.; Amthauer, H.; Furth, C. Reconstructed spatial resolution and contrast recovery with Bayesian penalized likelihood reconstruction (Q.Clear) for FDG-PET compared to time-of-flight (TOF) with point spread function (PSF). *EJNMMI Phys.* **2020**, *7*, 2. [CrossRef] [PubMed]
42. Bettinardi, V.; Castiglioni, I.; De Bernardi, E.; Gilardi, M.C. PET quantification: Strategies for partial volume correction. *Clin. Transl. Imaging* **2014**, *2*, 199–218. [CrossRef]
43. Hofheinz, F.; Langner, J.; Petr, J.; Beuthien-Baumann, B.; Oehme, L.; Steinbach, J.; Kotzerke, J.; van den Hoff, J. A method for model-free partial volume correction in oncological PET. *EJNMMI Res.* **2012**, *2*, 16. [CrossRef]
44. Surti, S.; Karp, J.S. Update on latest advances in time-of-flight PET. *Phys. Med.* **2020**, *80*, 251–258. [CrossRef] [PubMed]

45. Pan, T.; Einstein, S.A.; Kappadath, S.C.; Grogg, K.S.; Lois Gomez, C.; Alessio, A.M.; Hunter, W.C.; El Fakhri, G.; Kinahan, P.E.; Mawlawi, O.R. Performance evaluation of the 5-Ring GE Discovery MI PET/CT system using the national electrical manufacturers association NU 2-2012 Standard. *Med. Phys.* **2019**, *46*, 3025–3033. [CrossRef]
46. Reynés-Llompart, G.; Gámez-Cenzano, C.; Romero-Zayas, I.; Rodríguez-Bel, L.; Vercher-Conejero, J.L.; Martí-Climent, J.M. Performance Characteristics of the Whole-Body Discovery IQ PET/CT System. *J. Nucl. Med.* **2017**, *58*, 1155–1161. [CrossRef]
47. Van Sluis, J.; de Jong, J.; Schaar, J.; Noordzij, W.; van Snick, P.; Dierckx, R.; Borra, R.; Willemsen, A.; Boellaard, R. Performance Characteristics of the Digital Biograph Vision PET/CT System. *J. Nucl. Med.* **2019**, *60*, 1031–1036. [CrossRef]
48. Rausch, I.; Cal-González, J.; Dapra, D.; Gallowitsch, H.J.; Lind, P.; Beyer, T.; Minear, G. Performance evaluation of the Biograph mCT Flow PET/CT system according to the NEMA NU2-2012 standard. *EJNMMI Phys.* **2015**, *2*, 26. [CrossRef]
49. Conti, M. Focus on time-of-flight PET: The benefits of improved time resolution. *Eur. J. Nucl. Med. Mol. Imaging* **2011**, *38*, 1147–1157. [CrossRef]
50. Bailey, D.; Meikle, S.; Jones, T. Effective sensitivity in 3D PET: The impact of detector dead time on 3D system performance. *IEEE Trans. Nucl. Sci.* **1997**, *44*, 1180–1185. [CrossRef]
51. Cherry, S.R.; Jones, T.; Karp, J.S.; Qi, J.; Moses, W.W.; Badawi, R.D. Total-Body PET: Maximizing Sensitivity to Create New Opportunities for Clinical Research and Patient Care. *J. Nucl. Med.* **2018**, *59*, 3–12. [CrossRef] [PubMed]
52. Rausch, I.; Ruiz, A.; Valverde-Pascual, I.; Cal-González, J.; Beyer, T.; Carrio, I. Performance Evaluation of the Vereos PET/CT System According to the NEMA NU2-2012 Standard. *J. Nucl. Med.* **2019**, *60*, 561–567. [CrossRef] [PubMed]
53. Fuentes-Ocampo, F.; López-Mora, D.A.; Flotats, A.; Paillahueque, G.; Camacho, V.; Duch, J.; Fernández, A.; Domènech, A.; Estorch, M.; Carrió, I. Digital vs. analog PET/CT: Intra-subject comparison of the SUVmax in target lesions and reference regions. *Eur. J. Nucl. Med. Mol. Imaging* **2019**, *46*, 1745–1750. [CrossRef] [PubMed]
54. Hsu, D.F.C.; Ilan, E.; Peterson, W.T.; Uribe, J.; Lubberink, M.; Levin, C.S. Studies of a Next-Generation Silicon-Photomultiplier-Based Time-of-Flight PET/CT System. *J. Nucl. Med.* **2017**, *58*, 1511–1518. [CrossRef] [PubMed]
55. Zhang, J.; Maniawski, P.; Knopp, M.V. Performance evaluation of the next generation solid-state digital photon counting PET/CT system. *EJNMMI Res.* **2018**, *8*, 97. [CrossRef]
56. Oddstig, J.; Brolin, G.; Trägårdh, E.; Minarik, D. Head-to-head comparison of a Si-photomultiplier-based and a conventional photomultiplier-based PET-CT system. *EJNMMI Phys.* **2021**, *8*, 19. [CrossRef]
57. Kinahan, P.E.; Townsend, D.W.; Beyer, T.; Sashin, D. Attenuation correction for a combined 3D PET/CT scanner. *Med. Phys.* **1998**, *25*, 2046–2053. [CrossRef]
58. Boellaard, R.; Rausch, I.; Beyer, T.; Delso, G.; Yaqub, M.; Quick, H.H.; Sattler, B. Quality control for quantitative multicenter whole-body PET/MR studies: A NEMA image quality phantom study with three current PET/MR systems. *Med. Phys.* **2015**, *42*, 5961–5969. [CrossRef]
59. Mackewn, J.E.; Stirling, J.; Jeljeli, S.; Gould, S.M.; Johnstone, R.I.; Merida, I.; Pike, L.C.; McGinnity, C.J.; Beck, K.; Howes, O.; et al. Practical issues and limitations of brain attenuation correction on a simultaneous PET-MR scanner. *EJNMMI Phys.* **2020**, *7*, 24. [CrossRef]
60. Schäfer, J.F.; Gatidis, S.; Schmidt, H.; Gückel, B.; Bezrukov, I.; Pfannenberg, C.A.; Reimold, M.; Ebinger, M.; Fuchs, J.; Claussen, C.D.; et al. Simultaneous whole-body PET/MR imaging in comparison to PET/CT in pediatric oncology: Initial results. *Radiology* **2014**, *273*, 220–231. [CrossRef]
61. Beyer, T.; Lassen, M.L.; Boellaard, R.; Delso, G.; Yaqub, M.; Sattler, B.; Quick, H.H. Investigating the state-of-the-art in whole-body MR-based attenuation correction: An intra-individual, inter-system, inventory study on three clinical PET/MR systems. *Magma* **2016**, *29*, 75–87. [CrossRef]
62. Samarin, A.; Burger, C.; Wollenweber, S.D.; Crook, D.W.; Burger, I.A.; Schmid, D.T.; von Schulthess, G.K.; Kuhn, F.P. PET/MR imaging of bone lesions—Implications for PET quantification from imperfect attenuation correction. *Eur. J. Nucl. Med. Mol. Imaging* **2012**, *39*, 1154–1160. [CrossRef] [PubMed]
63. Ziegler, S.; Braun, H.; Ritt, P.; Hocke, C.; Kuwert, T.; Quick, H.H. Systematic evaluation of phantom fluids for simultaneous PET/MR hybrid imaging. *J. Nucl. Med.* **2013**, *54*, 1464–1471. [CrossRef] [PubMed]
64. Rausch, I.; Valladares, A.; Sundar, L.K.S.; Beyer, T.; Hacker, M.; Meyerspeer, M.; Unger, E. Standard MRI-based attenuation correction for PET/MRI phantoms: A novel concept using MRI-visible polymer. *EJNMMI Phys.* **2021**, *8*, 18. [CrossRef]
65. Heusch, P.; Buchbender, C.; Beiderwellen, K.; Nensa, F.; Hartung-Knemeyer, V.; Lauenstein, T.C.; Bockisch, A.; Forsting, M.; Antoch, G.; Heusner, T.A. Standardized uptake values for [^{18}F] FDG in normal organ tissues: Comparison of whole-body PET/CT and PET/MRI. *Eur. J. Radiol.* **2013**, *82*, 870–876. [CrossRef] [PubMed]
66. Al-Nabhani, K.Z.; Syed, R.; Michopoulou, S.; Alkalbani, J.; Afaq, A.; Panagiotidis, E.; O'Meara, C.; Groves, A.; Ell, P.; Bomanji, J. Qualitative and quantitative comparison of PET/CT and PET/MR imaging in clinical practice. *J. Nucl. Med.* **2014**, *55*, 88–94. [CrossRef]
67. Kaalep, A.; Sera, T.; Oyen, W.; Krause, B.J.; Chiti, A.; Liu, Y.; Boellaard, R. EANM/EARL FDG-PET/CT accreditation - Summary results from the first 200 accredited imaging systems. *Eur. J. Nucl. Med. Mol. Imaging* **2018**, *45*, 412–422. [CrossRef]
68. Sokoloff, L.; Reivich, M.; Kennedy, C.; Des Rosiers, M.H.; Patlak, C.S.; Pettigrew, K.D.; Sakurada, O.; Shinohara, M. The [^{14}C]deoxyglucose method for the measurement of local cerebral glucose utilization: Theory, procedure, and normal values in the conscious and anesthetized albino rat. *J. Neurochem.* **1977**, *28*, 897–916. [CrossRef]

69. van den Hoff, J.; Oehme, L.; Schramm, G.; Maus, J.; Lougovski, A.; Petr, J.; Beuthien-Baumann, B.; Hofheinz, F. The PET-derived tumor-to-blood standard uptake ratio (SUR) is superior to tumor SUV as a surrogate parameter of the metabolic rate of FDG. *EJNMMI Res.* **2013**, *3*, 77. [CrossRef]
70. Kramer, G.M.; Frings, V.; Hoetjes, N.; Hoekstra, O.S.; Smit, E.F.; de Langen, A.J.; Boellaard, R. Repeatability of Quantitative Whole-Body ^{18}F-FDG PET/CT Uptake Measures as Function of Uptake Interval and Lesion Selection in Non-Small Cell Lung Cancer Patients. *J. Nucl. Med.* **2016**, *57*, 1343–1349. [CrossRef]
71. van den Hoff, J.; Lougovski, A.; Schramm, G.; Maus, J.; Oehme, L.; Petr, J.; Beuthien-Baumann, B.; Kotzerke, J.; Hofheinz, F. Correction of scan time dependence of standard uptake values in oncological PET. *EJNMMI Res.* **2014**, *4*, 18. [CrossRef]
72. Wang, R.; Chen, H.; Fan, C. Impacts of time interval on ^{18}F-FDG uptake for PET/CT in normal organs: A systematic review. *Medicine* **2018**, *97*, e13122. [CrossRef]
73. Chin, B.B.; Green, E.D.; Turkington, T.G.; Hawk, T.C.; Coleman, R.E. Increasing uptake time in FDG-PET: Standardized uptake values in normal tissues at 1 versus 3 h. *Mol. Imaging Biol.* **2009**, *11*, 118–122. [CrossRef]
74. Ringheim, A.; Campos Neto, G.C.; Anazodo, U.; Cui, L.; da Cunha, M.L.; Vitor, T.; Martins, K.M.; Miranda, A.C.C.; de Barboza, M.F.; Fuscaldi, L.L.; et al. Kinetic modeling of ^{68}Ga-PSMA-11 and validation of simplified methods for quantification in primary prostate cancer patients. *EJNMMI Res.* **2020**, *10*, 12. [CrossRef]
75. Ilan, E.; Sandström, M.; Velikyan, I.; Sundin, A.; Eriksson, B.; Lubberink, M. Parametric Net Influx Rate Images of ^{68}Ga-DOTATOC and ^{68}Ga-DOTATATE: Quantitative Accuracy and Improved Image Contrast. *J. Nucl. Med.* **2017**, *58*, 744–749. [CrossRef] [PubMed]
76. Trägårdh, E.; Minarik, D.; Almquist, H.; Bitzén, U.; Garpered, S.; Hvittfelt, E.; Olsson, B.; Oddstig, J. Impact of acquisition time and penalizing factor in a block-sequential regularized expectation maximization reconstruction algorithm on a Si-photomultiplier-based PET-CT system for ^{18}F-FDG. *EJNMMI Res.* **2019**, *9*, 64. [CrossRef] [PubMed]
77. Masuda, Y.; Kondo, C.; Matsuo, Y.; Uetani, M.; Kusakabe, K. Comparison of imaging protocols for ^{18}F-FDG PET/CT in overweight patients: Optimizing scan duration versus administered dose. *J. Nucl. Med.* **2009**, *50*, 844–848. [CrossRef]
78. Pilz, J.; Hehenwarter, L.; Zimmermann, G.; Rendl, G.; Schweighofer-Zwink, G.; Beheshti, M.; Pirich, C. Feasibility of equivalent performance of 3D TOF [^{18}F]-FDG PET/CT with reduced acquisition time using clinical and semiquantitative parameters. *EJNMMI Res.* **2021**, *11*, 44. [CrossRef] [PubMed]
79. Alberts, I.; Sachpekidis, C.; Prenosil, G.; Viscione, M.; Bohn, K.P.; Mingels, C.; Shi, K.; Afshar-Oromieh, A.; Rominger, A. Digital PET/CT allows for shorter acquisition protocols or reduced radiopharmaceutical dose in [^{18}F]-FDG PET/CT. *Ann. Nucl. Med.* **2021**, *35*, 485–492. [CrossRef] [PubMed]
80. Sher, A.; Lacoeuille, F.; Fosse, P.; Vervueren, L.; Cahouet-Vannier, A.; Dabli, D.; Bouchet, F.; Couturier, O. For avid glucose tumors, the SUV peak is the most reliable parameter for [^{18}F]FDG-PET/CT quantification, regardless of acquisition time. *EJNMMI Res.* **2016**, *6*, 21. [CrossRef] [PubMed]
81. Sonni, I.; Baratto, L.; Park, S.; Hatami, N.; Srinivas, S.; Davidzon, G.; Gambhir, S.S.; Iagaru, A. Initial experience with a SiPM-based PET/CT scanner: Influence of acquisition time on image quality. *EJNMMI Phys.* **2018**, *5*, 9. [CrossRef] [PubMed]
82. Hausmann, D.; Dinter, D.J.; Sadick, M.; Brade, J.; Schoenberg, S.O.; Büsing, K. The impact of acquisition time on image quality in whole-body ^{18}F-FDG PET/CT for cancer staging. *J. Nucl. Med. Technol.* **2012**, *40*, 255–258. [CrossRef]
83. Werner, M.K.; Parker, J.A.; Kolodny, G.M.; English, J.R.; Palmer, M.R. Respiratory gating enhances imaging of pulmonary nodules and measurement of tracer uptake in FDG PET/CT. *AJR Am. J. Roentgenol.* **2009**, *193*, 1640–1645. [CrossRef]
84. Frood, R.; Prestwich, R.; Tsoumpas, C.; Murray, P.; Franks, K.; Scarsbrook, A. Effectiveness of Respiratory-gated Positron Emission Tomography/Computed Tomography for Radiotherapy Planning in Patients with Lung Carcinoma—A Systematic Review. *Clin. Oncol. R. Coll. Radiol.* **2018**, *30*, 225–232. [CrossRef] [PubMed]
85. Grootjans, W.; de Geus-Oei, L.F.; Meeuwis, A.P.; van der Vos, C.S.; Gotthardt, M.; Oyen, W.J.; Visser, E.P. Amplitude-based optimal respiratory gating in positron emission tomography in patients with primary lung cancer. *Eur. Radiol.* **2014**, *24*, 3242–3250. [CrossRef]
86. Suenaga, Y.; Kitajima, K.; Aoki, H.; Okunaga, T.; Kono, A.; Matsumoto, I.; Fukumoto, T.; Tanaka, K.; Sugimura, K. Respiratory-gated ^{18}F-FDG PET/CT for the diagnosis of liver metastasis. *Eur. J. Radiol.* **2013**, *82*, 1696–1701. [CrossRef] [PubMed]
87. Schulz, A.; Godt, J.C.; Dormagen, J.B.; Holtedahl, J.E.; Bogsrud, T.V.; Labori, K.J.; Kløw, N.E.; Bach-Gansmo, T. Respiratory gated PET/CT of the liver: A novel method and its impact on the detection of colorectal liver metastases. *Eur. J. Radiol.* **2015**, *84*, 1424–1431. [CrossRef]
88. Smeets, E.M.M.; Withaar, D.S.; Grootjans, W.; Hermans, J.J.; van Laarhoven, K.; de Geus-Oei, L.F.; Gotthardt, M.; Aarntzen, E. Optimal respiratory-gated [^{18}F]FDG PET/CT significantly impacts the quantification of metabolic parameters and their correlation with overall survival in patients with pancreatic ductal adenocarcinoma. *EJNMMI Res.* **2019**, *9*, 24. [CrossRef]
89. Pépin, A.; Daouk, J.; Bailly, P.; Hapdey, S.; Meyer, M.E. Management of respiratory motion in PET/computed tomography: The state of the art. *Nucl. Med. Commun.* **2014**, *35*, 113–122. [CrossRef]
90. Lassen, M.L.; Kwiecinski, J.; Slomka, P.J. Gating Approaches in Cardiac PET Imaging. *PET Clin.* **2019**, *14*, 271–279. [CrossRef]
91. Rubeaux, M.; Doris, M.K.; Alessio, A.; Slomka, P.J. Enhancing Cardiac PET by Motion Correction Techniques. *Curr. Cardiol. Rep.* **2017**, *19*, 14. [CrossRef]
92. Rogasch, J.M.M.; Boellaard, R.; Pike, L.; Borchmann, P.; Johnson, P.; Wolf, J.; Barrington, S.F.; Kobe, C. Moving the goalposts while scoring—the dilemma posed by new PET technologies. *Eur. J. Nucl. Med. Mol. Imaging* **2021**, *48*, 2696–2710. [CrossRef]

93. Aide, N.; Lasnon, C.; Kesner, A.; Levin, C.S.; Buvat, I.; Iagaru, A.; Hermann, K.; Badawi, R.D.; Cherry, S.R.; Bradley, K.M.; et al. New PET technologies—Embracing progress and pushing the limits. *Eur. J. Nucl. Med. Mol. Imaging* **2021**, *48*, 2711–2726. [CrossRef]
94. Surti, S. Update on time-of-flight PET imaging. *J. Nucl. Med.* **2015**, *56*, 98–105. [CrossRef]
95. Rogasch, J.M.; Steffen, I.G.; Hofheinz, F.; Großer, O.S.; Furth, C.; Mohnike, K.; Hass, P.; Walke, M.; Apostolova, I.; Amthauer, H. The association of tumor-to-background ratios and SUVmax deviations related to point spread function and time-of-flight F18-FDG-PET/CT reconstruction in colorectal liver metastases. *EJNMMI Res.* **2015**, *5*, 31. [CrossRef] [PubMed]
96. Li, C.Y.; Klohr, S.; Sadick, H.; Weiss, C.; Hoermann, K.; Schoenberg, S.O.; Sadick, M. Effect of time-of-flight technique on the diagnostic performance of ^{18}F-FDG PET/CT for assessment of lymph node metastases in head and neck squamous cell carcinoma. *J. Nucl. Med. Technol.* **2014**, *42*, 181–187. [CrossRef]
97. Rogasch, J.M.; Hofheinz, F.; Lougovski, A.; Furth, C.; Ruf, J.; Großer, O.S.; Mohnike, K.; Hass, P.; Walke, M.; Amthauer, H.; et al. The influence of different signal-to-background ratios on spatial resolution and F18-FDG-PET quantification using point spread function and time-of-flight reconstruction. *EJNMMI Phys.* **2014**, *1*, 12. [CrossRef]
98. Rapisarda, E.; Bettinardi, V.; Thielemans, K.; Gilardi, M.C. Image-based point spread function implementation in a fully 3D OSEM reconstruction algorithm for PET. *Phys. Med. Biol.* **2010**, *55*, 4131–4151. [CrossRef] [PubMed]
99. Akamatsu, G.; Mitsumoto, K.; Taniguchi, T.; Tsutsui, Y.; Baba, S.; Sasaki, M. Influences of point-spread function and time-of-flight reconstructions on standardized uptake value of lymph node metastases in FDG-PET. *Eur. J. Radiol.* **2014**, *83*, 226–230. [CrossRef]
100. Quak, E.; Le Roux, P.Y.; Hofman, M.S.; Robin, P.; Bourhis, D.; Callahan, J.; Binns, D.; Desmonts, C.; Salaun, P.Y.; Hicks, R.J.; et al. Harmonizing FDG PET quantification while maintaining optimal lesion detection: Prospective multicentre validation in 517 oncology patients. *Eur. J. Nucl. Med. Mol. Imaging* **2015**, *42*, 2072–2082. [CrossRef] [PubMed]
101. Kaalep, A.; Sera, T.; Rijnsdorp, S.; Yaqub, M.; Talsma, A.; Lodge, M.A.; Boellaard, R. Feasibility of state of the art PET/CT systems performance harmonisation. *Eur. J. Nucl. Med. Mol. Imaging* **2018**, *45*, 1344–1361. [CrossRef] [PubMed]
102. Kaalep, A.; Burggraaff, C.N.; Pieplenbosch, S.; Verwer, E.E.; Sera, T.; Zijlstra, J.; Hoekstra, O.S.; Oprea-Lager, D.E.; Boellaard, R. Quantitative implications of the updated EARL 2019 PET-CT performance standards. *EJNMMI Phys.* **2019**, *6*, 28. [CrossRef] [PubMed]
103. Houdu, B.; Lasnon, C.; Licaj, I.; Thomas, G.; Do, P.; Guizard, A.V.; Desmonts, C.; Aide, N. Why harmonization is needed when using FDG PET/CT as a prognosticator: Demonstration with EARL-compliant SUV as an independent prognostic factor in lung cancer. *Eur. J. Nucl. Med. Mol. Imaging* **2019**, *46*, 421–428. [CrossRef] [PubMed]
104. Mumcuoğlu, E.U.; Leahy, R.M.; Cherry, S.R. Bayesian reconstruction of PET images: Methodology and performance analysis. *Phys. Med. Biol.* **1996**, *41*, 1777–1807. [CrossRef]
105. Ahn, S.; Ross, S.G.; Asma, E.; Miao, J.; Jin, X.; Cheng, L.; Wollenweber, S.D.; Manjeshwar, R.M. Quantitative comparison of OSEM and penalized likelihood image reconstruction using relative difference penalties for clinical PET. *Phys. Med. Biol.* **2015**, *60*, 5733–5751. [CrossRef]
106. Ahn, S.; Fessler, J.A. Globally convergent image reconstruction for emission tomography using relaxed ordered subsets algorithms. *IEEE Trans. Med. Imaging* **2003**, *22*, 613–626. [CrossRef]
107. Teoh, E.J.; McGowan, D.R.; Macpherson, R.E.; Bradley, K.M.; Gleeson, F.V. Phantom and Clinical Evaluation of the Bayesian Penalized Likelihood Reconstruction Algorithm Q.Clear on an LYSO PET/CT System. *J. Nucl. Med.* **2015**, *56*, 1447–1452. [CrossRef]
108. Lindström, E.; Sundin, A.; Trampal, C.; Lindsjö, L.; Ilan, E.; Danfors, T.; Antoni, G.; Sörensen, J.; Lubberink, M. Evaluation of Penalized-Likelihood Estimation Reconstruction on a Digital Time-of-Flight PET/CT Scanner for ^{18}F-FDG Whole-Body Examinations. *J. Nucl. Med.* **2018**, *59*, 1152–1158. [CrossRef]
109. Te Riet, J.; Rijnsdorp, S.; Roef, M.J.; Arends, A.J. Evaluation of a Bayesian penalized likelihood reconstruction algorithm for low-count clinical ^{18}F-FDG PET/CT. *EJNMMI Phys.* **2019**, *6*, 32. [CrossRef]
110. Wu, Z.; Qin, Z.; Huang, B.; Guo, B.; Hao, X.; Wu, P.; Zhao, B.; Xie, J.; Li, S. Improved Absolute Quantification using Bayesian Penalized Likelihood Reconstruction on a Digital PET/CT—Towards True Uptake Measurement. *Res. Sq.* **2021**. [CrossRef]
111. Howard, B.A.; Morgan, R.; Thorpe, M.P.; Turkington, T.G.; Oldan, J.; James, O.G.; Borges-Neto, S. Comparison of Bayesian penalized likelihood reconstruction versus OS-EM for characterization of small pulmonary nodules in oncologic PET/CT. *Ann. Nucl. Med.* **2017**, *31*, 623–628. [CrossRef]
112. Messerli, M.; Stolzmann, P.; Egger-Sigg, M.; Trinckauf, J.; D'Aguanno, S.; Burger, I.A.; von Schulthess, G.K.; Kaufmann, P.A.; Huellner, M.W. Impact of a Bayesian penalized likelihood reconstruction algorithm on image quality in novel digital PET/CT: Clinical implications for the assessment of lung tumors. *EJNMMI Phys.* **2018**, *5*, 27. [CrossRef] [PubMed]
113. Otani, T.; Hosono, M.; Kanagaki, M.; Onishi, Y.; Matsubara, N.; Kawabata, K.; Kimura, H. Evaluation and Optimization of a New PET Reconstruction Algorithm, Bayesian Penalized Likelihood Reconstruction, for Lung Cancer Assessment According to Lesion Size. *AJR Am. J. Roentgenol.* **2019**, *213*, W50–W56. [CrossRef] [PubMed]
114. Reader, A.J.; Corda, G.; Mehranian, A.; Costa-Luis, C.d.; Ellis, S.; Schnabel, J.A. Deep Learning for PET Image Reconstruction. *IEEE Trans. Radiat. Plasma Med. Sci.* **2021**, *5*, 1–25. [CrossRef]
115. Aschoff, P.; Plathow, C.; Beyer, T.; Lichy, M.P.; Erb, G.; Öksüz, M.; Claussen, C.D.; Pfannenberg, C. Multiphase contrast-enhanced CT with highly concentrated contrast agent can be used for PET attenuation correction in integrated PET/CT imaging. *Eur. J. Nucl. Med. Mol. Imaging* **2012**, *39*, 316–325. [CrossRef] [PubMed]

116. Behrendt, F.F.; Temur, Y.; Verburg, F.A.; Palmowski, M.; Krohn, T.; Pietsch, H.; Kuhl, C.K.; Mottaghy, F.M. PET/CT in lung cancer: Influence of contrast medium on quantitative and clinical assessment. *Eur. Radiol.* **2012**, *22*, 2458–2464. [CrossRef]
117. Yau, Y.Y.; Chan, W.S.; Tam, Y.M.; Vernon, P.; Wong, S.; Coel, M.; Chu, S.K. Application of intravenous contrast in PET/CT: Does it really introduce significant attenuation correction error? *J. Nucl. Med.* **2005**, *46*, 283–291.
118. Rebière, M.; Verburg, F.A.; Palmowski, M.; Krohn, T.; Pietsch, H.; Kuhl, C.K.; Mottaghy, F.M.; Behrendt, F.F. Multiphase CT scanning and different intravenous contrast media concentrations in combined F-18-FDG PET/CT: Effect on quantitative and clinical assessment. *Eur. J. Radiol.* **2012**, *81*, e862–e869. [CrossRef]
119. Berthelsen, A.K.; Holm, S.; Loft, A.; Klausen, T.L.; Andersen, F.; Højgaard, L. PET/CT with intravenous contrast can be used for PET attenuation correction in cancer patients. *Eur. J. Nucl. Med. Mol. Imaging* **2005**, *32*, 1167–1175. [CrossRef]
120. Nakamoto, Y.; Chin, B.B.; Kraitchman, D.L.; Lawler, L.P.; Marshall, L.T.; Wahl, R.L. Effects of nonionic intravenous contrast agents at PET/CT imaging: Phantom and canine studies. *Radiology* **2003**, *227*, 817–824. [CrossRef]
121. Voltin, C.A.; Mettler, J.; Boellaard, R.; Kuhnert, G.; Dietlein, M.; Borchmann, P.; Drzezga, A.; Kobe, C. Quantitative assessment of ^{18}F-FDG PET in patients with Hodgkin lymphoma: Is it significantly affected by contrast-enhanced computed tomography attenuation correction? *Nucl. Med. Commun.* **2019**, *40*, 249–257. [CrossRef] [PubMed]
122. Berger, K.L.; Nicholson, S.A.; Dehdashti, F.; Siegel, B.A. FDG PET evaluation of mucinous neoplasms: Correlation of FDG uptake with histopathologic features. *AJR Am. J. Roentgenol.* **2000**, *174*, 1005–1008. [CrossRef] [PubMed]
123. Kang, D.E.; White, R.L., Jr.; Zuger, J.H.; Sasser, H.C.; Teigland, C.M. Clinical use of fluorodeoxyglucose F 18 positron emission tomography for detection of renal cell carcinoma. *J. Urol.* **2004**, *171*, 1806–1809. [CrossRef] [PubMed]
124. Vesselle, H.; Salskov, A.; Turcotte, E.; Wiens, L.; Schmidt, R.; Jordan, C.D.; Vallières, E.; Wood, D.E. Relationship between non-small cell lung cancer FDG uptake at PET, tumor histology, and Ki-67 proliferation index. *J. Thorac. Oncol.* **2008**, *3*, 971–978. [CrossRef]
125. Ioannidis, J.P.; Lau, J. ^{18}F-FDG PET for the diagnosis and grading of soft-tissue sarcoma: A meta-analysis. *J. Nucl. Med.* **2003**, *44*, 717–724.
126. Liu, I.J.; Zafar, M.B.; Lai, Y.H.; Segall, G.M.; Terris, M.K. Fluorodeoxyglucose positron emission tomography studies in diagnosis and staging of clinically organ-confined prostate cancer. *Urology* **2001**, *57*, 108–111. [CrossRef]
127. Hofman, M.S.; Lawrentschuk, N.; Francis, R.J.; Tang, C.; Vela, I.; Thomas, P.; Rutherford, N.; Martin, J.M.; Frydenberg, M.; Shakher, R.; et al. Prostate-specific membrane antigen PET-CT in patients with high-risk prostate cancer before curative-intent surgery or radiotherapy (proPSMA): A prospective, randomised, multicentre study. *Lancet* **2020**, *395*, 1208–1216. [CrossRef]
128. Naswa, N.; Sharma, P.; Gupta, S.K.; Karunanithi, S.; Reddy, R.M.; Patnecha, M.; Lata, S.; Kumar, R.; Malhotra, A.; Bal, C. Dual tracer functional imaging of gastroenteropancreatic neuroendocrine tumors using ^{68}Ga-DOTA-NOC PET-CT and ^{18}F-FDG PET-CT: Competitive or complimentary? *Clin. Nucl. Med.* **2014**, *39*, e27–e34. [CrossRef]
129. Dunet, V.; Pomoni, A.; Hottinger, A.; Nicod-Lalonde, M.; Prior, J.O. Performance of ^{18}F-FET versus ^{18}F-FDG-PET for the diagnosis and grading of brain tumors: Systematic review and meta-analysis. *Neuro-Oncology* **2016**, *18*, 426–434. [CrossRef]
130. Chen, H.; Pang, Y.; Wu, J.; Zhao, L.; Hao, B.; Wu, J.; Wei, J.; Wu, S.; Zhao, L.; Luo, Z.; et al. Comparison of [^{68}Ga]Ga-DOTA-FAPI-04 and [^{18}F] FDG PET/CT for the diagnosis of primary and metastatic lesions in patients with various types of cancer. *Eur. J. Nucl. Med. Mol. Imaging* **2020**, *47*, 1820–1832. [CrossRef]
131. Fendler, W.P.; Calais, J.; Eiber, M.; Simko, J.P.; Kurhanewicz, J.; Santos, R.D.; Feng, F.Y.; Reiter, R.E.; Rettig, M.B.; Nickols, N.G.; et al. False positive PSMA PET for tumor remnants in the irradiated prostate and other interpretation pitfalls in a prospective multi-center trial. *Eur. J. Nucl. Med. Mol. Imaging* **2021**, *48*, 501–508. [CrossRef] [PubMed]
132. Barbosa, F.; Queiroz, M.; Nunes, R.; Costa, L.; Zaniboni, E.; Marin, J.; Cerri, G.; Buchpiguel, C. Nonprostatic diseases on PSMA PET imaging: A spectrum of benign and malignant findings. *Cancer Imaging* **2020**, *20*, 23. [CrossRef] [PubMed]
133. Hofman, M.S.; Lau, W.F.; Hicks, R.J. Somatostatin receptor imaging with ^{68}Ga DOTATATE PET/CT: Clinical utility, normal patterns, pearls, and pitfalls in interpretation. *Radiographics* **2015**, *35*, 500–516. [CrossRef] [PubMed]
134. Zheng, S.; Lin, R.; Chen, S.; Zheng, J.; Lin, Z.; Zhang, Y.; Xue, Q.; Chen, Y.; Zhang, J.; Lin, K.; et al. Characterization of the benign lesions with increased ^{68}Ga-FAPI-04 uptake in PET/CT. *Ann. Nucl. Med.* **2021**, *35*, 1312–1320. [CrossRef] [PubMed]
135. Atterton-Evans, V.; Turner, J.; Vivanti, A.; Robertson, T. Variances of dietary preparation for suppression of physiological ^{18}F-FDG myocardial uptake in the presence of cardiac sarcoidosis: A systematic review. *J. Nucl. Cardiol. Off. Publ. Am. Soc. Nucl. Cardiol.* **2020**, *27*, 481–489. [CrossRef] [PubMed]
136. Rouzet, F.; Chequer, R.; Benali, K.; Lepage, L.; Ghodbane, W.; Duval, X.; Iung, B.; Vahanian, A.; Le Guludec, D.; Hyafil, F. Respective performance of ^{18}F-FDG PET and radiolabeled leukocyte scintigraphy for the diagnosis of prosthetic valve endocarditis. *J. Nucl. Med.* **2014**, *55*, 1980–1985. [CrossRef] [PubMed]
137. Scholtens, A.M.; Swart, L.E.; Verberne, H.J.; Tanis, W.; Lam, M.G.; Budde, R.P. Confounders in FDG-PET/CT Imaging of Suspected Prosthetic Valve Endocarditis. *JACC Cardiovasc. Imaging* **2016**, *9*, 1462–1465. [CrossRef]
138. Mathieu, C.; Mikaïl, N.; Benali, K.; Iung, B.; Duval, X.; Nataf, P.; Jondeau, G.; Hyafil, F.; Le Guludec, D.; Rouzet, F. Characterization of ^{18}F-Fluorodeoxyglucose Uptake Pattern in Noninfected Prosthetic Heart Valves. *Circ. Cardiovasc. Imaging* **2017**, *10*, e005585. [CrossRef]
139. Sohns, J.M.; Bavendiek, U.; Ross, T.L.; Bengel, F.M. Targeting Cardiovascular Implant Infection: Multimodality and Molecular Imaging. *Circ. Cardiovasc. Imaging* **2017**, *10*, e005376. [CrossRef]

140. Thackeray, J.T.; Derlin, T.; Haghikia, A.; Napp, L.C.; Wang, Y.; Ross, T.L.; Schäfer, A.; Tillmanns, J.; Wester, H.J.; Wollert, K.C.; et al. Molecular Imaging of the Chemokine Receptor CXCR4 After Acute Myocardial Infarction. *JACC Cardiovasc. Imaging* **2015**, *8*, 1417–1426. [CrossRef]
141. Takemiya, K.; Ning, X.; Seo, W.; Wang, X.; Mohammad, R.; Joseph, G.; Titterington, J.S.; Kraft, C.S.; Nye, J.A.; Murthy, N.; et al. Novel PET and Near Infrared Imaging Probes for the Specific Detection of Bacterial Infections Associated with Cardiac Devices. *JACC Cardiovasc. Imaging* **2019**, *12*, 875–886. [CrossRef] [PubMed]
142. Fin, L.; Bailly, P.; Daouk, J.; Meyer, M.E. A practical way to improve contrast-to-noise ratio and quantitation for statistical-based iterative reconstruction in whole-body PET imaging. *Med. Phys.* **2009**, *36*, 3072–3079. [CrossRef] [PubMed]
143. Trägårdh, E.; Minarik, D.; Brolin, G.; Bitzén, U.; Olsson, B.; Oddstig, J. Optimization of [^{18}F]PSMA-1007 PET-CT using regularized reconstruction in patients with prostate cancer. *EJNMMI Phys.* **2020**, *7*, 31. [CrossRef] [PubMed]
144. Geismar, J.H.; Stolzmann, P.; Sah, B.R.; Burger, I.A.; Seifert, B.; Delso, G.; von Schulthess, G.K.; Veit-Haibach, P.; Husmann, L. Intra-individual comparison of PET/CT with different body weight-adapted FDG dosage regimens. *Acta Radiol. Open* **2015**, *4*, 2047981614560076. [CrossRef] [PubMed]
145. EANM Research Ltd. (EARL) Publications and Guidelines. Available online: https://earl.eanm.org/guidelines-and-publications/ (accessed on 11 August 2021).
146. Teräs, M.; Tolvanen, T.; Johansson, J.J.; Williams, J.J.; Knuuti, J. Performance of the new generation of whole-body PET/CT scanners: Discovery STE and Discovery VCT. *Eur. J. Nucl. Med. Mol. Imaging* **2007**, *34*, 1683–1692. [CrossRef]
147. Wickham, F.; McMeekin, H.; Burniston, M.; McCool, D.; Pencharz, D.; Skillen, A.; Wagner, T. Patient-specific optimisation of administered activity and acquisition times for ^{18}F-FDG PET imaging. *EJNMMI Res.* **2017**, *7*, 3. [CrossRef]
148. Jakoby, B.W.; Bercier, Y.; Conti, M.; Casey, M.E.; Bendriem, B.; Townsend, D.W. Physical and clinical performance of the mCT time-of-flight PET/CT scanner. *Phys. Med. Biol.* **2011**, *56*, 2375–2389. [CrossRef]
149. Prenosil, G.A.; Sari, H.; Fürstner, M.; Afshar-Oromieh, A.; Shi, K.; Rominger, A.; Hentschel, M. Performance Characteristics of the Biograph Vision Quadra PET/CT system with long axial field of view using the NEMA NU 2-2018 Standard. *J. Nucl. Med.* **2021**. [CrossRef]
150. Spencer, B.A.; Berg, E.; Schmall, J.P.; Omidvari, N.; Leung, E.K.; Abdelhafez, Y.G.; Tang, S.; Deng, Z.; Dong, Y.; Lv, Y.; et al. Performance Evaluation of the uEXPLORER Total-Body PET/CT Scanner Based on NEMA NU 2-2018 with Additional Tests to Characterize PET Scanners with a Long Axial Field of View. *J. Nucl. Med.* **2021**, *62*, 861–870. [CrossRef]
151. Halpern, B.S.; Dahlbom, M.; Quon, A.; Schiepers, C.; Waldherr, C.; Silverman, D.H.; Ratib, O.; Czernin, J. Impact of patient weight and emission scan duration on PET/CT image quality and lesion detectability. *J. Nucl. Med.* **2004**, *45*, 797–801.
152. Halpern, B.S.; Dahlbom, M.; Auerbach, M.A.; Schiepers, C.; Fueger, B.J.; Weber, W.A.; Silverman, D.H.; Ratib, O.; Czernin, J. Optimizing imaging protocols for overweight and obese patients: A lutetium orthosilicate PET/CT study. *J. Nucl. Med.* **2005**, *46*, 603–607. [PubMed]
153. Sekine, T.; Delso, G.; Zeimpekis, K.G.; de Galiza Barbosa, F.; ter Voert, E.E.G.W.; Huellner, M.; Veit-Haibach, P. Reduction of ^{18}F-FDG Dose in Clinical PET/MR Imaging by Using Silicon Photomultiplier Detectors. *Radiology* **2017**, *286*, 249–259. [CrossRef] [PubMed]
154. López-Mora, D.A.; Flotats, A.; Fuentes-Ocampo, F.; Camacho, V.; Fernández, A.; Ruiz, A.; Duch, J.; Sizova, M.; Domènech, A.; Estorch, M.; et al. Comparison of image quality and lesion detection between digital and analog PET/CT. *Eur. J. Nucl. Med. Mol. Imaging* **2019**, *46*, 1383–1390. [CrossRef] [PubMed]
155. Baratto, L.; Toriihara, A.; Hatami, N.; Aparici, C.M.; Davidzon, G.; Levin, C.S.; Iagaru, A. Results of a Prospective Trial to Compare ^{68}Ga-DOTA-TATE with SiPM-Based PET/CT vs. Conventional PET/CT in Patients with Neuroendocrine Tumors. *Diagnostics* **2021**, *11*, 992. [CrossRef]
156. Minamimoto, R.; Levin, C.; Jamali, M.; Holley, D.; Barkhodari, A.; Zaharchuk, G.; Iagaru, A. Improvements in PET Image Quality in Time of Flight (TOF) Simultaneous PET/MRI. *Mol. Imaging Biol.* **2016**, *18*, 776–781. [CrossRef]
157. Akamatsu, G.; Ishikawa, K.; Mitsumoto, K.; Taniguchi, T.; Ohya, N.; Baba, S.; Abe, K.; Sasaki, M. Improvement in PET/CT image quality with a combination of point-spread function and time-of-flight in relation to reconstruction parameters. *J. Nucl. Med.* **2012**, *53*, 1716–1722. [CrossRef]
158. Taniguchi, T.; Akamatsu, G.; Kasahara, Y.; Mitsumoto, K.; Baba, S.; Tsutsui, Y.; Himuro, K.; Mikasa, S.; Kidera, D.; Sasaki, M. Improvement in PET/CT image quality in overweight patients with PSF and TOF. *Ann. Nucl. Med.* **2015**, *29*, 71–77. [CrossRef]
159. Surti, S.; Scheuermann, J.; El Fakhri, G.; Daube-witherspoon, M.E.; Lim, R.; Abi-Hatem, N.; Moussallem, E.; Benard, F.; Mankoff, D.; Karp, J.S. Impact of time-of-flight PET on whole-body oncologic studies: A human observer lesion detection and localization study. *J. Nucl. Med.* **2011**, *52*, 712–719. [CrossRef]
160. El Fakhri, G.; Surti, S.; Trott, C.M.; Scheuermann, J.; Karp, J.S. Improvement in lesion detection with whole-body oncologic time-of-flight PET. *J. Nucl. Med.* **2011**, *52*, 347–353. [CrossRef]
161. Schaefferkoetter, J.; Casey, M.; Townsend, D.; El Fakhri, G. Clinical impact of time-of-flight and point response modeling in PET reconstructions: A lesion detection study. *Phys. Med. Biol.* **2013**, *58*, 1465–1478. [CrossRef]
162. Aklan, B.; Oehmigen, M.; Beiderwellen, K.; Ruhlmann, M.; Paulus, D.H.; Jakoby, B.W.; Ritt, P.; Quick, H.H. Impact of Point-Spread Function Modeling on PET Image Quality in Integrated PET/MR Hybrid Imaging. *J. Nucl. Med.* **2016**, *57*, 78–84. [CrossRef] [PubMed]

163. Kadrmas, D.J.; Casey, M.E.; Conti, M.; Jakoby, B.W.; Lois, C.; Townsend, D.W. Impact of time-of-flight on PET tumor detection. *J. Nucl. Med.* **2009**, *50*, 1315–1323. [CrossRef] [PubMed]
164. Kurita, Y.; Ichikawa, Y.; Nakanishi, T.; Tomita, Y.; Hasegawa, D.; Murashima, S.; Hirano, T.; Sakuma, H. The value of Bayesian penalized likelihood reconstruction for improving lesion conspicuity of malignant lung tumors on ^{18}F-FDG PET/CT: Comparison with ordered subset expectation maximization reconstruction incorporating time-of-flight model and point spread function correction. *Ann. Nucl. Med.* **2020**, *34*, 272–279. [CrossRef] [PubMed]
165. Jansen, B.H.E.; Jansen, R.W.; Wondergem, M.; Srbljin, S.; de Klerk, J.M.H.; Lissenberg-Witte, B.I.; Vis, A.N.; van Moorselaar, R.J.A.; Boellaard, R.; Hoekstra, O.S.; et al. Lesion Detection and Interobserver Agreement with Advanced Image Reconstruction for ^{18}F-DCFPyL PET/CT in Patients with Biochemically Recurrent Prostate Cancer. *J. Nucl. Med.* **2020**, *61*, 210–216. [CrossRef]
166. Andersen, F.L.; Klausen, T.L.; Loft, A.; Beyer, T.; Holm, S. Clinical evaluation of PET image reconstruction using a spatial resolution model. *Eur. J. Radiol.* **2013**, *82*, 862–869. [CrossRef]
167. Panin, V.Y.; Kehren, F.; Michel, C.; Casey, M. Fully 3-D PET reconstruction with system matrix derived from point source measurements. *IEEE Trans. Med. Imaging* **2006**, *25*, 907–921. [CrossRef]
168. Caribé, P.; Koole, M.; D'Asseler, Y.; Van Den Broeck, B.; Vandenberghe, S. Noise reduction using a Bayesian penalized-likelihood reconstruction algorithm on a time-of-flight PET-CT scanner. *EJNMMI Phys.* **2019**, *6*, 22. [CrossRef]
169. Guo, B.; Wu, Z.; Zhao, B.; Huang, B.; Li, X.; Zhao, J.; Li, Y. Quantification Accuracy Using Bayesian Penalized Likelihood Based Reconstruction on ^{68}Ga PET-CT. *J. Nucl. Med.* **2020**, *61* (Suppl. S1), 162.
170. Lindström, E.; Velikyan, I.; Regula, N.; Alhuseinalkhudhur, A.; Sundin, A.; Sörensen, J.; Lubberink, M. Regularized reconstruction of digital time-of-flight ^{68}Ga-PSMA-11 PET/CT for the detection of recurrent disease in prostate cancer patients. *Theranostics* **2019**, *9*, 3476–3484. [CrossRef]
171. Chicheportiche, A.; Goshen, E.; Godefroy, J.; Grozinsky-Glasberg, S.; Oleinikov, K.; Meirovitz, A.; Gross, D.J.; Ben-Haim, S. Can a penalized-likelihood estimation algorithm be used to reduce the injected dose or the acquisition time in ^{68}Ga-DOTATATE PET/CT studies? *EJNMMI Phys.* **2021**, *8*, 13. [CrossRef]
172. Kirchner, J.; O'Donoghue, J.A.; Becker, A.S.; Ulaner, G.A. Improved image reconstruction of ^{89}Zr-immunoPET studies using a Bayesian penalized likelihood reconstruction algorithm. *EJNMMI Phys.* **2021**, *8*, 6. [CrossRef] [PubMed]
173. Teoh, E.J.; McGowan, D.R.; Bradley, K.M.; Belcher, E.; Black, E.; Gleeson, F.V. Novel penalised likelihood reconstruction of PET in the assessment of histologically verified small pulmonary nodules. *Eur. Radiol.* **2016**, *26*, 576–584. [CrossRef] [PubMed]
174. Schwyzer, M.; Martini, K.; Benz, D.C.; Burger, I.A.; Ferraro, D.A.; Kudura, K.; Treyer, V.; von Schulthess, G.K.; Kaufmann, P.A.; Huellner, M.W.; et al. Artificial intelligence for detecting small FDG-positive lung nodules in digital PET/CT: Impact of image reconstructions on diagnostic performance. *Eur. Radiol.* **2020**, *30*, 2031–2040. [CrossRef]
175. Björsdorff, M.; Oddstig, J.; Karindotter-Borgendahl, N.; Almquist, H.; Zackrisson, S.; Minarik, D.; Trägårdh, E. Impact of penalizing factor in a block-sequential regularized expectation maximization reconstruction algorithm for ^{18}F-fluorocholine PET-CT regarding image quality and interpretation. *EJNMMI Phys.* **2019**, *6*, 5. [CrossRef] [PubMed]
176. Ly, J.; Minarik, D.; Edenbrandt, L.; Wollmer, P.; Trägårdh, E. The use of a proposed updated EARL harmonization of ^{18}F-FDG PET-CT in patients with lymphoma yields significant differences in Deauville score compared with current EARL recommendations. *EJNMMI Res.* **2019**, *9*, 65. [CrossRef]
177. Reynés-Llompart, G.; Sabaté-Llobera, A.; Llinares-Tello, E.; Martí-Climent, J.M.; Gámez-Cenzano, C. Image quality evaluation in a modern PET system: Impact of new reconstructions methods and a radiomics approach. *Sci. Rep.* **2019**, *9*, 10640. [CrossRef]
178. Salvadori, J.; Imbert, L.; Perrin, M.; Karcher, G.; Lamiral, Z.; Marie, P.-Y.; Verger, A. Head-to-head comparison of image quality between brain ^{18}F-FDG images recorded with a fully digital versus a last-generation analog PET camera. *EJNMMI Res.* **2019**, *9*, 61. [CrossRef]
179. Reynés-Llompart, G.; Gámez-Cenzano, C.; Vercher-Conejero, J.L.; Sabaté-Llobera, A.; Calvo-Malvar, N.; Martí-Climent, J.M. Phantom, clinical, and texture indices evaluation and optimization of a penalized-likelihood image reconstruction method (Q.Clear) on a BGO PET/CT scanner. *Med. Phys.* **2018**, *45*, 3214–3222. [CrossRef]
180. Zhang, Y.Q.; Hu, P.C.; Wu, R.Z.; Gu, Y.S.; Chen, S.G.; Yu, H.J.; Wang, X.Q.; Song, J.; Shi, H.C. The image quality, lesion detectability, and acquisition time of ^{18}F-FDG total-body PET/CT in oncological patients. *Eur. J. Nucl. Med. Mol. Imaging* **2020**, *47*, 2507–2515. [CrossRef]
181. Aide, N.; Lasnon, C.; Veit-Haibach, P.; Sera, T.; Sattler, B.; Boellaard, R. EANM/EARL harmonization strategies in PET quantification: From daily practice to multicentre oncological studies. *Eur. J. Nucl. Med. Mol. Imaging* **2017**, *44*, 17–31. [CrossRef]
182. Lasnon, C.; Desmonts, C.; Quak, E.; Gervais, R.; Do, P.; Dubos-Arvis, C.; Aide, N. Harmonizing SUVs in multicentre trials when using different generation PET systems: Prospective validation in non-small cell lung cancer patients. *Eur. J. Nucl. Med. Mol. Imaging* **2013**, *40*, 985–996. [CrossRef]
183. Khalaf, M.; Abdel-Nabi, H.; Baker, J.; Shao, Y.; Lamonica, D.; Gona, J. Relation between nodule size and ^{18}F-FDG-PET SUV for malignant and benign pulmonary nodules. *J. Hematol. Oncol.* **2008**, *1*, 13. [CrossRef]
184. Schmidt-Hansen, M.; Baldwin, D.R.; Hasler, E.; Zamora, J.; Abraira, V.; Roqué, I.F.M. PET-CT for assessing mediastinal lymph node involvement in patients with suspected resectable non-small cell lung cancer. *Cochrane Database Syst. Rev.* **2014**, *2014*, Cd009519. [CrossRef]
185. Kunikowska, J.; Matyskiel, R.; Toutounchi, S.; Grabowska-Derlatka, L.; Koperski, L.; Królicki, L. What parameters from ^{18}F-FDG PET/CT are useful in evaluation of adrenal lesions? *Eur. J. Nucl. Med. Mol. Imaging* **2014**, *41*, 2273–2280. [CrossRef] [PubMed]

186. Shin, D.S.; Shon, O.J.; Han, D.S.; Choi, J.H.; Chun, K.A.; Cho, I.H. The clinical efficacy of ^{18}F-FDG-PET/CT in benign and malignant musculoskeletal tumors. *Ann. Nucl. Med.* **2008**, *22*, 603–609. [CrossRef] [PubMed]
187. Pauleit, D.; Floeth, F.; Hamacher, K.; Riemenschneider, M.J.; Reifenberger, G.; Müller, H.-W.; Zilles, K.; Coenen, H.H.; Langen, K.-J. O-(2-[^{18}F]fluoroethyl)-l-tyrosine PET combined with MRI improves the diagnostic assessment of cerebral gliomas. *Brain* **2005**, *128*, 678–687. [CrossRef]
188. Hasenclever, D.; Kurch, L.; Mauz-Körholz, C.; Elsner, A.; Georgi, T.; Wallace, H.; Landman-Parker, J.; Moryl-Bujakowska, A.; Cepelová, M.; Karlén, J.; et al. qPET—A quantitative extension of the Deauville scale to assess response in interim FDG-PET scans in lymphoma. *Eur. J. Nucl. Med. Mol. Imaging* **2014**, *41*, 1301–1308. [CrossRef]
189. de Langen, A.J.; Vincent, A.; Velasquez, L.M.; van Tinteren, H.; Boellaard, R.; Shankar, L.K.; Boers, M.; Smit, E.F.; Stroobants, S.; Weber, W.A.; et al. Repeatability of ^{18}F-FDG uptake measurements in tumors: A metaanalysis. *J. Nucl. Med.* **2012**, *53*, 701–708. [CrossRef] [PubMed]
190. Kumar, V.; Nath, K.; Berman, C.G.; Kim, J.; Tanvetyanon, T.; Chiappori, A.A.; Gatenby, R.A.; Gillies, R.J.; Eikman, E.A. Variance of SUVs for FDG-PET/CT is greater in clinical practice than under ideal study settings. *Clin. Nucl. Med.* **2013**, *38*, 175–182. [CrossRef]
191. Lodge, M.A. Repeatability of SUV in Oncologic ^{18}F-FDG PET. *J. Nucl. Med.* **2017**, *58*, 523–532. [CrossRef]
192. Vanderhoek, M.; Perlman, S.B.; Jeraj, R. Impact of the definition of peak standardized uptake value on quantification of treatment response. *J. Nucl. Med.* **2012**, *53*, 4–11. [CrossRef] [PubMed]
193. Vanderhoek, M.; Perlman, S.B.; Jeraj, R. Impact of different standardized uptake value measures on PET-based quantification of treatment response. *J. Nucl. Med.* **2013**, *54*, 1188–1194. [CrossRef] [PubMed]
194. Wahl, R.L.; Jacene, H.; Kasamon, Y.; Lodge, M.A. From RECIST to PERCIST: Evolving Considerations for PET response criteria in solid tumors. *J. Nucl. Med.* **2009**, *50* (Suppl. S1), 122s–150s. [CrossRef]
195. Tahari, A.K.; Paidpally, V.; Chirindel, A.; Wahl, R.L.; Subramaniam, R.M. Two-time-point FDG PET/CT: Liver SULmean repeatability. *AJR Am. J. Roentgenol.* **2015**, *204*, 402–407. [CrossRef]
196. Lee, P.; Bazan, J.G.; Lavori, P.W.; Weerasuriya, D.K.; Quon, A.; Le, Q.T.; Wakelee, H.A.; Graves, E.E.; Loo, B.W. Metabolic tumor volume is an independent prognostic factor in patients treated definitively for non-small-cell lung cancer. *Clin. Lung Cancer* **2012**, *13*, 52–58. [CrossRef] [PubMed]
197. Dosani, M.; Yang, R.; McLay, M.; Wilson, D.; Liu, M.; Yong-Hing, C.J.; Hamm, J.; Lund, C.R.; Olson, R.; Schellenberg, D. Metabolic tumour volume is prognostic in patients with non-small-cell lung cancer treated with stereotactic ablative radiotherapy. *Curr. Oncol.* **2019**, *26*, e57–e63. [CrossRef] [PubMed]
198. Han, S.; Kim, H.; Kim, Y.J.; Suh, C.H.; Woo, S. Prognostic Value of Volume-Based Metabolic Parameters of ^{18}F-FDG PET/CT in Uterine Cervical Cancer: A Systematic Review and Meta-Analysis. *AJR Am. J. Roentgenol.* **2018**, *211*, 1112–1121. [CrossRef]
199. Erdogan, M.; Erdemoglu, E.; Evrimler, Ş.; Hanedan, C.; Şengül, S.S. Prognostic value of metabolic tumor volume and total lesion glycolysis assessed by ^{18}F-FDG PET/CT in endometrial cancer. *Nucl. Med. Commun.* **2019**, *40*, 1099–1104. [CrossRef]
200. Wen, W.; Xuan, D.; Hu, Y.; Li, X.; Liu, L.; Xu, D. Prognostic value of maximum standard uptake value, metabolic tumor volume, and total lesion glycolysis of positron emission tomography/computed tomography in patients with breast cancer: A systematic review and meta-analysis. *PLoS ONE* **2019**, *14*, e0225959. [CrossRef] [PubMed]
201. Chung, H.H.; Kim, J.W.; Han, K.H.; Eo, J.S.; Kang, K.W.; Park, N.H.; Song, Y.S.; Chung, J.K.; Kang, S.B. Prognostic value of metabolic tumor volume measured by FDG-PET/CT in patients with cervical cancer. *Gynecol. Oncol.* **2011**, *120*, 270–274. [CrossRef]
202. Zschaeck, S.; Li, Y.; Lin, Q.; Beck, M.; Amthauer, H.; Bauersachs, L.; Hajiyianni, M.; Rogasch, J.; Ehrhardt, V.H.; Kalinauskaite, G.; et al. Prognostic value of baseline [^{18}F]-fluorodeoxyglucose positron emission tomography parameters MTV, TLG and asphericity in an international multicenter cohort of nasopharyngeal carcinoma patients. *PLoS ONE* **2020**, *15*, e0236841. [CrossRef]
203. Pak, K.; Cheon, G.J.; Nam, H.Y.; Kim, S.J.; Kang, K.W.; Chung, J.K.; Kim, E.E.; Lee, D.S. Prognostic value of metabolic tumor volume and total lesion glycolysis in head and neck cancer: A systematic review and meta-analysis. *J. Nucl. Med.* **2014**, *55*, 884–890. [CrossRef] [PubMed]
204. Seifert, R.; Kessel, K.; Schlack, K.; Weber, M.; Herrmann, K.; Spanke, M.; Fendler, W.P.; Hadaschik, B.; Kleesiek, J.; Schäfers, M.; et al. PSMA PET total tumor volume predicts outcome of patients with advanced prostate cancer receiving [^{177}Lu]Lu-PSMA-617 radioligand therapy in a bicentric analysis. *Eur. J. Nucl. Med. Mol. Imaging* **2021**, *48*, 1200–1210. [CrossRef]
205. Kitao, T.; Hirata, K.; Shima, K.; Hayashi, T.; Sekizawa, M.; Takei, T.; Ichimura, W.; Harada, M.; Kondo, K.; Tamaki, N. Reproducibility and uptake time dependency of volume-based parameters on FDG-PET for lung cancer. *BMC Cancer* **2016**, *16*, 576. [CrossRef]
206. Nestle, U.; Kremp, S.; Schaefer-Schuler, A.; Sebastian-Welsch, C.; Hellwig, D.; Rübe, C.; Kirsch, C.M. Comparison of different methods for delineation of ^{18}F-FDG PET-positive tissue for target volume definition in radiotherapy of patients with non-Small cell lung cancer. *J. Nucl. Med.* **2005**, *46*, 1342–1348. [PubMed]
207. Ilyas, H.; Mikhaeel, N.G.; Dunn, J.T.; Rahman, F.; Møller, H.; Smith, D.; Barrington, S.F. Defining the optimal method for measuring baseline metabolic tumour volume in diffuse large B cell lymphoma. *Eur. J. Nucl. Med. Mol. Imaging* **2018**, *45*, 1142–1154. [CrossRef]

208. Cottereau, A.S.; Hapdey, S.; Chartier, L.; Modzelewski, R.; Casasnovas, O.; Itti, E.; Tilly, H.; Vera, P.; Meignan, M.A.; Becker, S. Baseline Total Metabolic Tumor Volume Measured with Fixed or Different Adaptive Thresholding Methods Equally Predicts Outcome in Peripheral T Cell Lymphoma. *J. Nucl. Med.* **2017**, *58*, 276–281. [CrossRef]
209. Mettler, J.; Müller, H.; Voltin, C.A.; Baues, C.; Klaeser, B.; Moccia, A.; Borchmann, P.; Engert, A.; Kuhnert, G.; Drzezga, A.E.; et al. Metabolic Tumour Volume for Response Prediction in Advanced-Stage Hodgkin Lymphoma. *J. Nucl. Med.* **2018**. [CrossRef]
210. Furth, C.; Amthauer, H.; Hautzel, H.; Steffen, I.G.; Ruf, J.; Schiefer, J.; Schönberger, S.; Henze, G.; Grandt, R.; Hundsdoerfer, P.; et al. Evaluation of interim PET response criteria in paediatric Hodgkin's lymphoma—Results for dedicated assessment criteria in a blinded dual-centre read. *Ann. Oncol. Off. J. Eur. Soc. Med. Oncol.* **2011**, *22*, 1198–1203. [CrossRef]
211. Hofman, M.S.; Smeeton, N.C.; Rankin, S.C.; Nunan, T.; O'Doherty, M.J. Observer variation in interpreting ^{18}F-FDG PET/CT findings for lymphoma staging. *J. Nucl. Med.* **2009**, *50*, 1594–1597. [CrossRef]
212. Kluge, R.; Chavdarova, L.; Hoffmann, M.; Kobe, C.; Malkowski, B.; Montravers, F.; Kurch, L.; Georgi, T.; Dietlein, M.; Wallace, W.H.; et al. Inter-Reader Reliability of Early FDG-PET/CT Response Assessment Using the Deauville Scale after 2 Cycles of Intensive Chemotherapy (OEPA) in Hodgkin's Lymphoma. *PLoS ONE* **2016**, *11*, e0149072. [CrossRef] [PubMed]
213. Ceriani, L.; Barrington, S.; Biggi, A.; Malkowski, B.; Metser, U.; Versari, A.; Martelli, M.; Davies, A.; Johnson, P.W.; Zucca, E.; et al. Training improves the interobserver agreement of the expert positron emission tomography review panel in primary mediastinal B-cell lymphoma: Interim analysis in the ongoing International Extranodal Lymphoma Study Group-37 study. *Hematol. Oncol.* **2017**, *35*, 548–553. [CrossRef] [PubMed]
214. Fledelius, J.; Khalil, A.; Hjorthaug, K.; Frøkiær, J. Inter-observer agreement improves with PERCIST 1.0 as opposed to qualitative evaluation in non-small cell lung cancer patients evaluated with F-18-FDG PET/CT early in the course of chemo-radiotherapy. *EJNMMI Res.* **2016**, *6*, 71. [CrossRef] [PubMed]
215. Sørensen, J.S.; Vilstrup, M.H.; Holm, J.; Vogsen, M.; Bülow, J.L.; Ljungstrøm, L.; Braad, P.E.; Gerke, O.; Hildebrandt, M.G. Interrater Agreement and Reliability of PERCIST and Visual Assessment When Using ^{18}F-FDG-PET/CT for Response Monitoring of Metastatic Breast Cancer. *Diagnostics* **2020**, *10*, 1001. [CrossRef] [PubMed]
216. Rowe, S.P.; Pienta, K.J.; Pomper, M.G.; Gorin, M.A. Proposal for a Structured Reporting System for Prostate-Specific Membrane Antigen-Targeted PET Imaging: PSMA-RADS Version 1.0. *J. Nucl. Med.* **2018**, *59*, 479–485. [CrossRef]
217. Ceci, F.; Oprea-Lager, D.E.; Emmett, L.; Adam, J.A.; Bomanji, J.; Czernin, J.; Eiber, M.; Haberkorn, U.; Hofman, M.S.; Hope, T.A.; et al. E-PSMA: The EANM standardized reporting guidelines v1.0 for PSMA-PET. *Eur. J. Nucl. Med. Mol. Imaging* **2021**, *48*, 1626–1638. [CrossRef]
218. Eiber, M.; Herrmann, K.; Calais, J.; Hadaschik, B.; Giesel, F.L.; Hartenbach, M.; Hope, T.; Reiter, R.; Maurer, T.; Weber, W.A.; et al. Prostate Cancer Molecular Imaging Standardized Evaluation (PROMISE): Proposed miTNM Classification for the Interpretation of PSMA-Ligand PET/CT. *J. Nucl. Med.* **2018**, *59*, 469–478. [CrossRef]
219. Fanti, S.; Minozzi, S.; Morigi, J.J.; Giesel, F.; Ceci, F.; Uprimny, C.; Hofman, M.S.; Eiber, M.; Schwarzenbock, S.; Castellucci, P.; et al. Development of standardized image interpretation for ^{68}Ga-PSMA PET/CT to detect prostate cancer recurrent lesions. *Eur. J. Nucl. Med. Mol. Imaging* **2017**, *44*, 1622–1635. [CrossRef]
220. Werner, R.A.; Bundschuh, R.A.; Bundschuh, L.; Javadi, M.S.; Leal, J.P.; Higuchi, T.; Pienta, K.J.; Buck, A.K.; Pomper, M.G.; Gorin, M.A.; et al. Interobserver Agreement for the Standardized Reporting System PSMA-RADS 1.0 on ^{18}F-DCFPyL PET/CT Imaging. *J. Nucl. Med.* **2018**, *59*, 1857–1864. [CrossRef]
221. Fendler, W.P.; Calais, J.; Allen-Auerbach, M.; Bluemel, C.; Eberhardt, N.; Emmett, L.; Gupta, P.; Hartenbach, M.; Hope, T.A.; Okamoto, S.; et al. ^{68}Ga-PSMA-11 PET/CT Interobserver Agreement for Prostate Cancer Assessments: An International Multicenter Prospective Study. *J. Nucl. Med.* **2017**, *58*, 1617–1623. [CrossRef]
222. Demirci, E.; Akyel, R.; Caner, B.; Alan-Selçuk, N.; Güven-Meşe, Ş.; Ocak, M.; Kabasakal, L. Interobserver and intraobserver agreement on prostate-specific membrane antigen PET/CT images according to the miTNM and PSMA-RADS criteria. *Nucl. Med. Commun.* **2020**, *41*, 759–767. [CrossRef]
223. Derwael, C.; Lavergne, O.; Lovinfosse, P.; Nechifor, V.; Salvé, M.; Waltregny, D.; Hustinx, R.; Withofs, N. Interobserver agreement of [^{68}Ga]Ga-PSMA-11 PET/CT images interpretation in men with newly diagnosed prostate cancer. *EJNMMI Res.* **2020**, *10*, 15. [CrossRef] [PubMed]
224. Toriihara, A.; Nobashi, T.; Baratto, L.; Duan, H.; Moradi, F.; Park, S.; Hatami, N.; Aparici, C.M.; Davidzon, G.; Iagaru, A. Comparison of 3 Interpretation Criteria for ^{68}Ga-PSMA11 PET Based on Inter- and Intrareader Agreement. *J. Nucl. Med.* **2020**, *61*, 533–539. [CrossRef] [PubMed]
225. Khatri, W.; Chung, H.W.; Werner, R.A.; Leal, J.P.; Pienta, K.J.; Lodge, M.A.; Gorin, M.A.; Pomper, M.G.; Rowe, S.P. Effect of Point-Spread Function Reconstruction for Indeterminate PSMA-RADS-3A Lesions on PSMA-Targeted PET Imaging of Men with Prostate Cancer. *Diagnostics* **2021**, *11*, 665. [CrossRef] [PubMed]

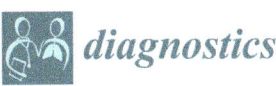

Article

Impact of the Noise Penalty Factor on Quantification in Bayesian Penalized Likelihood (Q.Clear) Reconstructions of ^{68}Ga-PSMA PET/CT Scans

Sjoerd Rijnsdorp [1,*], Mark J. Roef [2] and Albert J. Arends [1]

[1] Department of Medical Physics, Catharina Hospital Eindhoven, Michelangelolaan 2, 5623 EJ Eindhoven, The Netherlands; bertjan.arends@catharinaziekenhuis.nl
[2] Department of Nuclear Medicine, Catharina Hospital Eindhoven, Michelangelolaan 2, 5623 EJ Eindhoven, The Netherlands; mark.roef@catharinaziekenhuis.nl
* Correspondence: srijnsdorp@outlook.com

Citation: Rijnsdorp, S.; Roef, M.J.; Arends, A.J. Impact of the Noise Penalty Factor on Quantification in Bayesian Penalized Likelihood (Q.Clear) Reconstructions of ^{68}Ga-PSMA PET/CT Scans. *Diagnostics* **2021**, *11*, 847. https://doi.org/10.3390/diagnostics11050847

Academic Editor: Lioe-Fee de Geus-Oei

Received: 8 April 2021
Accepted: 4 May 2021
Published: 8 May 2021

Publisher's Note: MDPI stays neutral with regard to jurisdictional claims in published maps and institutional affiliations.

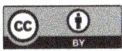

Copyright: © 2021 by the authors. Licensee MDPI, Basel, Switzerland. This article is an open access article distributed under the terms and conditions of the Creative Commons Attribution (CC BY) license (https://creativecommons.org/licenses/by/4.0/).

Abstract: Functional imaging with ^{68}Ga prostate-specific membrane antigen (PSMA) and positron emission tomography (PET) can fulfill an important role in treatment selection and adjustment in prostate cancer. This article focusses on quantitative assessment of ^{68}Ga-PSMA-PET. The effect of various parameters on standardized uptake values (SUVs) is explored, and an optimal Bayesian penalized likelihood (BPL) reconstruction is suggested. PET acquisitions of two phantoms consisting of a background compartment and spheres with diameter 4 mm to 37 mm, both filled with solutions of ^{68}Ga in water, were performed with a GE Discovery 710 PET/CT scanner. Recovery coefficients (RCs) in multiple reconstructions with varying noise penalty factors and acquisition times were determined and analyzed. Apparent recovery coefficients of spheres with a diameter smaller than 17 mm were significantly lower than those of spheres with a diameter of 17 mm and bigger ($p < 0.001$) for a tumor-to-background (T/B) ratio of 10:1 and a scan time of 10 min per bed position. With a T/B ratio of 10:1, the four largest spheres exhibit significantly higher RCs than those with a T/B ratio of 20:1 ($p < 0.0001$). For spheres with a diameter of 8 mm and less, alignment with the voxel grid potentially affects the RC. Evaluation of PET/CT scans using (semi-)quantitative measures such as SUVs should be performed with great caution, as SUVs are influenced by scanning and reconstruction parameters. Based on the evaluation of multiple reconstructions with different β of phantom scans, an intermediate β (600) is suggested as the optimal value for the reconstruction of clinical ^{68}Ga-PSMA PET/CT scans, considering that both detectability and reproducibility are relevant.

Keywords: ^{68}Ga-PSMA PET/CT; recovery coefficient; quantitative PET; Bayesian penalized likelihood

1. Introduction

Prostate cancer is the most frequent occurring malignancy in men. Global incidence in 2015 was estimated at over 1.6 million with prostate cancer having the highest incidence of all cancers in Western Europe, United States and Canada [1]. Many prostate cancers have a relatively indolent behavior and do not lead to significant medical complaints during the lifetime of a patient. However, patients may eventually progress to metastatic and/or castration-resistant prostate cancer (CRPC), which is considered an incurable and fatal stage of the disease. The optimal treatment for metastatic prostate cancer depends on characteristics of the tumor and of the patient, and may consist of multiple modalities including hormone therapy, chemotherapy, radiation therapy, and radionuclide therapy [2]. Selection and adjustment of a treatment is strongly dependent on treatment response. Therefore, there is a need for a tool that provides quantitative, lesion-specific and observer-independent response evaluation. Functional metabolic imaging with radiolabeled ^{68}Ga prostate-specific membrane antigen (PSMA) and positron emission tomography (PET) is potentially such a tool. Although there is a vast amount of literature on PSMA-PET in staging and restaging of prostate cancer, response evaluation using PSMA-PET is less well explored and a standardized quantitative approach still needs to be developed.

It is known that uptake measurements of radiolabeled tracers with in vivo PET are affected by many parameters, as demonstrated by experience with ^{18}F-fluor deoxyglucose (FDG), and standardization prior to application as response parameter is required [3]. For ^{18}F-FDG-PET, repeatabilities of around 10% on average and higher are reported [4–7]. Notwithstanding the differences in pharmacodynamics and pharmacokinetics between FDG and PSMA, this probably applies equally to PSMA-PET. Before quantification of PSMA uptake can be used as a biomarker or surrogate endpoint to identify response to treatment, and before we can design sufficiently powered response evaluation studies, a thorough understanding of parameters affecting the quantitative results is required. Uptake of FDG and PSMA differ due to pharmacodynamical differences [8–10]. Therefore, comparison of uptake measurements from scans with different ligands should be approached with caution.

The spatial resolution of PET imaging is limited due to inherent physical characteristics such as positron range and noncollinearity of annihilation photons. Combined with detector characteristics and image sampling effects caused by discretization of the continuous activity distribution by recording it in finite sized voxels, these result in spillover from structures with a high activity concentration to those with a low activity concentration and vice versa, referred to as partial volume effect (PVE) [11,12]. The PVE is particularly of interest when the object is smaller than 2–3 times the spatial resolution expressed by its full width at half maximum (FWHM) [13,14] which is typically around 4–5 mm for state-of-the-art PET/CT systems [15]. As prostate cancer recurrence often involves relatively small metastatic nodal lesions, these effects are of particular importance with respect to PSMA signal evaluation. Resolution recovery techniques such as point spread function (PSF) modelling can be applied in order to partly recover the true shape and uptake of these lesions. In this study, attention is given in particular to image reconstruction using a Bayesian penalized likelihood (BPL) algorithm which may be advantageous for the signal evaluation of such small lesions, due to better signal-to-noise ratios (SNRs) compared to standard reconstruction techniques.

A potentially relevant difference between ^{18}F-FDG-PET and ^{68}Ga-PSMA-PET is the positron energy. Positrons emitted by ^{68}Ga and ^{18}F have a mean energy of 0.88 MeV and 0.25 MeV [16] corresponding to mean ranges in water of 2.9 mm and 0.6 mm, respectively [17]. Higher positron energy negatively affects the spatial resolution, which is well described for high resolution preclinical PET scanners [18–20]. For small nodal lesions, the resulting blurring effect may have an effect on measured uptake values and lesion detectability. In addition, PSMA exhibits high specificity causing a high tumor-to-background (T/B) ratio which increases accuracy of quantification for larger lesions and visual detection of small lesions [21–23].

The BPL algorithm implemented by GE Healthcare (GE Healthcare, Chicago, IL, United States), Q.Clear, is an iterative reconstruction algorithm which enables users to define a noise penalty factor β. In contrast to ordered subset expectation maximization (OSEM [24]) reconstructions, penalized likelihood reconstructions can be run until full convergence leading to higher quantitative accuracy [25], improved lesion visual conspicuity and maximum standardized uptake value (SUV_{max}) in small nodules for low β [26] and a more consistent signal-to-noise ratio [27,28].

Although preferred image smoothness for visual assessment of PET studies is user dependent, suggestions for optimal β values are described in the literature for various types of PET/CT studies: a β of 400 for ^{18}F-FDG whole body PET/CT scans [29]; a β of 300 for BPL reconstructions of ^{18}F-fluciclovine scans for imaging of recurrent prostate cancer [30] and a β of 4000 for scans after administration of ^{90}Y for selective internal radiotherapy [31].

The aim of this study was to explore the effect of acquisition time and reconstruction parameters by providing recovery coefficients for various T/B ratios and sphere sizes, obtained from phantom studies with ^{68}Ga-PSMA while applying different β values, and to find an optimal β value for quantification as well as visual assessment of ^{68}Ga-PSMA PET/CT scans.

2. Materials and Methods

The Micro Hollow Sphere phantom (Data Spectrum Corporation, Durham, NC, United States) and the NEMA IEC Image Quality phantom (PTW, Freiburg, Germany) were used to obtain PET/CT images that could be assessed objectively and reproducibly. Both phantoms consist of a fillable background compartment and multiple hollow and fillable spheres with inner diameters 37, 28, 22, 17, 13 and 10 mm for the NEMA Image Quality phantom and 10, 8, 6, 5 and 4 mm for the Micro Hollow Sphere phantom, see Figure 1.

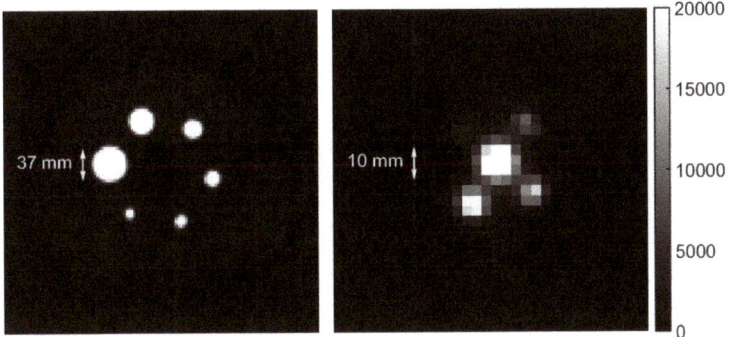

Figure 1. Transverse PET slices of the NEMA IEC Image Quality phantom (**left**) and the Micro Hollow Sphere phantom (**right**). The image of the Micro Hollow Sphere phantom is scaled up by a factor four with respect to that of the NEMA IEC Image Quality phantom to properly show the features. The dimensions of the largest sphere in the Micro Hollow Sphere phantom match with those of the smallest sphere in the NEMA IEC Image Quality phantom. As the voxel dimensions in the transverse plane are 2.73 by 2.73 mm, individual pixels can be clearly distinguished causing a seemingly low image resolution.

Both the background compartments and sets of spheres were filled with solutions of ^{68}Ga in water. To represent a patient scan, the ratio between the activity concentration of both solutions was based on reported T/B ratios for ^{68}Ga-PSMA diagnostic PET/CT scans one hour after administration of the radiopharmaceutical. A concise overview is given in Table 1. Based on these reports, the decision was made to perform two scans of the phantoms, one with a ratio of 20:1 and one with a ratio of 10:1 between the activity concentration in the spheres and the background compartment.

Table 1. Overview of T/B ratios in several studies concerning ^{68}Ga-PSMA PET/CT imaging. The T/B ratio was either computed with the tumor uptake and the SUV$_{mean}$ obtained from a region of interest (ROI) drawn in gluteal muscle [22,32,33] or tumor uptake and the SUV$_{mean}$ from adjacent healthy tissue [34].

	[32] Mean ± SD	[22] Median (Range)	[33] Mean ± SD (Range)	[34] Median (Range)
Lymph node metastases	21.0 ± 27.4		65.2 ± 65.7 (5.3–486.4)	12.2 (3.8–62.2)
Bone metastases	24.7 ± 34.2		84.4 ± 75.1 (3.8–355)	34 (6.8–40)
Local recurrences	15.7 ± 10.1		43.3 ± 33.5 (10.7–144.3)	
Axillary lymph nodes				3 (1.3–8.5)
Primary tumor				18.5 (6.7–92)
Other metastases	16.7 ± 14.1			
Total lesions	21.1 ± 27.4	18.8 (2.4–158.3)		7.8 (1.5–35)

2.1. Phantom Preparation and Scanning Procedure

Both phantoms were filled in a way similar to the one described in the 'Standard operating procedures for quality control' described in the EARL Accreditation Manual [35]. A solution with an activity concentration of 40 kBq/mL used to fill the spheres was prepared by adding 20 MBq ^{68}Ga to 500 mL of water (stock solution) and homogenized by extensive shaking. To obtain an activity concentration of 2 kBq/mL in the water-filled background compartments of known volumes, required amounts of ^{68}Ga were directly added to these volumes. The solutions in the background compartments were homogenized by shaking the phantoms extensively.

Subsequently, data were acquired with a GE Discovery 710 PET/CT scanner (GE Healthcare, Chicago, IL, USA). Both phantoms were scanned simultaneously. The long axes of both phantoms were aligned to coincide with the axis of the bore. The system was set to acquire data in list-mode to enable multiple reconstructions with different count statistics for both acquisitions. An acquisition time of 10 min per bed position was chosen, with a total of three bed positions per scan. The axial field of view was 15.7 cm and the overlap between subsequent bed positions was 23%. The bed positions were chosen in such a way that the spheres were not placed in the overlapping part of two bed positions.

Directly after the first scan, the activity concentrations in both background compartments were doubled by adding amounts of activity equal to those in step 1, to obtain a 10:1 ratio between the activity concentration in the spheres and the background compartments, correcting for radioactive decay. Again, the background compartments were homogenized by shaking the phantoms extensively. Exactly 68 min (one half-life of ^{68}Ga) after starting the acquisition of the first scan, a second acquisition with identical phantom placement and scanning parameters as described in step 2 was performed.

Using the acquired list-mode dataset, multiple iterative reconstructions were made for both scans. All data were corrected for attenuation, random events and scatter. Reconstructions were made with Q.Clear with varying β (300, 400, 450, 500, 600, 700, 800, 900 and 1000) including PSF modelling, for multiple simulated scan times (1, 2, 2.5, 5 and 10 min per bed position). As a reference, conventional iterative OSEM reconstructions with 2 iterations and 24 subsets, 6.4 mm Gaussian filter and 1:4:1 filter in axial direction with and without PSF modelling were obtained. All reconstructions used time-of-flight data and consisted of 2.73 × 2.73 × 3.27 mm^3 voxels and a 256 × 256-pixel matrix.

2.2. BPL Reconstructions

The Q.Clear algorithm introduces a noise control term $\beta R(x)$ to the objective function used in OSEM reconstructions, where β is the parameter controlling the strength and R(x) is defined as (1):

$$R(x) = \sum_{j=1}^{n_v} \sum_{k \in N_j} w_j w_k \frac{(x_j - x_k)^2}{(x_j + x_k) + \gamma |x_j - x_k|} \quad (1)$$

where n_v refers to the number of voxels, N_j is the set of neighboring voxels of voxel j, $w_j w_k$ is the weight of the local smoothing value which depends on the distance between voxels j and k, x is the activity in a voxel and γ is the parameter controlling edge preservation [36].

2.3. Background Variability

Background variability (BV) was determined for all reconstructions obtained, based on count statistics in a manually drawn region of interest (ROI) in the background, extended over multiple slices. Care was taken to neither include voxels near the edge of the phantom nor near the hot spheres in order to avoid a bias in the background volume of interest (VOI) due to partial volume effects.

The BV was calculated by (2):

$$BV = \frac{\sigma_{VOI}}{\mu_{VOI}} \quad (2)$$

where σ_{VOI} is the standard deviation of the number of counts in the VOI and μ_{VOI} is the mean number of counts in the VOI.

2.4. Activity Recovery Coefficients

The recovery coefficient was used as measure for the ratio between the apparent activity concentration and the true activity concentration in a VOI. Ideally, the RC is equal to 1 for all sphere diameters. In general, the recovery coefficient will gradually decrease for smaller sphere diameters.

RCs were obtained semi-automatically. First, the spheres were identified visually in the PET image. Subsequently a box was manually defined around the maximum voxel value for each sphere. Each box was constructed to fully include a sphere without inclusion of voxels of other spheres. In addition, a background VOI was manually defined in such a way that the boundaries were neither close to the phantom wall nor to the spheres, to ensure homogeneity and avoid partial volume effects.

Next, the maximum voxel value in each box corresponding to a sphere was obtained. The measured ratio $R_{meas,max}$ between the maximum activity concentration $C_{sphere,max}$ in a sphere and the average activity concentration in the manually drawn background VOI $C_{bg,avg}$ (equivalent to the T/B ratio in a patient scan, comparing maximum SUV to the background SUV), was defined as (3)

$$R_{meas,\,max} = \frac{C_{sphere,max}}{C_{bg,avg}} \qquad (3)$$

Using the location of the maximum voxel value of each sphere in the PET reconstruction, VOIs to determine the average voxel value in the sphere volume $C_{sphere,avg}$ were constructed automatically using a simple region growing algorithm including all voxels within a 3D isocontour at 50% of the maximum voxel intensity corrected for background [31]. These VOIs were used to calculate the measured ratio between the average activity concentration in the sphere and the background $R_{meas,avg}$ (equivalent to the T/B ratio in a patient scan, comparing mean SUV to the background SUV) (4).

$$R_{meas,\,avg} = \frac{C_{sphere,avg}}{C_{bg,avg}} \qquad (4)$$

The peak recovery coefficient RC_{peak} was also determined for each sphere by positioning a spherical contour with a 1.2 cm diameter such that the average voxel value within that sphere is maximized [3]. The measured ratio $R_{meas,peak}$ between the average activity concentration in the spherical VOI $C_{sphere,peak}$ and the background is equivalent to the SUV_{peak} in a patient scan (5):

$$R_{meas,peak} = \frac{C_{sphere,peak}}{C_{bg,avg}} \qquad (5)$$

As the actual ratio R between the activity concentration in the spheres and the activity concentration in the background compartments of the phantoms was known, RC_{max}, RC_{avg} and RC_{peak} could be calculated by (6)–(8):

$$RC_{max} = \frac{R_{meas,\,max}}{R} \qquad (6)$$

$$RC_{avg} = \frac{R_{meas,\,avg}}{R} \qquad (7)$$

$$RC_{peak} = \frac{R_{meas,peak}}{R} \qquad (8)$$

These RCs are therefore equivalent to the ratios between the observed maximum, average and peak T/B ratio and the true T/B ratio.

Statistical analysis was performed using a Student t-test for comparison of data in a single reconstruction and a paired t-test for assessment of differences between two reconstructions. A confidence level of 95% was used.

For each sphere, the RC_{avg} values calculated in multiple acquisitions (1 min, 2 min and 5 min per bed position, each with a T/B ratio of 10:1 and 20:1) were averaged and the coefficient of variation (COV) was assessed. The optimal β value was chosen based on reproducibility, i.e., low COV, and detectability, i.e., high recovery and low background variability.

3. Results

During the first acquisition, the actual ratios between the activity concentration in the spheres and the background compartments were 20.4:1 and 22.1:1 for the NEMA Image Quality phantom and the Micro Hollow Sphere phantom, respectively. After adding ^{68}Ga to the background compartments following the first scan, the second acquisition was performed with phantoms containing activity concentration ratios of 10.1:1 and 11.8:1, respectively.

3.1. Background Variability

Background variability was assessed for all available Q.Clear reconstructions. Regarding acquisition parameters, reconstructions from scans with longer acquisition times show lower BV overall due to the higher number of counts and background variability is similar for both scans with different T/B ratios as the background activity concentration is the same. Increasing β results in reconstructions with a lower BV due to the noise reducing effect. In a clinical setting, considering a limited acquisition time, a higher β to obtain less noisy images would be preferable.

3.2. Contrast Recovery

3.2.1. NEMA IEC Image Quality Phantom

For a T/B ratio of 10:1, a scan time of 10 min per bed position and a high level of noise tolerance (low β), a relatively constant RC_{avg} between 0.8 and 0.9 is found for the biggest four spheres. The RC_{avg} decreases significantly for spheres with a diameter smaller than 17 mm ($p < 0.001$). Increasing the β to 400 and higher and thus effectively smoothing the image, the decrease in RC_{avg} is already seen in the 17 mm-diameter spheres ($p < 0.05$). Shortening the acquisition time to the clinically used two minutes per bed position resulted in apparently higher average recovery coefficients (Figure 2a). The RC_{peak} of each of the three smallest spheres is lower than that of the three biggest spheres ($p < 0.001$) for both scan times. The higher apparent RCs in the shorter scan do not necessarily correlate with improved lesion detectability due to the increased noise levels.

For the acquisition with a T/B ratio of 20:1 and a scan time of 10 min per bed position, a similar trend was noted. For sphere diameters 17 mm and larger, the average recovery coefficient is similar for all Q.Clear reconstructions. The RC_{peak} of each of the three smallest spheres is lower than that of the three biggest spheres ($p < 0.001$). For the 10 and 13 mm-diameter spheres a spread developed, with a decrease in average recovery coefficient for increasing β. Reconstructions with data acquired for two minutes per bed position (Figure 2b) showed a similar pattern, but with a slightly higher RC_{avg} overall and a more pronounced spread in RC_{avg} for the 10 and 13 mm-diameter spheres.

The four largest spheres with a T/B ratio of 10:1 exhibit a significantly higher RC_{avg} and RC_{max} than those with a T/B ratio of 20:1 ($p < 0.0001$), for all reconstructions considered. For the three biggest spheres, RC_{peak} is similar for both T/B ratios.

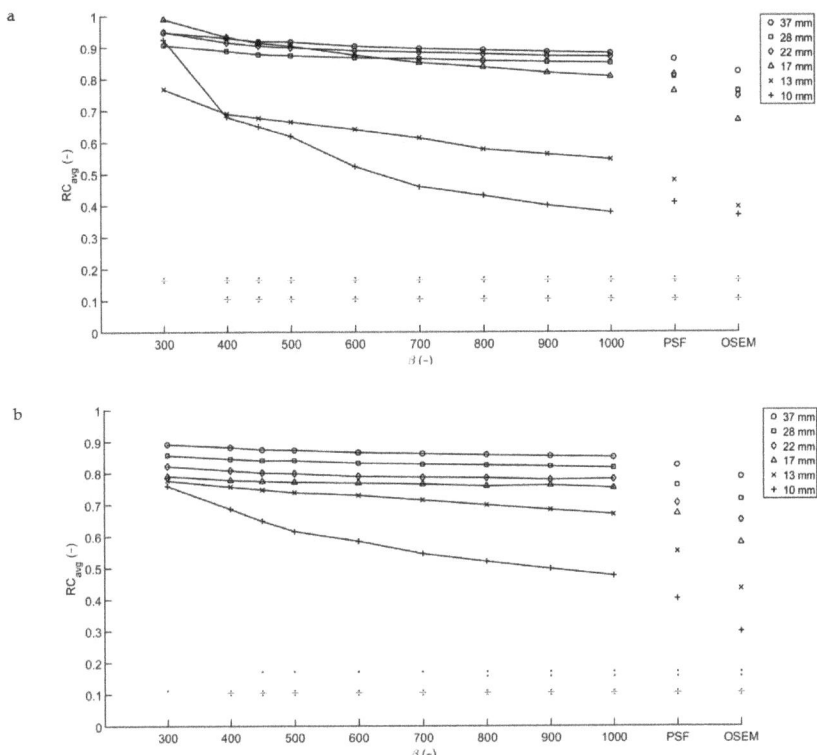

Figure 2. Recovery coefficients from the Image Quality phantom for multiple T/B ratios. RC$_{avg}$ for T/B ratio 10:1 (**a**) and 20:1 (**b**), with acquisition time per bed position of 2 min. The symbols in the lower part of both graphs denote the significance of the differences between the 13 mm sphere and the four biggest spheres (upper row) and the 10 mm sphere and the four biggest spheres (lower row). An obelus (÷) corresponds to $p < 0.001$, a colon to $p < 0.01$ and a single dot to $p < 0.05$.

3.2.2. Micro Hollow Sphere Phantom

The diameter of the largest sphere in the Micro Hollow Sphere phantom matches with that of the smallest sphere in the NEMA Image Quality phantom. Comparing the two, in general a higher average recovery coefficient is found for the sphere in the Micro Hollow Sphere phantom. These differences in recovery coefficient result from differences in the phantom geometry. An approximate correction factor was introduced to scale the RCs of the Micro Hollow Sphere phantom to those of the NEMA Image Quality phantom. The scaling factor was defined as the ratio between the RC of the matching spheres in the NEMA Image Quality phantom and the Micro Hollow Sphere phantom.

Recovery coefficients are provided for all spheres that could be semi-automatically segmented. For the smaller spheres, the apparent activity concentration in a sphere decreased to less than twice the background value due to the PVE. For these spheres, the region growing algorithm with a threshold 3D isocontour at 50% of the maximum voxel value failed to properly calculate an average recovery coefficient. An increase in β caused a decrease in apparent activity concentration in a sphere and therefore an increase in the number of spheres that could not be properly segmented. A lower T/B ratio also resulted in more difficulties in the segmentation process.

For both phantom scans performed, a large increase in RC$_{avg}$ for one of the spheres at lower β values was observed as can be seen for the scan with a T/B ratio of 10:1 in Figure 3.

Taking RC_{peak} as a quantitative measure, the obtained recovery coefficients appear to be more robust but lower than the RC_{avg}.

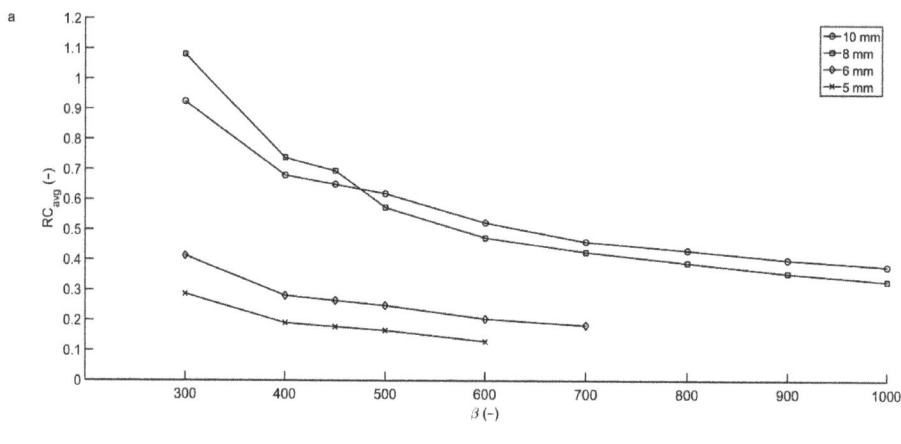

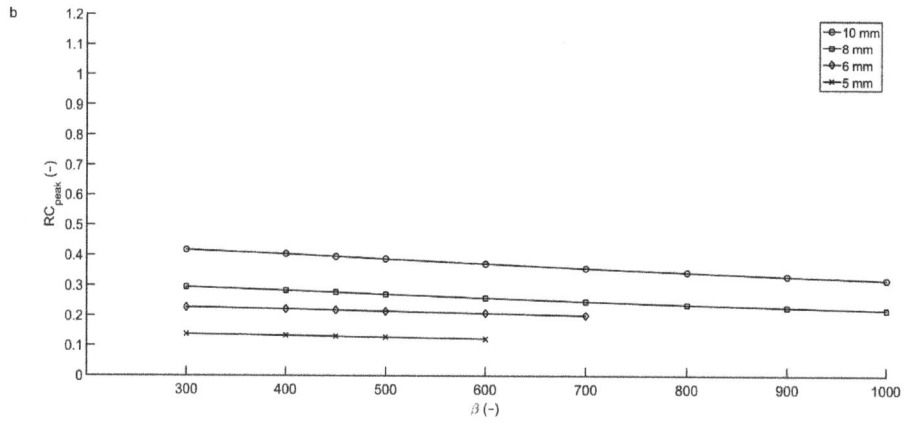

Figure 3. Average and peak recovery coefficients from the Micro Hollow Sphere phantom. For an acquisition time of two minutes per bed position, the apparent RC_{avg} (**a**) of the 8 mm sphere measured with T/B ratio 10:1 exceeds that of the bigger spheres for low β, as the center of this sphere happened to coincide with the center of a voxel. Taking RC_{peak} as a measure for the recovery coefficient (**b**), the recovery coefficients are lower, but more robust.

3.3. Reproducibility

For each sphere of the Image Quality phantom, the RC_{avg} calculated in the acquisitions with short, medium and long acquisition times (1, 2 and 5 min per bed position), and T/B ratios of 10:1 and 20:1 were averaged and the COV was determined to assess reproducibility considering varying scan parameters. Scans with acquisition times of 2.5 and 10 min per bed position were omitted as these results are similar to 2 and 5 min per bed position, respectively. As shown in Figure 4, the averaged RC_{avg} decreases as β increases, with the largest differences for the RC_{avg} of the smallest sphere. For the largest 4 spheres, the COV decreases as β increases. The COV for the 10 and 13 mm-diameter spheres exhibit an inverse opposite relation as differences in RC_{avg} between the two T/B ratios arise for increasing β. Due to the construction of the prior, the noise penalty term depends on the relative difference in values of adjacent voxels, with higher relative differences yielding better edge preservation. This mainly affects the voxels at the edge of a sphere and hence the RC_{max} and correspondingly the RC_{avg} of bigger spheres is less affected. For spheres consisting of only a few voxels, however, RC_{max} and RC_{avg} will slightly decrease. For the 10 mm-diameter sphere, the minimum COV is found at $\beta = 600$. For lower β values, the COV increases as a result of increasing RC_{avg} for shorter acquisition times. This increase corresponds to an increase in RC_{max} which is explained by the higher relative noise level for low count acquisitions. Again, the effect is most profound in small spheres as the number of counts within the region and the maximum number of counts collected in a voxel is smaller than in larger spheres.

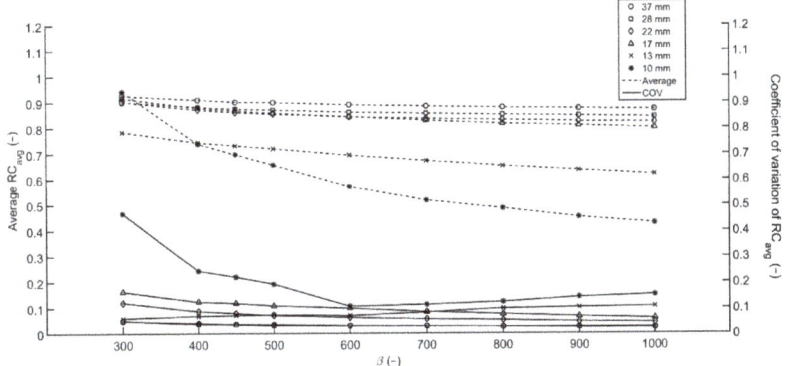

Figure 4. Averaged RC_{avg} and COV from the Image Quality phantom. Averaged RC_{avg} over 6 reconstructions with varying acquisition times per bed position (1, 2 and 5 min) and T/B ratios (10:1 and 20:1).

4. Discussion

Interpretation of SUV metrics is a valuable tool in the assessment of PET/CT scans, as clinically relevant parameters such as d'Amico risk classification, PSA plasma levels and Gleason score correlate significantly with SUV [37–39]. However, SUV is also affected by aspects inherent to the imaging method such as uptake time [40], reconstruction algorithm used and the use of PSF modelling [41,42], bed motion [43], use of breathing instructions [44,45], scan time [46] and scanner properties [47]. Therefore, caution is warranted when interpreting SUV for clinical evaluation of ^{68}Ga-PSMA PET/CT scans. Differences in pharmacokinetics and pharmacodynamics should be considered when comparing uptake values obtained from scans with different tracers.

Improved lesion conspicuity and increased SUV_{max} for Q.Clear reconstructions with low β are described in the literature [26]. Lowering the β corresponds to less noise suppression and therefore higher SUV_{max} values. For SUV measurements, low β values are found to be more accurate when considering the average uptake in a lesion.

This effect is noticed in phantom scans for measurements of the RC_{max} for both T/B ratios, all simulated acquisition times and all spheres considered in this study. As the RC_{avg} is dependent on the maximum voxel value, this effect is also present in the average recovery curves but less pronounced due to averaging over a larger number of voxels. The RCs exhibited by PSF and OSEM reconstructions are affected by the 6.4 mm Gaussian post-filter, which was chosen based on clinical reconstruction settings in our institute. Lowering or eliminating post-filtering, RCs will increase. On the other hand, even with the post-filter applied, noise levels based on the background variability measurements are higher for PSF and OSEM reconstructions than for any of the BPL reconstructions considered.

The higher recovery coefficients measured for shortened acquisition times are consistent with the increase in SNR. The maximum voxel uptake value is likely to increase when the number of counts is decreased, as the signal-to-noise ratio is proportional to the square root of the number of counts (9):

$$\frac{\text{Signal}}{\text{Noise}} \sim \sqrt{N} \qquad (9)$$

Therefore, both the average and the maximum apparent recovery coefficient increase when the number of counts taken into account in the reconstruction is decreased. This effect is less pronounced with increased β, due to the smaller noise tolerance and therefore smoother images from high β reconstructions. In general, caution is needed when comparing SUVs between two scans in which administered activity or scan times differ.

As the two phantoms used in this study were scanned simultaneously, acquisition of the bed position containing the spheres in the Micro Hollow Sphere phantom was started 10 min after acquisition of the bed position containing the spheres of the NEMA Image Quality phantom. Therefore, the activity concentrations in the Micro Hollow Sphere phantom were approximately 6% lower than those in the NEMA Image Quality phantom. The resulting decrease in the number of counts detected probably has a small effect on the maximum voxel value, and may contribute to the difference in recovery coefficients found in the NEMA Image Quality phantom and the Micro Hollow Sphere phantom.

Due to spill-out, RCs are affected by lesion size for smaller lesions. Looking at the sphere diameter at which the spheres' RC_{avg} deviates significantly from that of the larger spheres in the same reconstruction, a dependence on the β is noted. For higher β, the decrease in RC starts at larger diameters. The volume of each of the three smallest spheres considered in this article (33.51 mm^3, 65.45 mm^3 and 113.1 mm^3) is smaller than five voxels using the minimal voxel size of the used PET/CT scanner (24.37 mm^3). Coincidental high count rates in a single voxel, for example induced by a coincidental centering of a voxel amid a sphere, can induce a 3D isocontour at 50% of the maximum voxel value that consists of a single voxel. This will result in a positive RC bias, an overestimation of the recovery coefficient.

A large increase in average recovery coefficient observed for the 8 mm-diameter sphere for T/B ratio 10:1 and the 6 mm sphere for T/B ratio 20:1, most evident at low β, is worth mentioning. Detailed inspection of the reconstructions revealed that these spheres appeared to be coincidentally aligned with the reconstruction matrix. As the diameter of the spheres is smaller than three times the minimum voxel dimension, the exact position of the phantom defines the number of voxels over which the total number of counts from the sphere are distributed and therefore strongly influences the recovery coefficient. The effect can be enhanced by a coincidental high number of counts due to Poisson noise, which means the effect is more likely to be noticed for lower β, shorter acquisition times and lower activity concentrations. Taking RC_{peak} rather than RC_{avg} as a measure, the voxel sampling effects are eliminated leading to more robust results. However, as the 1.2 cm-diameter spherical VOI used for obtaining the RC_{peak} is larger than the hot spheres in the Micro Hollow Sphere phantom, this method incorporates background voxels in the VOI, leading to a lower RC. Therefore, in small lesions, SUV_{peak} cannot be used to discriminate between larger volumes with low uptake and smaller lesions with high uptake.

The findings from this study are comparable to those described in ^{18}F-FDG PET/CT studies. Improving contrast recovery for lower noise penalties in BPL reconstructions is well described by Teoh et al. [28,29] and similarities between the preferred β values for patient scans in this study and those recently described by Messerli et al. for ^{18}F-FDG are also noted [48]; the observation that voxel sampling influences measured uptake values is in line with results for ^{18}F-FDG PET/CT shown by Mansor et al. [49] and the observation that RCs decrease for increasing T/B ratio is described by Munk et al. [50]. These similarities are explained by the fact that, from a physics point of view, the main potentially relevant difference between use of ^{68}Ga and ^{18}F is the positron range.

For a PET system, the spatial resolution can be written as (10):

$$R_{sys} \approx \sqrt{R_{det}^2 + R_{range}^2 + R_{180}^2} \qquad (10)$$

where R_{sys} is the spatial resolution of the system, R_{det} is the contribution of the detectors, R_{range} is the contribution of the root mean square (RMS) positron range in water and R_{180} is the contribution of the noncollinearity of the annihilation photons [51]. Assuming a system resolution for ^{18}F of approximately 5 mm FWHM [15] and evaluating in the RMS positron ranges of 0.23 mm for ^{18}F and 1.2 mm for ^{68}Ga [52,53], it is evident that the increased positron range only yields an incremental increase in spatial resolution.

To summarize, comparison of SUV measures between different lesions or the same lesion in two different scans is not straightforward even when administration, scanning and reconstruction protocols are equal.

This finding is in line with the conclusion by previous authors that quantitative measures for small lesions in PSF reconstructed PET images can lead to misinterpretation as they vary with lesion size and are less reproducible [50].

Assessment of the reproducibility of RC_{avg} and detectability of lesions in terms of the COV, RC_{avg} and BV for different β suggests a value of 600 as an optimum when quantification as well as detection is of importance. Higher values yield impaired detectability as small lesions blur into the background. Lower values will lead to more accurate uptake measures and better detectability for small lesions. However, the introduction of additional noise will probably yield an increase in false-positives and lower reproducibility which is of particular importance for test–retest studies and follow-up scans.

5. Conclusions

Evaluation of PET/CT scans using (semi-)quantitative measures such as SUVs should be performed with great caution, as SUVs are influenced by scanning and reconstruction parameters. Based on the evaluation of multiple reconstructions with different β of phantom scans, an intermediate β (600) is suggested as the optimal value for the reconstruction of clinical ^{68}Ga-PSMA PET/CT scans, considering that both detectability and reproducibility are relevant.

Author Contributions: Conceptualization, S.R., M.J.R., A.J.A.; methodology, S.R., M.J.R., A.J.A.; formal analysis, S.R.; writing—original draft preparation, S.R., M.J.R., A.J.A.; writing—review and editing, S.R., M.J.R., A.J.A.; visualization, S.R.; All authors have read and agreed to the published version of the manuscript.

Funding: This research received no external funding.

Institutional Review Board Statement: Not applicable.

Informed Consent Statement: Not applicable.

Data Availability Statement: The data presented in this study are available on request from the corresponding author.

Conflicts of Interest: The authors declare no conflict of interest.

References

1. Global Burden of Disease Cancer Collaboration; Fitzmaurice, C.; Allen, C.; Barber, R.M.; Barregard, L.; Bhutta, Z.A.; Brenner, H.; Dicker, D.J.; Chimed-Orchir, O.; Dandona, R.; et al. Global, Regional, and National Cancer Incidence, Mortality, Years of Life Lost, Years Lived With Disability, and Disability-Adjusted Life-years for 32 Cancer Groups, 1990 to 2015. *JAMA Oncol.* **2017**, *3*, 524–548. [CrossRef]
2. Mottet, N.; Bellmunt, J.; Bolla, M.; Joniau, S.; Mason, M.; Matveev, V.; Schmid, H.-P.; Van der Kwast, T.; Wiegel, T.; Zattoni, F.; et al. EAU Guidelines on Prostate Cancer. Part II: Treatment of Advanced, Relapsing, and Castration-Resistant Prostate Cancer. *Eur. Urol.* **2011**, *59*, 572–583. [CrossRef]
3. Boellaard, R.; Delgado-Bolton, R.; Oyen, W.J.G.; Giammarile, F.; Tatsch, K.; Eschner, W.; Verzijlbergen, F.J.; Barrington, S.F.; Pike, L.C.; Weber, W.A.; et al. FDG PET/CT: EANM procedure guidelines for tumour imaging: Version 2.0. *Eur. J. Nucl. Med. Mol. Imaging* **2015**, *42*, 328–354. [CrossRef]
4. Fraum, T.J.; Fowler, K.J.; Crandall, J.P.; Laforest, R.A.; Salter, A.; An, H.; Jacobs, M.A.; Grigsby, P.W.; Dehdashti, F.; Wahl, R.L. Measurement Repeatability of 18F-FDG PET/CT Versus 18F-FDG PET/MRI in Solid Tumors of the Pelvis. *J. Nucl. Med.* **2019**, *60*, 1080–1086. [CrossRef] [PubMed]

5. Kurland, B.F.; Peterson, L.M.; Shields, A.T.; Lee, J.H.; Byrd, D.W.; Novakova-Jiresova, A.; Muzi, M.; Specht, J.M.; Mankoff, D.A.; Linden, H.M.; et al. Test–Retest Reproducibility of 18F-FDG PET/CT Uptake in Cancer Patients Within a Qualified and Calibrated Local Network. *J. Nucl. Med.* **2018**, *60*, 608–614. [CrossRef] [PubMed]
6. Kramer, G.M.; Frings, V.; Hoetjes, N.; Hoekstra, O.S.; Smit, E.F.; De Langen, A.J.; Boellaard, R. Repeatability of Quantitative Whole Body 18F-FDG PET/CT Uptake Measures as Function of Uptake Interval and Lesion Selection in Non-Small Cell Lung Cancer Patients. *J. Nucl. Med.* **2016**, *57*, 1343–1349. [CrossRef] [PubMed]
7. Velasquez, L.M.; Boellaard, R.; Kollia, G.; Hayes, W.; Hoekstra, O.S.; Lammertsma, A.A.; Galbraith, S.M. Repeatability of 18F-FDG PET in a Multicenter Phase I Study of Patients with Advanced Gastrointestinal Malignancies. *J. Nucl. Med.* **2009**, *50*, 1646–1654. [CrossRef] [PubMed]
8. Wang, B.; Liu, C.; Wei, Y.; Meng, J.; Zhang, Y.; Gan, H.; Xu, X.-P.; Wan, F.; Pan, J.; Ma, X.; et al. A Prospective Trial of 68Ga-PSMA and 18F-FDG PET/CT in Nonmetastatic Prostate Cancer Patients with an Early PSA Progression During Castration. *Clin. Cancer Res.* **2020**, *26*, 4551–4558. [CrossRef]
9. Zhou, X.; Li, Y.; Jiang, X.; Wang, X.; Chen, S.; Shen, T.; You, J.; Lu, H.; Liao, H.; Li, Z.; et al. Intra-Individual Comparison of 18F-PSMA-1007 and 18F-FDG PET/CT in the Evaluation of Patients With Prostate Cancer. *Front. Oncol.* **2021**, *10*. [CrossRef] [PubMed]
10. Kuyumcu, S.; Has-Simsek, D.; Iliaz, R.; Sanli, Y.; Buyukkaya, F.; Akyuz, F.; Turkmen, C. Evidence of Prostate-Specific Membrane Antigen Expression in Hepatocellular Carcinoma Using 68Ga-PSMA PET/CT. *Clin. Nucl. Med.* **2019**, *44*, 702–706. [CrossRef] [PubMed]
11. Moses, W.W. Fundamental limits of spatial resolution in PET. *Nucl. Instruments Methods Phys. Res. Sect. A Accel. Spectrometers, Detect. Assoc. Equip.* **2011**, *648*, S236–S240. [CrossRef]
12. Soret, M.; Bacharach, S.L.; Buvat, I. Partial-Volume Effect in PET Tumor Imaging. *J. Nucl. Med.* **2007**, *48*, 932–945. [CrossRef] [PubMed]
13. Kessler, R.M.; Ellis, J.R.; Eden, M. Analysis of Emission Tomographic Scan Data: Limitations Imposed by Resolution and Background. *J. Comput. Assist. Tomogr.* **1984**, *8*, 514–522. [CrossRef]
14. Hoffman, E.J.; Huang, S.-C.; Phelps, M.E. Quantitation in Positron Emission Computed Tomography. *J. Comput. Assist. Tomogr.* **1979**, *3*, 299–308. [CrossRef]
15. Van Der Vos, C.S.; Koopman, D.; Rijnsdorp, S.; Arends, A.J.; Boellaard, R.; Van Dalen, J.A.; Lubberink, M.; Willemsen, A.T.M.; Visser, E.P. Quantification, improvement, and harmonization of small lesion detection with state-of-the-art PET. *Eur. J. Nucl. Med. Mol. Imaging* **2017**, *44*, 4–16. [CrossRef]
16. Eckerman, K.; Endo, A. PREFACE. *Ann. ICRP* **2008**, *38*, 9–10. [CrossRef]
17. Bailey, D.L.; Townsend, D.W.; Valk, P.E.; Maisey, M.N. (Eds.) *Positron Emission Tomography – Basic Sciences*; Springer: London, UK, 2005.
18. Levin, C.S.; Hoffman, E.J. Calculation of positron range and its effect on the fundamental limit of positron emission tomography system spatial resolution. *Phys. Med. Biol.* **1999**, *44*, 781–799. [CrossRef] [PubMed]
19. Cal-Gonzalez, J.; Vaquero, J.J.; Herraiz, J.L.; Pérez-Liva, M.; Soto-Montenegro, M.L.; Peña-Zalbidea, S.; Desco, M.; Udías, J.M. Improving PET Quantification of Small Animal [68Ga]DOTA-Labeled PET/CT Studies by Using a CT-Based Positron Range Correction. *Mol. Imaging Biol.* **2018**, *20*, 584–593. [CrossRef]
20. Disselhorst, J.A.; Brom, M.; Laverman, P.; Slump, C.H.; Boerman, O.C.; Oyen, W.J.G.; Gotthardt, M.; Visser, E.P. Image-Quality Assessment for Several Positron Emitters Using the NEMA NU 4-2008 Standards in the Siemens Inveon Small-Animal PET Scanner. *J. Nucl. Med.* **2010**, *51*, 610–617. [CrossRef] [PubMed]
21. Prasad, V.; Steffen, I.G.; Diederichs, G.; Makowski, M.R.; Wust, P.; Brenner, W. Biodistribution of [68Ga]PSMA-HBED-CC in Patients with Prostate Cancer: Characterization of Uptake in Normal Organs and Tumour Lesions. *Mol. Imaging Biol.* **2016**, *18*, 428–436. [CrossRef] [PubMed]
22. Afshar-Oromieh, A.; Malcher, A.; Eder, M.; Eisenhut, M.; Linhart, H.G.; Hadaschik, B.A.; Holland-Letz, T.; Giesel, F.L.; Kratochwil, C.; Haufe, S.; et al. PET imaging with a [68Ga]gallium-labelled PSMA ligand for the diagnosis of prostate cancer: Biodistribution in humans and first evaluation of tumour lesions. *Eur. J. Nucl. Med. Mol. Imaging* **2013**, *40*, 486–495. [CrossRef]
23. Eder, M.; Schäfer, M.; Bauder-Wüst, U.; Hull, W.-E.; Wängler, C.; Mier, W.; Haberkorn, U.; Eisenhut, M. 68Ga-Complex Lipophilicity and the Targeting Property of a Urea-Based PSMA Inhibitor for PET Imaging. *Bioconjugate Chem.* **2012**, *23*, 688–697. [CrossRef]
24. Hudson, H.; Larkin, R. Accelerated image reconstruction using ordered subsets of projection data. *IEEE Trans. Med Imaging* **1994**, *13*, 601–609. [CrossRef] [PubMed]
25. Ahn, S.; Ross, S.G.; Asma, E.; Miao, J.; Jin, X.; Cheng, L.; Wollenweber, S.D.; Manjeshwar, R.M. Quantitative comparison of OSEM and penalized likelihood image reconstruction using relative difference penalties for clinical PET. *Phys. Med. Biol.* **2015**, *60*, 5733–5751. [CrossRef] [PubMed]
26. Howard, B.A.; Morgan, R.; Thorpe, M.P.; Turkington, T.G.; Oldan, J.; James, O.G.; Borges-Neto, S. Comparison of Bayesian penalized likelihood reconstruction versus OS-EM for characterization of small pulmonary nodules in oncologic PET/CT. *Ann. Nucl. Med.* **2017**, *31*, 623–628. [CrossRef] [PubMed]

27. Chilcott, A.K.; Bradley, K.M.; McGowan, D.R. Effect of a Bayesian Penalized Likelihood PET Reconstruction Compared With Ordered Subset Expectation Maximization on Clinical Image Quality Over a Wide Range of Patient Weights. *Am. J. Roentgenol.* **2018**, *210*, 153–157. [CrossRef]
28. Riet, J.T.; Rijnsdorp, S.; Roef, M.J.; Arends, A.J. Evaluation of a Bayesian penalized likelihood reconstruction algorithm for low-count clinical 18F-FDG PET/CT. *EJNMMI Phys.* **2019**, *6*, 1–14. [CrossRef]
29. Teoh, E.J.; McGowan, D.R.; MacPherson, R.E.; Bradley, K.M.; Gleeson, F.V. Phantom and Clinical Evaluation of the Bayesian Penalized Likelihood Reconstruction Algorithm Q.Clear on an LYSO PET/CT System. *J. Nucl. Med.* **2015**, *56*, 1447–1452. [CrossRef]
30. Teoh, E.J.; McGowan, D.R.; Schuster, D.M.; Tsakok, M.T.; Gleeson, F.V.; Bradley, K.M. Bayesian penalised likelihood reconstruction (Q.Clear) of 18F-fluciclovine PET for imaging of recurrent prostate cancer: Semi-quantitative and clinical evaluation. *Br. J. Radiol.* **2018**. [CrossRef]
31. Rowley, L.M.; Bradley, K.M.; Boardman, P.; Hallam, A.; McGowan, D.R. Optimization of Image Reconstruction for 90 Y Selective Internal Radiotherapy on a Lutetium Yttrium Orthosilicate PET/CT System Using a Bayesian Penalized Likelihood Reconstruction Algorithm. *J. Nucl. Med.* **2017**, *58*, 658–664. [CrossRef]
32. Berliner, C.; Tienken, M.; Frenzel, T.; Kobayashi, Y.; Helberg, A.; Kirchner, U.; Klutmann, S.; Beyersdorff, D.; Budäus, L.; Wester, H.-J.; et al. Detection rate of PET/CT in patients with biochemical relapse of prostate cancer using [68Ga]PSMA I&T and comparison with published data of [68Ga]PSMA HBED-CC. *Eur. J. Nucl. Med. Mol. Imaging* **2016**, *44*, 670–677. [CrossRef]
33. Schmuck, S.; Nordlohne, S.; Von Klot, C.-A.; Henkenberens, C.; Sohns, J.M.; Christiansen, H.; Wester, H.-J.; Ross, T.L.; Bengel, F.M.; Derlin, T. Comparison of standard and delayed imaging to improve the detection rate of [68Ga]PSMA I&T PET/CT in patients with biochemical recurrence or prostate-specific antigen persistence after primary therapy for prostate cancer. *Eur. J. Nucl. Med. Mol. Imaging* **2017**, *44*, 960–968. [CrossRef] [PubMed]
34. Sahlmann, C.-O.; Meller, B.; Bouter, C.; Ritter, C.O.; Ströbel, P.; Lotz, J.; Trojan, L.; Meller, J.; Hijazi, S. Biphasic 68Ga-PSMA-HBED-CC-PET/CT in patients with recurrent and high-risk prostate carcinoma. *Eur. J. Nucl. Med. Mol. Imaging* **2015**, *43*, 898–905. [CrossRef]
35. EARL Accreditation Manual Version 2.1 (Oct 2020). Available online: http://earl.eanm.org/html/img/pool/MASTER_EARL_Manual_Oct2020_2.1.pdf (accessed on 5 May 2021).
36. Nuyts, J.; Beque, D.; Dupont, P.; Mortelmans, L. A concave prior penalizing relative differences for maximum-a-posteriori reconstruction in emission tomography. *IEEE Trans. Nucl. Sci.* **2002**, *49*, 56–60. [CrossRef]
37. D'Amico, A.V.; Whittington, R.; Malkowicz, S.B.; Schultz, D.; Blank, K.; Broderick, G.A.; Tomaszewski, J.E.; Renshaw, A.A.; Kaplan, I.; Beard, C.J.; et al. Biochemical Outcome After Radical Prostatectomy, External Beam Radiation Therapy, or Interstitial Radiation Therapy for Clinically Localized Prostate Cancer. *JAMA* **1998**, *280*, 969–974. [CrossRef]
38. Koerber, S.A.; Utzinger, M.T.; Kratochwil, C.; Kesch, C.; Haefner, M.F.; Katayama, S.; Mier, W.; Iagaru, A.H.; Herfarth, K.; Haberkorn, U.; et al. 68Ga-PSMA-11 PET/CT in Newly Diagnosed Carcinoma of the Prostate: Correlation of Intraprostatic PSMA Uptake with Several Clinical Parameters. *J. Nucl. Med.* **2017**, *58*, 1943–1948. [CrossRef]
39. Sachpekidis, C.; Bäumer, P.; Kopka, K.; Hadaschik, B.A.; Hohenfellner, M.; Kopp-Schneider, A.; Haberkorn, U.; Dimitrakopoulou-Strauss, A. 68Ga-PSMA PET/CT in the evaluation of bone metastases in prostate cancer. *Eur. J. Nucl. Med. Mol. Imaging* **2018**, *45*, 904–912. [CrossRef]
40. Beheshti, M.; Paymani, Z.; Brilhante, J.; Geinitz, H.; Gehring, D.; Leopoldseder, T.; Wouters, L.; Pirich, C.; Loidl, W.; Langsteger, W. Optimal time-point for 68Ga-PSMA-11 PET/CT imaging in assessment of prostate cancer: Feasibility of sterile cold-kit tracer preparation? *Eur. J. Nucl. Med. Mol. Imaging* **2018**, *45*, 1188–1196. [CrossRef]
41. Lindström, E.; Sundin, A.; Trampal, C.; Lindsjö, L.; Ilan, E.; Danfors, T.; Antoni, G.; Sörensen, J.; Lubberink, M. Evaluation of Penalized-Likelihood Estimation Reconstruction on a Digital Time-of-Flight PET/CT Scanner for18F-FDG Whole-Body Examinations. *J. Nucl. Med.* **2018**, *59*, 1152–1158. [CrossRef] [PubMed]
42. Wagner, T.; Gellee, S.; Page, J.; Sanghera, B.; Payoux, P. Impact of the Point Spread Function on Maximum Standardized Uptake Value Measurements in Patients with Pulmonary Cancer. *World J. Nucl. Med.* **2014**, *13*, 128–131. [CrossRef]
43. Yamashita, S.; Yamamoto, H.; Nakaichi, T.; Yoneyama, T.; Yokoyama, K. Comparison of image quality between step-and-shoot and continuous bed motion techniques in whole-body 18F-fluorodeoxyglucose positron emission tomography with the same acquisition duration. *Ann. Nucl. Med.* **2017**, *31*, 686–695. [CrossRef] [PubMed]
44. Bärwolf, R.; Zirnsak, M.; Freesmeyer, M. Breath-hold and free-breathing F-18-FDG-PET/CT in malignant melanoma—detection of additional tumoral foci and effects on quantitative parameters. *Med.* **2017**, *96*, e5882. [CrossRef] [PubMed]
45. Li, G.; Schmidtlein, C.R.; Burger, I.A.; Ridge, C.A.; Solomon, S.B.; Humm, J.L. Assessing and accounting for the impact of respiratory motion on FDG uptake and viable volume for liver lesions in free-breathing PET using respiration-suspended PET images as reference. *Med Phys.* **2014**, *41*, 091905. [CrossRef] [PubMed]
46. Akamatsu, G.; Ikari, Y.; Nishida, H.; Nishio, T.; Ohnishi, A.; Maebatake, A.; Sasaki, M.; Senda, M. Influence of Statistical Fluctuation on Reproducibility and Accuracy of SUVmax and SUVpeak: A Phantom Study. *J. Nucl. Med. Technol.* **2015**, *43*, 222–226. [CrossRef] [PubMed]
47. Boellaard, R.; Krak, N.C.; Hoekstra, O.S.; A Lammertsma, A. Effects of noise, image resolution, and ROI definition on the accuracy of standard uptake values: A simulation study. *J. Nucl. Med.* **2004**, *45*, 1519–1527.

48. Messerli, M.; Stolzmann, P.; Egger-Sigg, M.; Trinckauf, J.; D'Aguanno, S.; Burger, I.A.; Von Schulthess, G.K.; Kaufmann, P.A.; Huellner, M.W. Impact of a Bayesian penalized likelihood reconstruction algorithm on image quality in novel digital PET/CT: Clinical implications for the assessment of lung tumors. *EJNMMI Phys.* **2018**, *5*, 1–13. [CrossRef]
49. Mansor, S.; Pfaehler, E.; Heijtel, D.; Lodge, M.A.; Boellaard, R.; Yaqub, M. Impact of PET/CT system, reconstruction protocol, data analysis method, and repositioning on PET/CT precision: An experimental evaluation using an oncology and brain phantom. *Med Phys.* **2017**, *44*, 6413–6424. [CrossRef]
50. Munk, O.L.; Tolbod, L.P.; Hansen, S.B.; Bogsrud, T.V. Point-spread function reconstructed PET images of sub-centimeter lesions are not quantitative. *EJNMMI Phys.* **2017**, *4*, 5. [CrossRef]
51. Cherry, S.R.; Sorenson, J.A.; Phelps, M.E. Physics in Nuclear Medicine, 4th ed.Saunders: Philadelphia, PA, USA, 2012.
52. Derenzo, S.E. Precision measurement of annihilation point spread distributions for medically important positron emitters. In Proceedings of the 5th International Conference on Positron Annihilation, Lake Yamanaka, Japan, 8–11 April 1979.
53. Derenzo, S.E. Mathematical Removal of Positron Range Blurring in High Resolution Tomography. *IEEE Trans. Nucl. Sci.* **1986**, *33*, 565–569. [CrossRef]

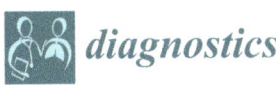

Article

Compensating Positron Range Effects of Ga-68 in Preclinical PET Imaging by Using Convolutional Neural Network: A Monte Carlo Simulation Study

Ching-Ching Yang [1,2]

1. Department of Medical Imaging and Radiological Sciences, Kaohsiung Medical University, Kaohsiung 807, Taiwan; cyang@kmu.edu.tw
2. Department of Medical Research, Kaohsiung Medical University Chung-Ho Memorial Hospital, Kaohsiung 807, Taiwan

Abstract: This study aimed to investigate the feasibility of positron range correction based on three different convolutional neural network (CNN) models in preclinical PET imaging of Ga-68. The first model (CNN1) was originally designed for super-resolution recovery, while the second model (CNN2) and the third model (CNN3) were originally designed for pseudo CT synthesis from MRI. A preclinical PET scanner and 30 phantom configurations were modeled in Monte Carlo simulations, where each phantom configuration was simulated twice, once for Ga-68 (CNN input images) and once for back-to-back 511-keV gamma rays (CNN output images) with a 20 min emission scan duration. The Euclidean distance was used as the loss function to minimize the difference between CNN input and output images. According to our results, CNN3 outperformed CNN1 and CNN2 qualitatively and quantitatively. With regard to qualitative observation, it was found that boundaries in Ga-68 images became sharper after correction. As for quantitative analysis, the recovery coefficient (RC) and spill-over ratio (SOR) were increased after correction, while no substantial increase in coefficient of variation of RC (CV_{RC}) or coefficient of variation of SOR (CV_{SOR}) was observed. Overall, CNN3 should be a good candidate architecture for positron range correction in Ga-68 preclinical PET imaging.

Keywords: Ga-68 preclinical PET imaging; positron range correction; convolutional neural network

1. Introduction

Positron emission tomography (PET) is widely recognized as a powerful imaging technique for in vivo quantification and localization of physiological and pathophysiological functions. Furthermore, PET imaging allows to follow the progression of human diseases in transgenic and knockout mice noninvasively, so it has been used to study the effectiveness of new drugs or treatments [1–3]. Due to the small size of experimental animals, high spatial resolution is mandatory in preclinical PET system, which is associated with positron physics, scanner design, data correction, and the reconstruction algorithm [4,5]. Among various positron emission radioisotopes, F-18 is by far the most widely used radionuclide. Nevertheless, with the increasing interest in theranostic approaches for cancer treatment, radioisotopes other than F-18 are also considered in PET imaging, such as Ga-68 [6–8]. Using Ga-68 labeled tracers for diagnostics can be effectively followed by targeted radionuclide therapy performed using the same tracer labeled with Lu-177. Since Ga-68 PET imaging is used to determine the therapeutic protocols with Lu-177, the dose delivered to targets and organs at risk through Lu-177 radionuclide therapy is affected by the imaging performance of Ga-68 PET [9–11]. The mean positron energy of Ga-68 is 0.83 MeV, which results in a mean positron range of 3.5 mm. Hence, the spatial resolution of PET imaging is inferior with Ga-68 compared to F-18 [12]. Improving spatial resolution through positron range correction would increase the accuracy of Ga-68 PET-based treatment planning.

Convolutional neural network (CNN) has been applied in several medical imaging areas, and various architectures have been developed for different tasks [13]. This study aimed to investigate the feasibility of positron range correction based on three different CNN models in preclinical PET imaging of Ga-68. The first CNN model (CNN1) used in this study was originally designed to recover high resolution image from low resolution input image, while the second CNN model (CNN2) and the third CNN model (CNN3) were originally designed to convert MRI into pseudo CT. The image data for CNN training and testing were generated by Monte Carlo simulation to prevent experimental errors while realistically modeling the positron range effects.

2. Materials and Methods

2.1. Monte Carlo Simulation Toolkit

Monte Carlo simulation was performed by using GATE (GEANT4 Application for Tomographic Emission) version 6.0.0 [14]. GATE comprises four layers of codes, which is GEANT4 in the innermost layer, followed by the core layer, application layer, and user layer. GEANT4, a toolkit for the simulation of the passage of particles through matter based on Monte Carlo method, has been proven to be a proper tool for simulation of positron transportation. In GATE, the scanner geometry, particle type, position, energy, physical interactions of particles with matter and run process were defined by using a scripted language at the user layer to output descriptive data in the form of random number for running simulation using GEANT4.

2.2. Preclinical PET System

A FLEX Triumph PET/CT scanner (Gamma Medica-Ideas, Nortridge, CA, USA) was modeled by using the cylindrical PET system in GATE, which was comprised of 5 hierarchic levels: world cylindrical PET, r sector, module, crystal, layer, to produce and store the hit information that generates the singles and the coincidences of the simulation. The preclinical PET scanner investigated in this study includes 180 detector blocks that are arranged into 48 rings, and each block contains an 8×8 array of BGO crystals of $2.3 \times 2.3 \times 10$ mm^3. This configuration covers a transaxial field-of-view (FOV) of 10 cm and an axial FOV of 11.6 cm. PET data were simulated with a 250- to 750-keV energy window and 12-ns timing window in listmode format, which were consequently assigned into 3D sinograms. The sinograms were Fourier rebinned first and then reconstructed using 2D ordered subsets expectation maximization with 4 iterations and 10 subsets. The voxel size used for PET reconstruction was $0.4 \times 0.4 \times 0.4$ mm^3.

2.3. Phantom Design

The phantoms shown in Figure 1 were constructed in GATE Monte Carlo simulation by using the voxelized source and voxelized phantom to define the activity distribution and photon attenuation, respectively. $PHAN_{brain}$ was the Hoffman 3D brain phantom. Figure 1a–c demonstrate the axial, coronal, and sagittal view of $PHAN_{brain}$. To increase the dataset size and diversity for CNN training, $PHAN_{brain}$ was slightly modified to generate 20 phantom configurations (2 translations × 2 rotations × 5 deformations), where each of them was filled with activity of 3.7×10^6 Bq. $PHAN_{5rod}$ was a cylinder of dimeter 50 mm, length of 80 mm and containing 5 rods with diameters of 2, 4, 6, 8, 10 mm. Figure 1d demonstrates the axial view of $PHAN_{5rod}$. The target-to-background ratio (TBR) was set at 0, 2, 4, 5, 8, 10, 16, 20 to generate 8 phantom configurations, where the rod inserts within $PHAN_{5rod}$ were filled with activity concentration of 1.69×10^6 Bq/mL. $PHAN_{1sphere}$ was a cylinder of diameter 50 mm, length of 80 mm and containing a 10-mm-diameter sphere. Figure 1e demonstrates the axial view of $PHAN_{1sphere}$. The sphere within $PHAN_{1sphere}$ was filled with water (i.e., cold sphere), while the cylinder was filled with activity concentration of 1.69×10^6 Bq/mL. $PHAN_{20rod}$ was an elliptical cylinder of major axis 55 mm, minor axis of 50 mm, length of 80 mm, and containing 20 rods with 2, 3, 4, 5 mm diameter. Figure 1f demonstrates the axial view of $PHAN_{20rod}$. The white rod inserts within $PHAN_{20rod}$ were filled with activity concentration of 1.69×10^6 Bq/mL, while the gray rod inserts were filled with activity concentration of 8.44×10^5 Bq/mL. Overall, a total of 30 phantom configurations were modeled in GATE Monte Carlo simulation, where each phantom configuration was simulated twice with a 20 min emission scan duration, once for Ga-68 (CNN input images) and once for back-to-back 511-keV gamma rays (CNN output images).

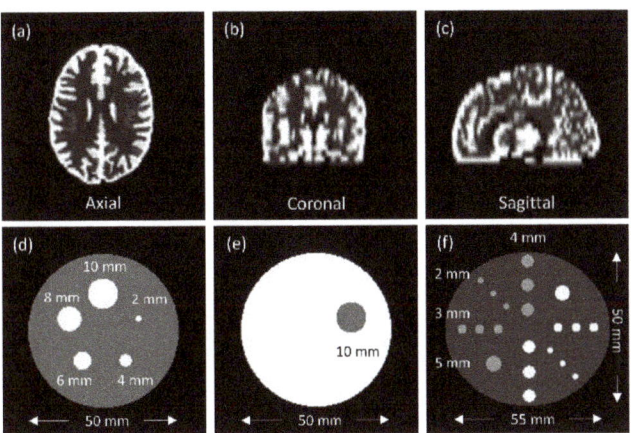

Figure 1. $PHAN_{brain}$ in (**a**) axial plane, (**b**) coronal plane, (**c**) sagittal plane, and the central axial slice of (**d**) $PHAN_{5rod}$, (**e**) $PHAN_{1sphere}$, (**f**) $PHAN_{20rod}$.

2.4. CNN Models for Positron Range Correction

Figure 2 shows the architectures of CNN models used in this study to compensate positron range effects of Ga-68 in preclinical PET imaging. CNN1 was a 3-layered model proposed by Dong et al. for super-resolution recovery [15]. CNN2 was a 4-layered model proposed by Nie et al. for pseudo CT synthesis from MRI [16]. CNN3 was the deeply supervised nets (DSN) version of CNN2 to supervise features at each convolutional stage, enabled by layer-wise dense connections in both backbone networks and prediction layers [17]. Because the error distribution was expected to be Gaussian, the root mean square error (RMSE), i.e., the Euclidean distance, was used as the loss function to minimize the difference between Ga-68 PET images and the corresponding gamma source images. Using RMSE as the loss function favors a high peak signal-to-noise ratio (PSNR). The input images were prepared as 32×32-pixel sub-images randomly cropped from the original image. To avoid border effects, all the convolutional layers have no padding, and the network produces an output image with 20×20 matrix size for CNN1 and 18×18 matrix size for CNN2 and CNN3. The training datasets were sub-images extracted from the PET images of 16 $PHAN_{brain}$ and 4 $PHAN_{5rod}$ (TBR = 0, 4, 5, 8) with a stride of 14. The testing datasets were sub-images extracted from the PET images of 4 $PHAN_{brain}$ (other than those used in CNN training) and 4 $PHAN_{5rod}$ (TBR = 2, 10, 16, 20) with a stride of 21. The training and testing datasets provide roughly 111,078 and 25,774 sub-images, respectively. The filter weights of each layer were initialized by using Xavier initialization, which could automatically determine the scale of initialization based on the number of input and output neurons [18]. All biases were initialized with zero. The models were trained using stochastic gradient descent with mini-batch size of 128, learning rate of 0.01 and momentum of 0.9. The CNN models were built, trained and tested by using Caffe (Convolutional Architecture for Fast Feature Embedding) CNN platform (version 1.0.0-rc5 with CUDA 8.0.61) on an Ubuntu server (version 16.04.4 LTS) with two RTX 2080 (NVIDIA, Santa Clara, CA, USA) graphics cards [19].

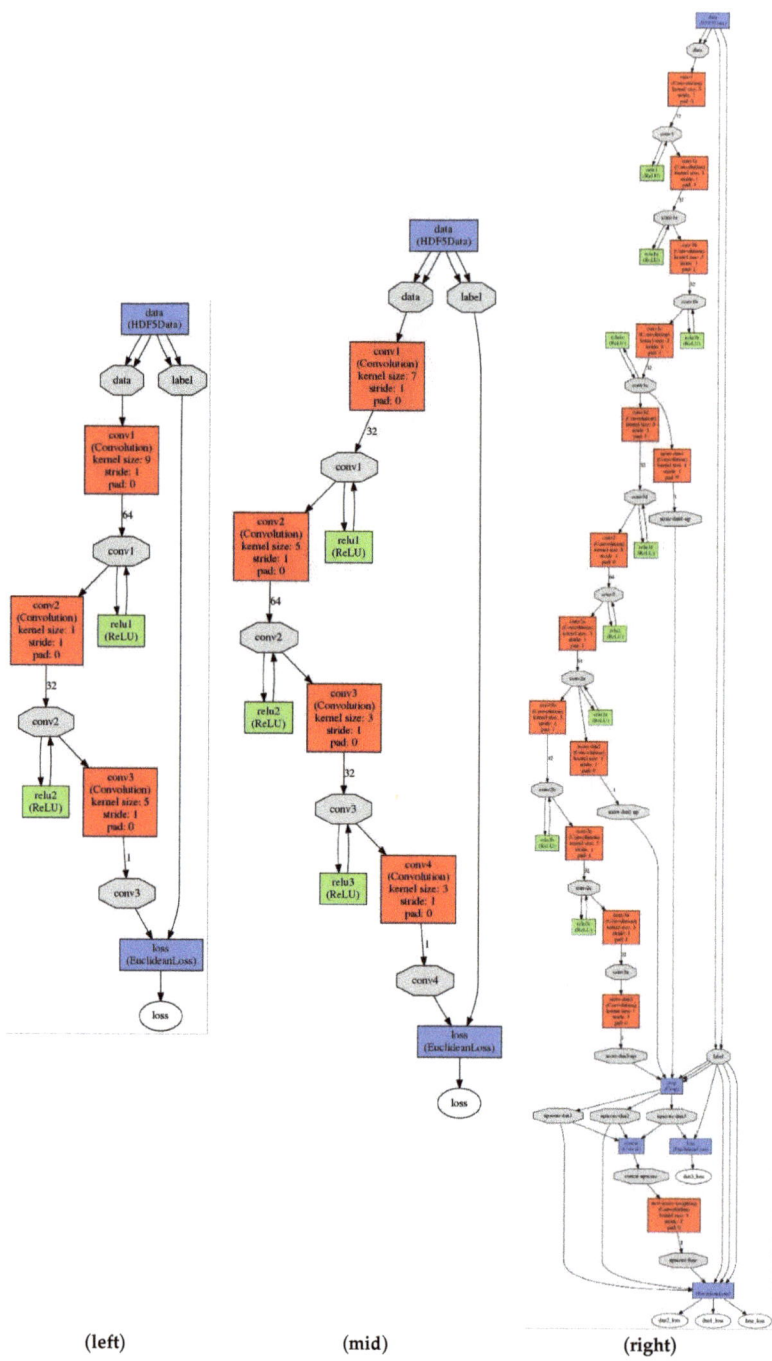

Figure 2. The architectures of CNN1 (**left**), CNN2 (**mid**) and CNN3 (**right**).

2.5. Quantitative Analysis

The difference between Ga-68 PET images corrected by CNN-based positron range correction (I_{PRC}) and the corresponding gamma source images (I_{gamma}) was quantified by calculating the RMSE and PSNR:

$$\text{RMSE} = \sqrt{\frac{\sum_{i=1}^{V}\left(I_{gamma} - I_{PRC}\right)^2}{V}} \tag{1}$$

where V is the number of voxels within the whole image,

$$\text{PSNR} = 20\log_{10}\frac{I_{max}}{\text{RMSE}} \tag{2}$$

where I_{max} is the maximum intensity value of the image. RMSE and PSNR provide a measure of image quality over the whole image.

The ability of Ga-68 PET images (I_{Ga68}), I_{gamma}, and I_{PRC} to recover contrast in small targets was quantified by calculating the recovery coefficient (RC), which was defined as:

$$\text{RC} = \frac{\text{AVG}_{target}}{\text{AVG}_{uniform}} \tag{3}$$

where AVG_{target} is the average of a small target, and $\text{AVG}_{uniform}$ is the average of a uniform region. The coefficient of variation of RC (CV_{RC}) was defined as:

$$CV_{RC} = \sqrt{\left(\frac{\text{SD}_{target}}{\text{AVG}_{target}}\right)^2 + \left(\frac{\text{SD}_{uniform}}{\text{AVG}_{uniform}}\right)^2} \tag{4}$$

where SD_{target} is the standard deviation of a small target, and $\text{SD}_{uniform}$ is the standard deviation of a uniform region. To calculate AVG_{target} and SD_{target}, the image slices of PHAN_{5rod} over the central 50 mm length were averaged to obtain one average image, which was used to determine the voxel coordinate with maximum intensity for each rod. The pixel coordinates were then used to create a line profile along the axial direction. The AVG_{target} and SD_{target} were the average and standard deviation of pixel values in the line profile. As for $\text{AVG}_{uniform}$ and $\text{SD}_{uniform}$, the image slices of $\text{PHAN}_{1sphere}$ over the central 50 mm length were averaged to obtain one average image. A circular region-of-interest (ROI) with 10 mm diameter was placed on the cylinder of the average image to calculate $\text{AVG}_{uniform}$ and $\text{SD}_{uniform}$, corresponding to the average and standard deviation within the circular ROI, respectively.

The spill-over of activity in I_{Ga68}, I_{gamma} and I_{PRC} was quantified by calculating the spill-over ratio (SOR), which was defined as:

$$\text{SOR} = \frac{\text{AVG}_{cold}}{\text{AVG}_{hot}} \tag{5}$$

where AVG_{cold} is the average of a cold spot, and AVG_{hot} is the average of a hot spot. The coefficient of variation of SOR (CV_{SOR}) was defined as:

$$CV_{SOR} = \sqrt{\left(\frac{\text{SD}_{cold}}{\text{AVG}_{cold}}\right)^2 + \left(\frac{\text{SD}_{hot}}{\text{AVG}_{hot}}\right)^2} \tag{6}$$

where SD_{cold} is the standard deviation of a cold spot, and SD_{hot} is the standard deviation of a hot spot. A 10-mm-diameter ROI was placed on the cold sphere of $\text{PHAN}_{1sphere}$ in the slice of the sphere center to calculate AVG_{cold} and SD_{cold}, corresponding to the average and standard deviation within the cold ROI, respectively. For the same image slice, a 10-mm-diameter ROI was placed on the cylinder of $\text{PHAN}_{1sphere}$ to calculate AVG_{hot} and SD_{hot}, corresponding to the average and standard deviation within the hot ROI, respectively.

3. Results

Figure 3 demonstrates I_{gamma}, I_{Ga68}, and Ga-68 PET images after positron range correction based on CNN1 (I_{PRC}^{CNN1}), CNN2 (I_{PRC}^{CNN2}) and CNN3 (I_{PRC}^{CNN3}) of PHAN$_{brain}$. With naked eye observation, boundaries in Ga-68 PET images became sharper after correction. Figure 4 demonstrates I_{gamma}, I_{Ga68}, I_{PRC}^{CNN1}, I_{PRC}^{CNN2}, I_{PRC}^{CNN3} of PHAN$_{5rod}$ with TBR = 0 and 10. The 2-mm rod in PHAN$_{5rod}$ with TBR = 0 that was barely seen in I_{Ga68} became visible in I_{PRC}^{CNN2} and I_{PRC}^{CNN3}. The RMSE and PSNR between I_{gamma} and I_{PRC} are shown in Figure 5a for PHAN$_{brain}$ and Figure 5b for PHAN$_{5rod}$ with TBR = 10. Lower RMSEs and higher PSNRs were observed in Figure 5b than those in Figure 5a. For either phantom configuration, the lowest RMSE and the highest PSNR were found in CNN3-based correction, followed by CNN2- and CNN1-based correction.

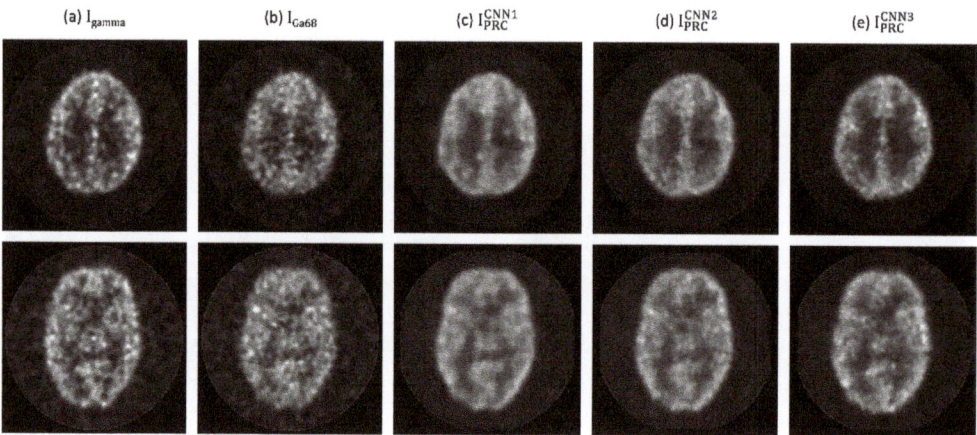

Figure 3. (a) I_{gamma}, (b) I_{Ga68}, (c) I_{PRC}^{CNN1}, (d) I_{PRC}^{CNN2}, (e) I_{PRC}^{CNN3} of PHAN$_{brain}$ at 2 different axial slices (**top row** and **bottom row**).

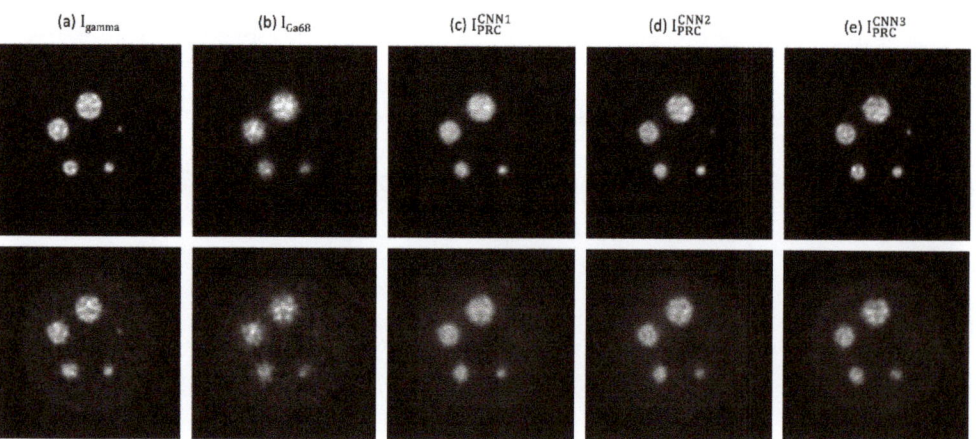

Figure 4. (a) I_{gamma}, (b) I_{Ga68}, (c) I_{PRC}^{CNN1}, (d) I_{PRC}^{CNN2}, (e) I_{PRC}^{CNN3} of PHAN$_{5rod}$ with TBR = 0 (**top row**) and TBR = 10 (**bottom row**).

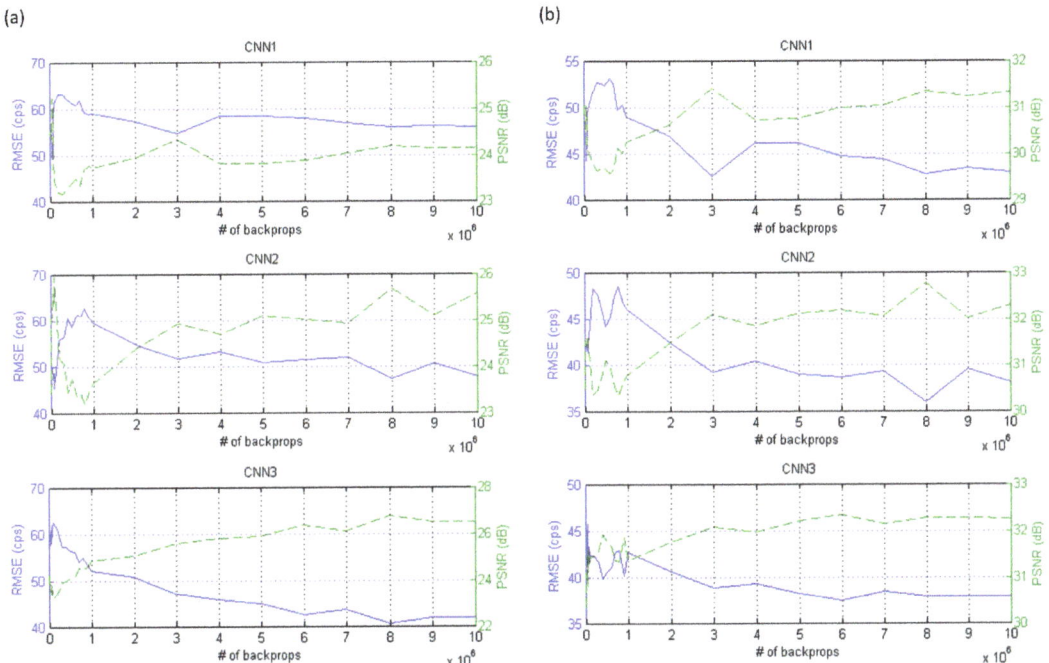

Figure 5. RMSE (solid line, left axis) and PSNR (dashed line, right axis) between I_{gamma} and I_{PRC} for (**a**) $PHAN_{brain}$ and (**b**) $PHAN_{5rod}$ with TBR = 10 (**top row**: CNN1-based correction; **mid row**: CNN2-based correction; **bottom row**: CNN3-based correction).

The RCs of I_{gamma}, I_{Ga68}, I_{PRC}^{CNN1}, I_{PRC}^{CNN2}, I_{PRC}^{CNN3} are shown in Figure 6a for $PHAN_{5rod}$ with TBR = 0 and Figure 6b for $PHAN_{5rod}$ with TBR = 10. The RCs of positron range corrected images were higher in TBR = 0 than those in TBR = 10 for 4- and 6-mm rods, while the difference was less obvious in 8- and 10-mm rods. Among three corrected images, the highest RCs were observed in I_{PRC}^{CNN3} for 6-, 8-, and 10-mm rods in TBR = 0, while the highest RC for 4-mm rod was observed in I_{PRC}^{CNN2}. With regard to TBR = 10, the highest RCs were observed in I_{PRC}^{CNN3} for 4-, 6-, and 8-mm rods, while the highest RC for 10-mm rod was observed in I_{PRC}^{CNN2}. The CV_{RCS} of I_{gamma}, I_{Ga68}, I_{PRC}^{CNN1}, I_{PRC}^{CNN2}, I_{PRC}^{CNN3} were shown in Figure 7a for $PHAN_{5rod}$ with TBR = 0 and Figure 7b for $PHAN_{5rod}$ with TBR = 10. The CV_{RCS} of positron range corrected images were lower in TBR = 0 than those in TBR = 10 for 4-, 6-, 8-, and 10-mm rods. Among three corrected images, the CV_{RCS} of I_{PRC}^{CNN1} were slight lower than those from I_{PRC}^{CNN2} and I_{PRC}^{CNN3} for either phantom configuration.

With regard to the spillover effect determined by using $PHAN_{1sphere}$, the SORs of I_{gamma}, I_{Ga68}, I_{PRC}^{CNN1}, I_{PRC}^{CNN2}, I_{PRC}^{CNN3} were 0.017, 0.026, 0.021, 0.020, and 0.020, respectively, while the corresponding CV_{SORS} were 0.454, 0.424, 0.406, 0.416, and 0.441. Figure 8 demonstrates I_{Ga68}, I_{PRC}^{CNN1}, I_{PRC}^{CNN2}, I_{PRC}^{CNN3} of $PHAN_{20rod}$ and comparison of intensity profiles through the dashed line. Sharper boundaries were observed in 4- and 5-mm rods after positron range correction. On the other hand, the image quality improvement was limited in 2- and 3-mm rods, except for the 3-mm rod with 8.44×10^5 Bq/mL in I_{PRC}^{CNN2} and I_{PRC}^{CNN3}.

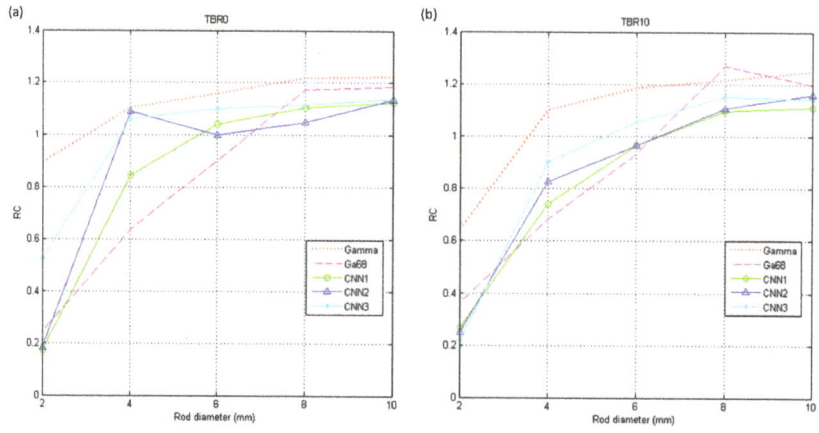

Figure 6. RC of I_{gamma}, I_{Ga68}, I_{PRC}^{CNN1}, I_{PRC}^{CNN2}, I_{PRC}^{CNN3} using $PHAN_{5rod}$ with (**a**) TBR = 0 and (**b**) TBR = 10.

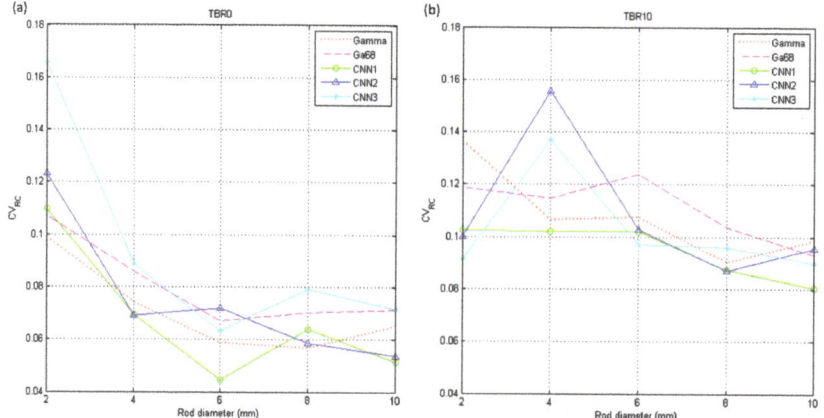

Figure 7. CV_{RC} of I_{gamma}, I_{Ga68}, I_{PRC}^{CNN1}, I_{PRC}^{CNN2}, I_{PRC}^{CNN3} using $PHAN_{5rod}$ with (**a**) TBR = 0 and (**b**) TBR = 10.

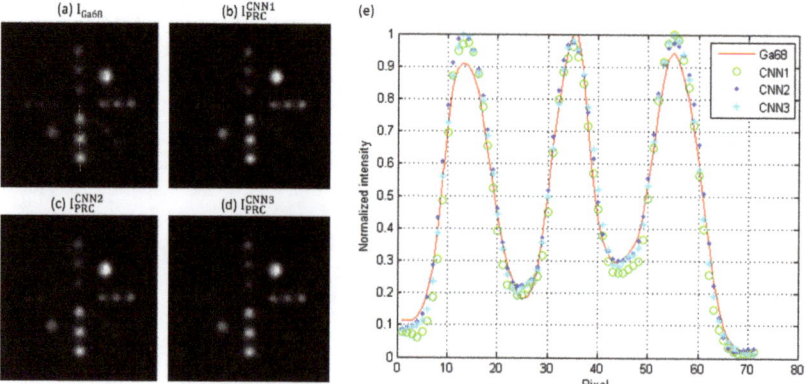

Figure 8. (**a**) I_{Ga68}, (**b**) I_{PRC}^{CNN1}, (**c**) I_{PRC}^{CNN2}, (**d**) I_{PRC}^{CNN3} of $PHAN_{20rod}$ and (**e**) comparison of intensity profiles through the dashed line in (**a**).

4. Discussion

The quantitative capabilities of PET are confounded by a number of degrading factors, whereas the most prominent factors are low signal-to-noise ratio and intrinsically limited spatial resolution [20]. Tumor-targeted theranostic approaches have high lesion-to-background ratio. For example, PET imaging with Ga-68 labeled somatostatin analogues shows high affinity for tumors expressing somatostatin receptors [7,8]. However, the image blurring caused by the positron range effect of Ga-68 may impact the accuracy of treatment planning based on Ga-68 PET imaging. Fourier devolution techniques have been applied to compensate the positron range effects in PET imaging [21], which inspired us to investigate the possibility of using CNN methods for positron range correction. According to Herraiz et al. [22], their study published in 2021 was the first work to successfully combine deep learning and positron range correction in a coherent framework. In our opinion, more studies are needed in this field. Hence, we investigated the feasibility of positron range correction based on three different CNN models in preclinical PET imaging of Ga-68.

Song et al. have presented a work to recover high-resolution PET image from its low-resolution version by using CNN-based approaches for F-18 FDG exams [23]. A 3-layer CNN model proposed by Dong et al. [15], i.e., CNN1, and a 20-layer CNN model proposed by Kim et al. [24] were adapted in their work. The low-resolution images used as the CNN inputs were acquired with Siemens HR+ scanner, while the high-resolution images used as the CNN labels were acquired with Siemens HRRT scanner, a high-resolution dedicated brain PET scanner. Two simulation studies using the BrainWeb digital phantom and a clinical patient study were conducted. They concluded that adding additional channels that extract anatomical features from MRI could improve the performance of CNN-based resolution recovery methods, whereas deep CNNs outperform shallow CNNs. Since the positron range effect would result in image blurring, it is intuitively reasonable to expect that CNN models designed for resolution recovery may be potential candidate for positron range correction in Ga-68 PET imaging. Hence, CNN1 was adapted in our study.

Herraiz et al. have presented a work which adapts the U-Net network to correct positron range effects of Ga-68 in preclinical PET imaging [22]. In their work, the input data to CNN were Ga-68 images, while the label data were the F-18 images. The PET images for CNN training and testing were generated by using the Monte Carlo simulator MCGPU-PET to model data acquisition in an Inveon PET/CT scanner. Their results demonstrated that their proposed method was able to restore the PET images going from 60% up to 95% while maintain low noise levels. They concluded that it is sufficient to use PET images without the corresponding CT as input for the neural network, and including not only the reference slice but also some additional neighbor slices could improve the CNN-based positron range correction method. In our opinion, Herraiz et al. demonstrated that CNN models suitable for positron range correction were not only limited to those designed for resolution recovery, because the U-Net network was originally designed for image segmentation [25]. Positron range correction is inherently an ill-posed problem, because there are multiple Ga-68 activity distributions that may correspond to the same blurred image. Pseudo CT synthesis from MRI is also proposed to solve ill-posed problem, because there are multiple MRI values that may correspond to the same CT value. It was hypothesized that CNN models designed for pseudo CT synthesis from MRI may be potential candidate for positron range correction, so CNN2 and CNN3 were adapted in our study.

In Reference [22], it was assumed that the reconstruction method already incorporated positron range correction for F-18, and their image data for CNN training, testing, and validation were generated from numerical models of mice from a repository. In this work, the CNN output images were back-to-back 511-keV gamma rays, which were not affected by the positron range effects. Hence, our method can be used in PET scanners without F-18 positron range correction. NEMA performance measurements have been well accepted by the manufacturers, and most major companies now specify their product performance in terms of these standardized and traceable specifications. This approach to performance documentation facilitates quantitative comparison of cameras by the user with the assurance that all reported values are measured in the same way and, therefore, are directly comparable [26,27]. Hence, a modified NEMA protocol was used in this study to evaluate the performance of CNN-based positron range correction in terms of resolution recovery and spill-over. Our results demonstrated that the image quality of Ga-68 images was improved after positron range correction based on the 3 CNN models investigated in this work, while CNN3 outperformed CNN1 and CNN2 qualitatively and quantitatively. With regard to qualitative observation, it was found that boundaries in Ga-68 images became sharper after correction (see Figures 3, 4 and 8). As for quantitative analysis, the RC and SOR were increased after correction, while no substantial increase in CV_{RC} or CV_{SOR} was observed. Overall, CNN3 should be a good candidate architecture for positron range correction in Ga-68 preclinical PET imaging.

Several limitations to this study need to be acknowledged. First, the data acquisition, processing and reconstruction approaches can influence the study results. The protocol parameters used in this study were suggested by the manufacturers and are currently employed in a real scanner installed in our institution. Second, all images were generated from Monte Carlo simulations. Since it is difficult to obtain PET images without positron range effect from real experiments, Monte Carlo simulation was used to generate Ga-68 images and corresponding gamma source images for CNN training and testing. Third, the impact of image blurring caused by positron range effect on the accuracy of treatment planning based on Ga-68 was not investigated. Assessments of the proposed methods in real Ga-68 images and the resulting impact on treatment planning for Lu-177 radionuclide therapy need to be further investigated.

5. Conclusions

This study investigated the feasibility of positron range correction based on three different CNN models in preclinical PET imaging of Ga-68. CNN1 was a model originally designed for super-resolution recovery, while CNN2 and CNN3 were models originally designed for pseudo CT synthesis from MRI. Monte Carlo simulation was used to generate Ga-68 images and corresponding gamma source images for CNN training and testing. According to our results, CNN3 outperformed CNN1 and CNN2 qualitatively and quantitatively. With regard to qualitative observation, it was found that boundaries in Ga-68 images became sharper after correction. As for quantitative analysis, the RC and SOR were increased after correction, while no substantial increase in CV_{RC} or CV_{SOR} was observed. Overall, CNN3 should be a good candidate architecture for positron range correction in Ga-68 preclinical PET imaging.

Funding: This research was supported in part by a grant from the Ministry of Science and Technology in Taiwan (MOST110-2314-B-037-076).

Conflicts of Interest: The author declares no conflict of interest.

References

1. Herfert, K.; Mannheim, J.G.; Kuebler, L.; Marciano, S.; Amend, M.; Parl, C.; Napieczynska, H.; Maier, F.M.; Vega, S.C.; Pichler, B.J. Quantitative Rodent Brain Receptor Imaging. *Mol. Imaging Biol.* **2020**, *22*, 223–244. [CrossRef] [PubMed]
2. Wierstra, P.; Sandker, G.; Aarntzen, E.; Gotthardt, M.; Adema, G.; Bussink, J.; Raavé, R.; Heskamp, S. Tracers for non-invasive radionuclide imaging of immune checkpoint expression in cancer. *EJNMMI Radiopharm. Chem.* **2019**, *4*, 29. [CrossRef] [PubMed]
3. Walter, M.A.; Hildebrandt, I.J.; Hacke, K.; Kesner, A.L.; Kelly, O.; Lawson, G.W.; Phelps, M.E.; Czernin, J.; Weber, W.A.; Schiestl, R.H. Small-animal PET/CT for monitoring the development and response to chemotherapy of thymic lymphoma in Trp53−/− mice. *J. Nucl. Med. Off. Publ. Soc. Nucl. Med.* **2010**, *51*, 1285–1292. [CrossRef] [PubMed]
4. Moses, W.W. Fundamental Limits of Spatial Resolution in PET. *Nucl. Instrum. Methods Phys. Res. Sect. A* **2011**, *648*, S236–S240. [CrossRef] [PubMed]
5. Kuntner, C.; Stout, D. Quantitative preclinical PET imaging: Opportunities and challenges. *Front. Phys.* **2014**, *2*, 12. [CrossRef]
6. Payolla, F.; Massabni, A.; Orvig, C. Radiopharmaceuticals for diagnosis in nuclear medicine: A short review. *Eclética Química J.* **2019**, *44*, 11–19. [CrossRef]
7. Baum, R.P.; Kulkarni, H.R. THERANOSTICS: From Molecular Imaging Using Ga-68 Labeled Tracers and PET/CT to Personalized Radionuclide Therapy—The Bad Berka Experience. *Theranostics* **2012**, *2*, 437–447. [CrossRef] [PubMed]

8. Emmett, L.; Willowson, K.; Violet, J.; Shin, J.; Blanksby, A.; Lee, J. Lutetium (177) PSMA radionuclide therapy for men with prostate cancer: A review of the current literature and discussion of practical aspects of therapy. *J. Med. Radiat. Sci.* **2017**, *64*, 52–60. [CrossRef]
9. St. James, S.; Bednarz, B.; Benedict, S.; Buchsbaum, J.C.; Dewaraja, Y.; Frey, E.; Hobbs, R.; Grudzinski, J.; Roncali, E.; Sgouros, G.; et al. Current Status of Radiopharmaceutical Therapy. *Int. J. Radiat. Oncol. Biol. Phys.* **2021**, *109*, 891–901. [CrossRef]
10. Malcolm, J.; Falzone, N.; Lee, B.Q.; Vallis, K.A. Targeted Radionuclide Therapy: New Advances for Improvement of Patient Management and Response. *Cancers* **2019**, *11*, 268. [CrossRef] [PubMed]
11. Lassmann, M.; Eberlein, U. The Relevance of Dosimetry in Precision Medicine. *J. Nucl. Med. Off. Publ. Soc. Nucl. Med.* **2018**, *59*, 1494–1499. [CrossRef] [PubMed]
12. Conti, M.; Eriksson, L. Physics of pure and non-pure positron emitters for PET: A review and a discussion. *EJNMMI Phys.* **2016**, *3*, 8. [CrossRef] [PubMed]
13. Arabi, H.; AkhavanAllaf, A.; Sanaat, A.; Shiri, I.; Zaidi, H. The promise of artificial intelligence and deep learning in PET and SPECT imaging. *Phys. Med.* **2021**, *83*, 122–137. [CrossRef] [PubMed]
14. Jan, S.; Santin, G.; Strul, D.; Staelens, S.; Assié, K.; Autret, D.; Avner, S.; Barbier, R.; Bardiès, M.; Bloomfield, P.M.; et al. GATE: A simulation toolkit for PET and SPECT. *Phys. Med. Biol.* **2004**, *49*, 4543–4561. [CrossRef] [PubMed]
15. Dong, C.; Loy, C.C.; He, K.; Tang, X. Image Super-Resolution Using Deep Convolutional Networks. *IEEE Trans. Pattern Anal. Mach. Intell.* **2016**, *38*, 295–307. [CrossRef] [PubMed]
16. Nie, D.; Cao, X.; Gao, Y.; Wang, L.; Shen, D. Estimating CT Image from MRI Data Using 3D Fully Convolutional Networks. In Proceedings of the Deep Learning and Data Labeling for Medical Applications: First International Workshop, LABELS 2016, and Second International Workshop, DLMIA 2016, Held in Conjunction with MICCAI 2016, Athens, Greece, 21 October 2016; pp. 170–178. [CrossRef]
17. Lee, C.-Y.; Xie, S.; Gallagher, P.; Zhang, Z.; Tu, Z. Deeply-Supervised Nets. *arXiv* **2014**, arXiv:1409.5185.
18. Glorot, X.; Bengio, Y. Understanding the difficulty of training deep feedforward neural networks. In Proceedings of the Thirteenth International Conference on Artificial Intelligence and Statistics, Sardinia, Italy, 13–15 May 2010; pp. 249–256.
19. Jia, Y.; Shelhamer, E.; Donahue, J.; Karayev, S.; Long, J.; Girshick, R.; Guadarrama, S.; Darrell, T. Caffe: Convolutional Architecture for Fast Feature Embedding. In Proceedings of the 2014 ACM Conference on Multimedia, New York, NY, USA, 3–7 November 2014. [CrossRef]
20. Rogasch, J.M.M.; Hofheinz, F.; Lougovski, A.; Furth, C.; Ruf, J.; Großer, O.S.; Mohnike, K.; Hass, P.; Walke, M.; Amthauer, H.; et al. The influence of different signal-to-background ratios on spatial resolution and F18-FDG-PET quantification using point spread function and time-of-flight reconstruction. *EJNMMI Phys.* **2014**, *1*, 12. [CrossRef]
21. Derenzo, S.E. Mathematical Removal of Positron Range Blurring in High Resolution Tomography. *IEEE Trans. Nucl. Sci.* **1986**, *33*, 565–569. [CrossRef]
22. Herraiz, J.L.; Bembibre, A.; López-Montes, A. Deep-Learning Based Positron Range Correction of PET Images. *Appl. Sci.* **2021**, *11*, 266. [CrossRef]
23. Song, T.A.; Chowdhury, S.R.; Yang, F.; Dutta, J. Super-Resolution PET Imaging Using Convolutional Neural Networks. *IEEE Trans. Comput. Imaging* **2020**, *6*, 518–528. [CrossRef] [PubMed]
24. Kim, J.; Lee, J.K.; Lee, K.M. Accurate Image Super-Resolution Using Very Deep Convolutional Networks. In Proceedings of the 2016 IEEE Conference on Computer Vision and Pattern Recognition (CVPR), Las Vegas, NV, USA, 27–30 June 2016; pp. 1646–1654.
25. Ronneberger, O.; Fischer, P.; Brox, T. U-Net: Convolutional Networks for Biomedical Image Segmentation. *arXiv* **2015**, arXiv:1505.04597.
26. Raff, U.; Spitzer, V.M.; Hendee, W.R. Practicality of NEMA performance specification measurements for user-based acceptance testing and routine quality assurance. *J. Nucl. Med. Off. Publ. Soc. Nucl. Med.* **1984**, *25*, 679–687.
27. Teuho, J.; Riehakainen, L.; Honkaniemi, A.; Moisio, O.; Han, C.; Tirri, M.; Liu, S.; Grönroos, T.J.; Liu, J.; Wan, L.; et al. Evaluation of image quality with four positron emitters and three preclinical PET/CT systems. *EJNMMI Res.* **2020**, *10*, 155. [CrossRef] [PubMed]

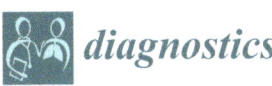

Article

Effects of Respiratory Motion on Y-90 PET Dosimetry for SIRT

Matthew D. Walker [1,*], Jonathan I. Gear [2], Allison J. Craig [2] and Daniel R. McGowan [1,3]

1. Department of Medical Physics and Clinical Engineering, Churchill Hospital, Oxford University Hospitals NHS Foundation Trust, Oxford OX3 7LE, UK; daniel.mcgowan@oncology.ox.ac.uk
2. Joint Department of Physics, The Royal Marsden NHS Foundation Trust and Institute of Cancer Research, Sutton SM2 5PT, UK; jonathan.gear@icr.ac.uk (J.I.G.); Allison.Craig@icr.ac.uk (A.J.C.)
3. Department of Oncology, University of Oxford, Old Road Campus Research Building, Oxford OX3 7DQ, UK
* Correspondence: matthew.walker@ouh.nhs.uk

Abstract: Respiratory motion degrades the quantification accuracy of PET imaging by blurring the radioactivity distribution. In the case of post-SIRT PET-CT verification imaging, respiratory motion can lead to inaccuracies in dosimetric measures. Using an anthropomorphic phantom filled with ^{90}Y at a range of clinically relevant activities, together with a respiratory motion platform performing realistic motions (10–15 mm amplitude), we assessed the impact of respiratory motion on PET-derived post-SIRT dosimetry. Two PET scanners at two sites were included in the assessment. The phantom experiments showed that device-driven quiescent period respiratory motion correction improved the accuracy of the quantification with statistically significant increases in both the mean contrast recovery (+5%, $p = 0.003$) and the threshold activities corresponding to the dose to 80% of the volume of interest (+6%, $p < 0.001$). Although quiescent period gating also reduces the number of counts and hence increases the noise in the PET image, its use is encouraged where accurate quantification of the above metrics is desired.

Keywords: PET-CT; respiratory motion; SIRT; dosimetry; Yttrium 90

Citation: Walker, M.D.; Gear, J.I.; Craig, A.J.; McGowan, D.R. Effects of Respiratory Motion on Y-90 PET Dosimetry for SIRT. *Diagnostics* 2022, 12, 194. https://doi.org/10.3390/diagnostics12010194

Academic Editors: Lioe-Fee de Geus-Oei and F.H.P. van Velden

Received: 29 November 2021
Accepted: 10 January 2022
Published: 14 January 2022

Publisher's Note: MDPI stays neutral with regard to jurisdictional claims in published maps and institutional affiliations.

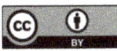

Copyright: © 2022 by the authors. Licensee MDPI, Basel, Switzerland. This article is an open access article distributed under the terms and conditions of the Creative Commons Attribution (CC BY) license (https://creativecommons.org/licenses/by/4.0/).

1. Introduction

Selective internal radiation therapy (SIRT) is a treatment option for patients with tumours in the liver that cannot be surgically resected. SIRT is most commonly used to treat liver metastases from colorectal cancer and hepatocellular carcinoma, and involves injection of ^{90}Y- or ^{166}Ho-microspheres into the hepatic arterial vasculature [1,2]. Although SIRT has been in clinical use for over 15 years, the benefits of this treatment remain unclear. A review of SIRT in randomized controlled trials found a lack of evidence for improved survival or quality of life for colorectal cancer patients with metastatic disease in the liver [3]. Investigations into the efficacy of SIRT have demonstrated the existence of a strong dose–response relationship [4–8]. Hence, a personalised, optimised approach ensuring adequate tumour-absorbed dose may be crucial to increase the efficacy of the technique and to allow demonstrable and significant treatment benefits.

SIRT dose-response studies generally use ^{90}Y PET imaging to provide estimates of tumour absorbed doses. Optimisation of the treatment, and dose verification, are hence reliant on accurate image-derived dosimetry [9]. Respiratory motion during the PET acquisition degrades the image quality. If left uncorrected, this leads to images with a blurring of the radioactivity distribution which will produce errors in dosimetry. In the case of SIRT, it is the motion of the liver that is of interest. This organ typically moves 10–26 mm cranio-caudally during normal respiration [10,11]. The purpose of the current investigation was to assess the effect of respiratory motion on tumour absorbed doses calculated from ^{90}Y PET images following SIRT, and to evaluate the benefits of respiratory motion correction for this application.

The probability of positron production during ^{90}Y decay is extremely low, making ^{90}Y a challenging radionuclide to image using PET [12]. Despite relatively high activities in the scanner's field of view (e.g., 0.5–3 GBq), the coincidence count-rate is low, hampering quantification. The quantitative accuracy of ^{90}Y PET in the absence of motion has been evaluated by several groups [13–16] including a multi-centre phantom evaluation [17]. The consistent findings are that modern time-of-flight (TOF) PET scanners provide accurate quantification of radioactivity concentrations in phantoms, subject to the expected errors arising from a limited spatial resolution. Simulations performed by Ausland et al. [18] predicted that the errors in tumour dose quantification caused by respiratory motion could be substantial. The effects of image noise, respiratory motion, and motion compensations for ^{90}Y SIRT have been considered by Siman et al. [19] who used short-duration images from the National Electrical Manufacturers Association (NEMA) International Electrotechnical Commission (IEC) body phantom, filled with ^{18}F, to mimic noisy ^{90}Y acquisitions. With no motion the quantification was found to be accurate, but large errors occurred when motion was applied (>50% for some dose measures), with these errors ameliorated by motion compensation (quiescent-period gating). Effects of respiratory motion have also been studied via simulation for pre-SIRT ^{99m}Tc MAA SPECT [20]. Siman et al. [19] suggested that further studies, using anthropomorphic phantoms, with ^{90}Y PET-CT studies, were needed to confirm the effectiveness of the motion compensation method. Our investigation addresses this by using clinically relevant activities of ^{90}Y within an anthropomorphic phantom specifically designed for evaluation of SIRT dosimetry [21]. The phantom was filled and imaged several times to provide a range of activities and contrast ratios. Furthermore, we acquired data on two time-of-flight PET scanners from different vendors, allowing interpretation of the results in a wider context as opposed to being scanner-/vendor-specific. Respiratory gating signals were obtained using external devices, as data driven respiratory gating in clinical use for ^{18}F and ^{68}Ga based PET [22,23] has yet to be robustly implemented for ^{90}Y PET [24].

2. Materials and Methods

2.1. Phantom Experiments

Experiments were performed on a Discovery D710 PET-CT scanner (GE; Milwaukee, WI, USA) and on a Biograph mCT (Siemens; Knoxville, TN, USA). The Abdo-Man^{TM} Phantom [21] was used as a test object throughout. This is a 3D-printed phantom of the abdomen, with a fillable liver compartment and fillable spherical inserts. The phantom was specifically designed to allow a SIRT-like radioactivity distribution to be generated within an object that mimics the lower-torso in terms of imaging characteristics (i.e., shape and density). Five inserts were placed within the liver region of the phantom, four of which were hollow fillable spheres of different diameter (10, 20, 30, 40 mm). The fifth insert was a 40 mm diameter sphere containing a 25 mm diameter solid inner sphere; this insert mimics the distribution of microspheres in the neovascular rim of a tumour that has a necrotic or poorly perfused core. Two of the spheres (the 40 mm with solid core, and the 20 mm diameter) were placed close to the superior end of the liver compartment. The 30 and 40 mm diameter spheres were close to the centre (in the superior-inferior direction) and the 10 mm diameter sphere was located near the inferior end of the compartment. All spheres were at least 10 mm from the boundaries of the liver compartment.

The phantom was filled with ^{90}Y on four different occasions for each scanner. Four different total activities were used for each scanner, in the range 0.7–3.2 GBq. The spheres were filled with radioactivity concentrations that were greater than the surrounding liver compartment. Two sphere-to-liver concentration ratios were tested, 4:1 and 8:1. The total activity, activity concentrations and concentration ratios were accurately measured during phantom filling, through use of accurate scales and dose calibrators with calibration factors for ^{90}Y that are traceable to the national standard.

The phantom was placed on the QUASAR^{TM} respiratory motion platform (Modus QA; London, ON, Canada), which was set to be either stationary or to move according to a typical respiratory waveform. The platform translated the phantom axially to simulate the cranio-caudal motion of the liver during respiration. The maximum displacement from the central position was set to be ±10 or ±15 mm. Data were hence acquired with maximum displacements between inhalation and exhalation of 0, 20 and 30 mm. The respiratory motion system includes a platform that moves vertically in-time with the axial displacement of the phantom. This platform allows attachment of external devices used for monitoring respiratory motion, from which respiratory gating signals are obtained. For data acquired on the Discovery D710, the Real-time Position Management™ (RPM) Respiratory Gating system (Varian Medical Systems; Palo Alto, CA, USA) was used to track the position of a marker that was placed on the chest-wall platform. The system uses an infrared video camera for this purpose. For acquisitions on the Biograph mCT, gating signals were provided by a pressure belt on the same platform (Anzai Medical Corp.; Tokyo, Japan).

Following a helical CT scan, PET data were acquired for 15 min at a single bed position which included all spherical inserts. This acquisition protocol matches our local acquisition protocol for post-SIRT verification imaging [25]. Additional PET datasets were acquired with the phantom in motion, with motion amplitudes of 10 mm and 15 mm. For acquisitions with 10 mm motion amplitude the duration was increased, when possible, to 45 min and the data processed into 3 × 15 min images. This provided additional data to increase the power of the study. The process was repeated at four phantom activities on both PET-CT scanners. The total number of 15 min duration sets of raw data was 32. Data were reconstructed to provide attenuation and scatter corrected PET images. Different image reconstruction algorithms were tested for the Discovery 710, one based on suggestions from the QUEST study [17] as optimal for quantitative ^{90}Y imaging, alongside a Bayesian penalized likelihood reconstruction. For the Discovery 710, the QUEST reconstruction was the manufacturer's 3D OSEM reconstruction (VPFX) including resolution recovery (SharpIR) and TOF data, with two iterations of 24 subsets, without any z-axis filtration and using a 256 × 256 matrix size (giving voxels of 2.7 × 2.7 × 3.3 mm^3). For the BPL (Q.Clear) reconstruction, a beta value of 1000 was used [25]. For the Biograph mCT, a local protocol was followed consisting of the manufacturer's 3D OSEM reconstruction (1 iteration, 21 subsets) including resolution recovery and time of flight (without post filtering). For the cases where motion was present, images were reconstructed with and without quiescent period respiratory gating (QPG) as implemented by the manufacturers, retaining approximately 50% of the acquired data within the quiescent phase [26]. For the Discovery 710, the gating is phase-based (Q.Static™), while for the Biograph mCT it is amplitude-based (HD•Chest™).

2.2. Image Analysis

The images were analysed at a single site using commercial software (Hybrid Viewer v5.1, Hermes Medical Solutions AB, Stockholm, Sweden). The quantitative accuracy of the data was first verified for the stationary phantom acquisitions. For each image, 7 spherical volumes of interest (VOI), each 2 cm in diameter, were placed within the (background) liver compartment. These regions were placed at least 1 cm from the walls of the compartment and the inserts and were expected to be free of partial volume effects. We hence expected the mean radioactivity concentrations to closely match the known activity concentration, as determined from radionuclide dose calibrator measurements during preparation of the phantom.

The effects of respiratory motion on dosimetric measures were assessed by investigating the accuracy of activity quantification for the spherical inserts. Spherical VOIs were placed on each of the inserts, with the VOI manually centred on the given sphere as observed in the PET image. The VOI diameters matched the inner diameters of the spheres. In the case of the sphere with a solid core, two VOIs were analysed: one pertaining to the hot outer shell (a 40 mm spherical VOI but with a central 25-mm diameter sphere excluded), and one 25 mm spherical VOI centred on the cold core. These VOIs were repeated with manual alignment on each image from the study, i.e., for the phantom stationary or moving, with or without motion compensation via respiratory gating. From the hot spheres, an activity concentration volume histogram (ACVH) was extracted alongside the VOI mean activity concentration (AC_{mean}). From these ACVHs, the dosimetric measure AC_{80} was extracted for summary analysis. AC_{80} is defined as the activity concentration threshold that incorporates 80% of voxels within the VOI. Although other thresholds can be used (e.g., AC_{50} as the median), we narrowed the current investigation to AC_{80} on the basis that we expect the mean or median dose to a tumour volume to have a weaker correlation with tumour response compared to AC_{80} [27], but higher thresholds such as AC_{90} to be more greatly affected by image noise. Results were converted to recovery percentages (i.e., the measured activity concentration as a percentage of the true activity concentration) to allow comparative analysis across the range of activity concentrations studied. The contrast recovery for the cold core was calculated as $Q_C = (1 - C_{core}/C_{shell}) \times 100\%$, where C_{core} is the VOI mean value of the cold core, and C_{shell} the VOI mean of the hot shell. Comparison of the results for the phantom in motion to those found with the phantom stationary, for the different sphere sizes, allowed the impact of respiratory motion and motion correction to be placed into perspective alongside the partial volume effect. Hence, the relative benefit of respiratory motion correction, in terms of impact on dosimetric measures, was assessed.

2.3. Statistical Analysis

The recovery coefficients from the four hot spherical inserts were used for a multiple linear regression analysis (IBM SPSS, v28) to determine which variables had a statistically significant impact on the measured recoveries. The impact of respiratory motion correction was further assessed by a paired, two-tailed t-test on the recovery coefficients from all inserts, comparing results from images with and without respiratory gating. The same test was applied to the AC_{80} values.

3. Results

The QUEST reconstruction for the Discovery 710 was found to be unsuitable for analyses at the voxel level and generation of an ACVH due to excessive noise. Hence, we focused our analysis on BPL images for this scanner.

The quantitative accuracy of the images determined from the background region in the stationary phantom acquisitions, expressed as the percentage recovery coefficient, was $100.0 \pm 7\%$ and $98.2 \pm 4\%$ (mean $\pm$ standard error) for the GE Discovery 710 (using BPL reconstruction) and the Siemens Biograph mCT, respectively. This verifies that the phantom filling and scanner calibrations were accurate for ^{90}Y. The quantification accuracy of the background region is presented in Figure 1.

A simple multi-linear model gave a reasonable fit to the recovery coefficients from the hot spheres, with the multiple correlation coefficient equalling 0.81 and the adjusted coefficient of determination being 0.65. The coefficients of the model were significantly different from zero for motion amplitude ($p < 0.001$) and motion correction (being on or off, $p = 0.003$). There was a dependence on the scanner ($p < 0.001$) and unsurprisingly on the sphere diameter ($p < 0.001$), the contrast ($p < 0.001$) and the phantom activity ($p < 0.001$). The model parameters confirmed an increased contrast recovery (+16% per cm) with increasing sphere diameter over the tested range of 1–4 cm. The application of 1–1.5 cm motion reduced the contrast (−11% per cm) which was partly compensated by motion correction being applied (+6.1% on average).

The paired-samples two-tailed t-test confirmed that the mean contrast recovery with quiescent period gating was significantly higher than without gating. For the Biograph mCT, the mean recovery coefficient, from all studies including motion and for all six VOI, was 55% without motion correction compared to 59% with respiratory gating ($p = 0.007$). For the Discovery 710, the corresponding values were 50% increasing to 55% with gating ($p = 0.003$). Similar findings were found when examining the AC_{80} values from the four hot spheres, where for the Biograph mCT the mean value of AC_{80} was 25% without motion correction compared to 29% with respiratory gating ($p < 0.001$). For the Discovery 710, the mean AC_{80} values were 23% and 29% for uncorrected motion and with respiratory gating respectively ($p < 0.001$).

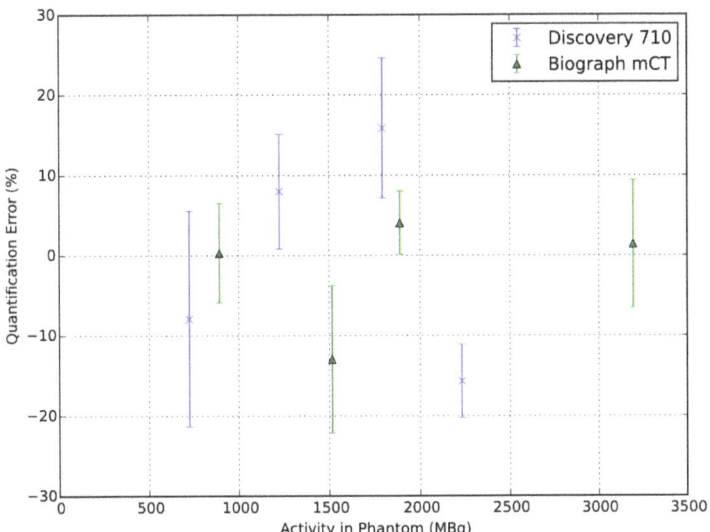

Figure 1. The quantification accuracy from the seven background regions in images from the Discovery 710 and Biograph mCT when the phantom was static. Error bars represent standard errors.

Example ^{90}Y PET images are shown in Figure 2, where the improvement in contrast provided by gating is apparent at the expense of increased noise.

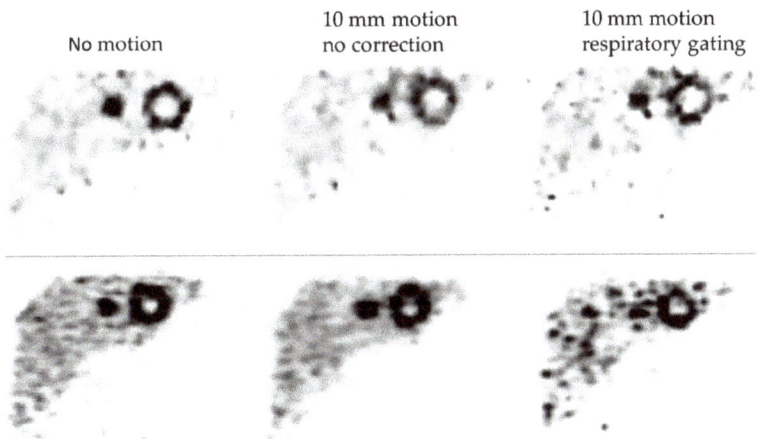

Figure 2. PET images (coronal slices) from the phantom with and without motion applied. The upper row of images is from the Discovery 710. The lower row is from the Biograph mCT. The grey scale maximum equals the true activity concentration in the hot spheres, with minimum at zero. The activity concentration ratio between the spheres and background was 8:1. For each scanner the images show a similar slice of the phantom while stationary, while in motion but without correction, and while in motion with quiescent period respiratory gating. The motion amplitude was 10 mm. The total activity in the phantom was 1.8 GBq for the Discovery and 1.9 GBq and Biograph. The slice contains the 40 mm insert with 25 mm cold core, as well as a 20 mm diameter sphere.

Averaged ACVHs are presented in Figure 3, for the case of the stationary and moving phantom with and without quiescent period gating. The recovery of the ^{90}Y activity within the spherical inserts is presented in Figure 4 for which data are grouped by scanner and contrast ratio, with the presented data being the average of the tests performed at similar contrast ratios. The impact from the partial-volume effect for the different spheres is provided by the no-motion data, which is seen alongside the results for respiratory motion and respiratory motion with gating. The AC_{80} values extracted from the ACVHs are similarly presented in Figure 5.

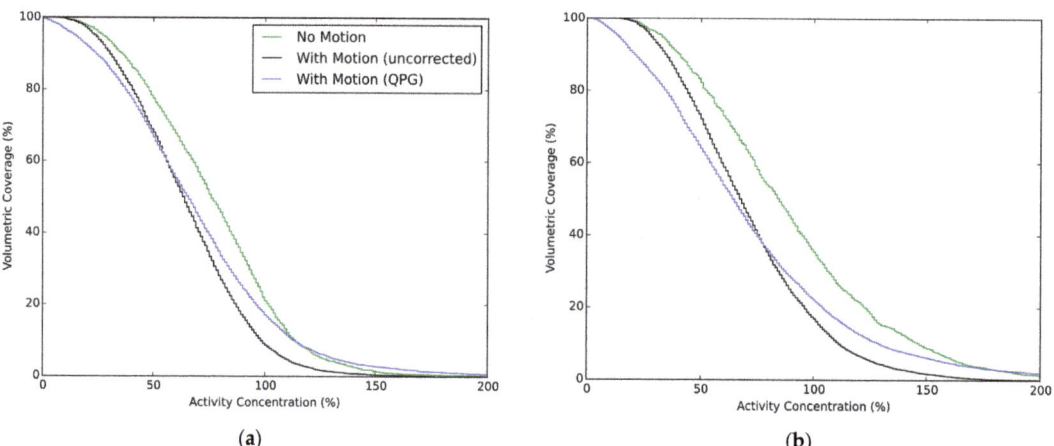

Figure 3. Activity concentration volume histograms for the 30 mm sphere. Each figure part shows the results for no motion, and when motion is present (10–15 mm amplitudes) either with or without quiescent period gating. Data are presented as the average ACVH for this sphere from the four phantom experiments on each scanner. (**a**) Discovery 710 (BPL reconstruction); (**b**) Biograph mCT.

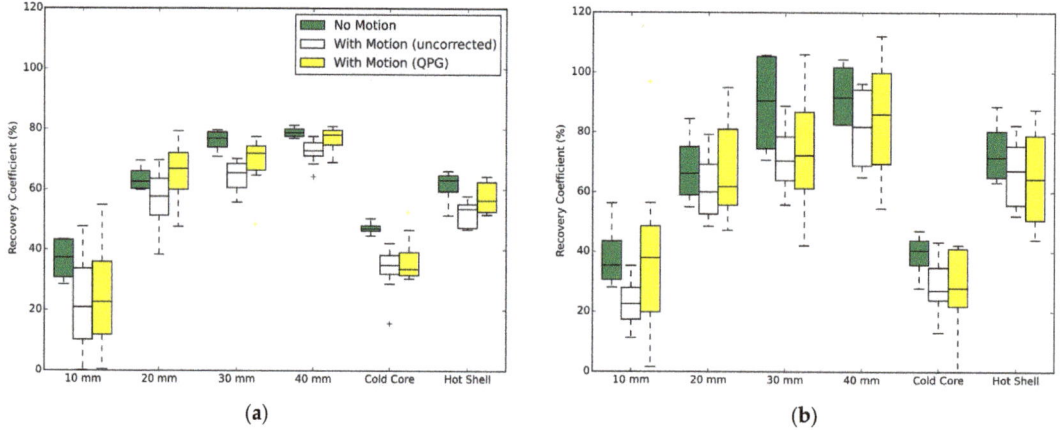

Figure 4. Contrast recoveries for different sphere diameters and types. Each figure part shows the results for no motion, and when motion is present (10–15 mm amplitudes) either with or without quiescent period gating. Combined datasets from four phantom experiments on each scanner. (**a**) Discovery 710 (BPL reconstruction); (**b**) Biograph mCT.

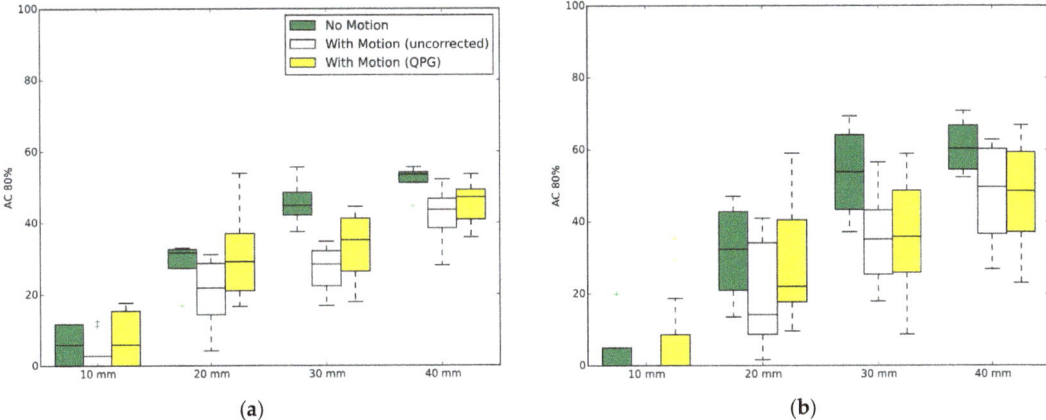

Figure 5. AC_{80} from different sphere diameters. Each figure part shows the results for no motion, and when motion is present (10–15 mm amplitudes) either with or without quiescent period gating. Combined datasets from four phantom experiments on each scanner. (**a**) Discovery 710 (BPL reconstruction); (**b**) Biograph mCT.

4. Discussion

Using an anthropomorphic phantom filled with ^{90}Y at clinically relevant activities placed on a respiratory motion platform, this investigation found that quiescent period respiratory gating leads to increased accuracy in measures of the activity concentration in both hot and cold features within a liver region. The study provided consistent results across a range of clinically relevant activities and at two contrast ratios, for two PET-CT scanners from different vendors. Our findings agree with expectations based on results from Siman et al. [19] who performed experiments using a less realistic phantom filled with a small amount of ^{18}F on a single scanner. Although we found statistically significant increases in quantification accuracy, we note the data had high variance and the absolute gains from the application of quiescent period gating were moderate. The impact of the partial volume effect, seen by the difference in quantitative measures between smaller and larger spheres, was generally larger than the impact of applying the respiratory motion correction for the features analysed in this study (diameters ranging from 1 to 4 cm). This can be seen visually in Figures 4 and 5 but was also evidenced by the coefficients of the multi-linear regression. A decrease in sphere diameter of 1 cm led to a larger decrease in contrast recovery (−16%) compared to respiratory motion of 1 cm amplitude (−11% and −5% for uncorrected data and for quiescent period gating, respectively).

In this study, and in agreement with Hou et al. [16], we noted that the QUEST reconstruction for the Discovery 710 was not suitable for a voxel-level analyses. We considered images with relatively high noise to be unsuitable for estimation of the distribution of activity concentrations within a region. This reconstruction should hence not be used when a dose-volume histogram analysis is to be performed. The quantitative accuracy of the QUEST reconstruction was, however, acceptable when assessed using the background region in the stationary phantom acquisitions, with a percentage recovery coefficient of $104 \pm 8\%$. As the QUEST images from the Discovery 710 were too noisy to be subjected to ACVH analysis our work focused on the BPL images for this scanner. A limitation of our study is that we only studied images with $\beta = 1000$ as chosen based on previous investigations [25]. In the case of a voxel level analysis aiming for accurate estimation of the distribution of activity concentrations (for accurate DVH generation), high β values that provide smoother images may be optimal [16]. Furthermore, our study investigated only one method of respiratory motion correction (device-driven quiescent period gating) without optimisation of the retained fraction, which was set at 50%. This method of correction was chosen due to the relative simplicity and wide availability of the technique. The aim of our study was, however, not to optimise imaging parameters, but to demonstrate the extent to which respiratory motion degrades quantification accuracy, and the extent to which commonly used quiescent period gating can mitigate these effects. In this regard, our study shows that respiratory gating can be beneficial. Despite reducing the statistical quality of the images when discarding 50% of the coincidences, the application of gating was of net benefit with more accurate quantification of both VOI means and dosimetric measures such as AC_{80}. However, we recognise the need for further investigations; for example, it would be useful from a practical point of view to define a minimum signal-to-noise ratio for the image (at the voxel level), below which the application of voxel-level dosimetric measures are not advised. Further development of methods for robust respiratory gating with retention of all (or most) counts in the case of ^{90}Y PET is also needed. This is an ongoing area of research for ^{18}F PET-CT imaging and the extension of methods, many of which use image registrations or other data-led techniques, to the case of low-count ^{90}Y PET presents a variety of challenges. Without such techniques the justification for respiratory gating is tempered by the increase in image noise and the detrimental impact this has on voxel-level, DVH-type analyses. Increased smoothing or regularization of the image reconstruction (e.g., by increasing the β value in BPL) could compensate for the increased noise but at the expense of reducing spatial resolution. Although ^{90}Y PET is challenging, we note that the current study did not utilise the most recent generation of long axial FOV, SiPM-based PET scanners. These offer significantly increased sensitivity through their extended axial coverage and reduced noise through improved time-of-flight capabilities, both of which make the newer scanners more suitable for gated ^{90}Y PET. The image quality for gated studies is also expected to improve if higher activities are present in the scanner's FOV. This study investigated the range of activities encountered at both sites (up to 3.2 GBq).

The use of respiratory gating is becoming more common, and it is noteworthy that in this patient population the additional radiation dose from a respiratory gated CT is likely justified given the poor prognosis of patients referred for SIRT. While data-driven respiratory gating methods for both ^{90}Y PET and CT are yet to be robustly implemented in clinical practice, it may be appropriate to perform device-based gating of both the PET and the CT components of post-SIRT therapy PET-CT verification imaging. Accurate alignment of CT and PET images within the quiescent phase has been shown to be important for quantification using ^{18}F and ^{68}Ga PET-CT [28], and this is expected to apply equally to ^{90}Y imaging.

As evidence mounts for a strong relationship between tumour dose and treatment response, the need for accurate dosimetry in SIRT also increases. While accurate dose estimation from pre-therapy imaging can be used to optimise treatment, post-therapy dosimetry can be used to verify the delivered dose and thus build the evidence base for the dose-response, allowing the treatment to be refined and to unravel the disease- and patient-related factors that may alter the dose thresholds for effective treatment.

5. Conclusions

Results from anthropomorphic phantom studies suggest that post-therapy SIRT PET-CT imaging is improved by quiescent period respiratory motion correction. Specifically, improved accuracy of tumour quantification and dosimetric measures are predicted.

Author Contributions: Conceptualization, M.D.W. and D.R.M.; methodology, M.D.W. and D.R.M.; investigation, M.D.W., J.I.G. and A.J.C.; writing—original draft preparation, M.D.W.; writing—review and editing, M.D.W., J.I.G., A.J.C. and D.R.M.; funding acquisition, D.R.M. All authors have read and agreed to the published version of the manuscript.

Funding: This research received no external funding. The APC was funded by Oxford University Hospitals NHS Foundation Trust.

Institutional Review Board Statement: Not applicable.

Informed Consent Statement: Not applicable.

Data Availability Statement: The data presented in this study are available on request from the corresponding author.

Acknowledgments: The radionuclides used for this research were provided by Sirtex, and the Abdo-man phantom was loaned from the Royal Marsden NHS Foundation Trust and Institute of Cancer Research.

Conflicts of Interest: The authors declare no conflict of interest.

References

1. Salem, R.; Thurston, K.G. Radioembolization with 90Yttrium Microspheres: A State-of-the-Art Brachytherapy Treatment for Primary and Secondary Liver Malignancies. Part 1: Technical and Methodologic Considerations. *J. Vasc. Interv. Radiol. JVIR* **2006**, *17*, 1251–1278. [CrossRef]
2. Coldwell, D.; Sangro, B.; Salem, R.; Wasan, H.; Kennedy, A. Radioembolization in the Treatment of Unresectable Liver Tumors: Experience across a Range of Primary Cancers. *Am. J. Clin. Oncol.* **2012**, *35*, 167–177. [CrossRef] [PubMed]
3. Townsend, A.R.; Chong, L.C.; Karapetis, C.; Price, T.J. Selective Internal Radiation Therapy for Liver Metastases from Colorectal Cancer. *Cancer Treat. Rev.* **2016**, *50*, 148–154. [CrossRef] [PubMed]
4. van den Hoven, A.F.; Rosenbaum, C.E.N.M.; Elias, S.G.; de Jong, H.W.A.M.; Koopman, M.; Verkooijen, H.M.; Alavi, A.; van den Bosch, M.A.A.J.; Lam, M.G.E.H. Insights into the Dose-Response Relationship of Radioembolization with Resin 90Y-Microspheres: A Prospective Cohort Study in Patients with Colorectal Cancer Liver Metastases. *J. Nucl. Med.* **2016**, *57*, 1014–1019. [CrossRef]
5. Fowler, K.J.; Maughan, N.M.; Laforest, R.; Saad, N.E.; Sharma, A.; Olsen, J.; Speirs, C.K.; Parikh, P.J. PET/MRI of Hepatic 90Y Microsphere Deposition Determines Individual Tumor Response. *Cardiovasc. Interv. Radiol.* **2016**, *39*, 855–864. [CrossRef]
6. Kao, Y.-H.; Steinberg, J.D.; Tay, Y.-S.; Lim, G.K.; Yan, J.; Townsend, D.W.; Budgeon, C.A.; Boucek, J.A.; Francis, R.J.; Cheo, T.S.; et al. Post-Radioembolization Yttrium-90 PET/CT—Part 2: Dose-Response and Tumor Predictive Dosimetry for Resin Microspheres. *EJNMMI Res.* **2013**, *3*, 57. [CrossRef] [PubMed]
7. Alsultan, A.A.; van Roekel, C.; Barentsz, M.W.; Smits, M.L.J.; Kunnen, B.; Koopman, M.; Braat, A.J.A.T.; Bruijnen, R.C.G.; de Keizer, B.; Lam, M.G.E.H. Dose-Response and Dose-Toxicity Relationships for Glass 90Y Radioembolization in Patients with Liver Metastases from Colorectal Cancer. *J. Nucl. Med.* **2021**, *62*, 1616–1623. [CrossRef]
8. Garin, E.; Tselikas, L.; Guiu, B.; Chalaye, J.; Edeline, J.; de Baere, T.; Assenat, E.; Tacher, V.; Robert, C.; Terroir-Cassou-Mounat, M.; et al. Personalised versus Standard Dosimetry Approach of Selective Internal Radiation Therapy in Patients with Locally Advanced Hepatocellular Carcinoma (DOSISPHERE-01): A Randomised, Multicentre, Open-Label Phase 2 Trial. *Lancet Gastroenterol. Hepatol.* **2021**, *6*, 17–29. [CrossRef]
9. Lea, W.B.; Tapp, K.N.; Tann, M.; Hutchins, G.D.; Fletcher, J.W.; Johnson, M.S. Microsphere Localization and Dose Quantification Using Positron Emission Tomography/CT Following Hepatic Intraarterial Radioembolization with Yttrium-90 in Patients with Advanced Hepatocellular Carcinoma. *J. Vasc. Interv. Radiol.* **2014**, *25*, 1595–1603. [CrossRef]
10. Balter, J.M.; Ten Haken, R.K.; Lawrence, T.S.; Lam, K.L.; Robertson, J.M. Uncertainties in CT-Based Radiation Therapy Treatment Planning Associated with Patient Breathing. *Int. J. Radiat. Oncol. Biol. Phys.* **1996**, *36*, 167–174. [CrossRef]
11. Clifford, M.A.; Banovac, F.; Levy, E.; Cleary, K. Assessment of Hepatic Motion Secondary to Respiration for Computer Assisted Interventions. *Comput. Aided Surg.* **2002**, *7*, 291–299. [CrossRef] [PubMed]
12. D'Arienzo, M. Emission of B+ Particles Via Internal Pair Production in the 0+–0+ Transition of 90Zr: Historical Background and Current Applications in Nuclear Medicine Imaging. *Atoms* **2013**, *1*, 2–12. [CrossRef]
13. van Elmpt, W.; Hamill, J.; Jones, J.; De Ruysscher, D.; Lambin, P.; Ollers, M. Optimal Gating Compared to 3D and 4D PET Reconstruction for Characterization of Lung Tumours. *Eur. J. Nucl. Med. Mol. Imaging* **2011**, *38*, 843–855. [CrossRef]
14. Carlier, T.; Willowson, K.P.; Fourkal, E.; Bailey, D.L.; Doss, M.; Conti, M. (90)Y-PET Imaging: Exploring Limitations and Accuracy under Conditions of Low Counts and High Random Fraction. *Med. Phys.* **2015**, *42*, 4295–4309. [CrossRef] [PubMed]
15. Rowley, L.M.; Bradley, K.M.; Boardman, P.; Hallam, A.; McGowan, D.R. Optimization of Image Reconstruction for 90Y Selective Internal Radiotherapy on a Lutetium Yttrium Orthosilicate PET/CT System Using a Bayesian Penalized Likelihood Reconstruction Algorithm. *J. Nucl. Med.* **2017**, *58*, 658–664. [CrossRef]
16. Hou, X.; Ma, H.; Esquinas, P.L.; Uribe, C.; Tolhurst, S.; Bénard, F.; Liu, D.; Rahmim, A.; Celler, A. Impact of Image Reconstruction Method on Dose Distributions Derived from 90Y PET Images: Phantom and Liver Radioembolization Patient Studies. *Phys. Med. Biol.* **2020**, *65*, 215022. [CrossRef] [PubMed]
17. Willowson, K.P.; Tapner, M.; QUEST Investigator Team; Bailey, D.L. A Multicentre Comparison of Quantitative (90)Y PET/CT for Dosimetric Purposes after Radioembolization with Resin Microspheres: The QUEST Phantom Study. *Eur. J. Nucl. Med. Mol. Imaging* **2015**, *42*, 1202–1222. [CrossRef] [PubMed]
18. Ausland, L.; Revheim, M.-E.; Skretting, A.; Stokke, C. Respiratory Motion during 90Yttrium PET Contributes to Underestimation of Tumor Dose and Overestimation of Normal Liver Tissue Dose. *Acta Radiol.* **2018**, *59*, 132–139. [CrossRef]
19. Siman, W.; Mawlawi, O.R.; Mikell, J.K.; Mourtada, F.; Kappadath, S.C. Effects of Image Noise, Respiratory Motion, and Motion Compensation on 3D Activity Quantification in Count-Limited PET Images. *Phys. Med. Biol.* **2017**, *62*, 448–464. [CrossRef]

20. Bastiaannet, R.; Viergever, M.A.; Jong, H.W.A.M. de Impact of Respiratory Motion and Acquisition Settings on SPECT Liver Dosimetry for Radioembolization. *Med. Phys.* **2017**, *44*, 5270–5279. [CrossRef]
21. Gear, J.I.; Cummings, C.; Craig, A.J.; Divoli, A.; Long, C.D.C.; Tapner, M.; Flux, G.D. Abdo-Man: A 3D-Printed Anthropomorphic Phantom for Validating Quantitative SIRT. *EJNMMI Phys.* **2016**, *3*, 17. [CrossRef]
22. Kesner, A.L.; Chung, J.H.; Lind, K.E.; Kwak, J.J.; Lynch, D.; Burckhardt, D.; Koo, P.J. Validation of Software Gating: A Practical Technology for Respiratory Motion Correction in PET. *Radiology* **2016**, *281*, 239–248. [CrossRef] [PubMed]
23. Walker, M.D.; Morgan, A.J.; Bradley, K.M.; McGowan, D.R. Data-Driven Respiratory Gating Outperforms Device-Based Gating for Clinical 18F-FDG PET/CT. *J. Nucl. Med.* **2020**, *61*, 1678–1683. [CrossRef]
24. Chiesa, C.; Sjogreen-Gleisner, K.; Walrand, S.; Strigari, L.; Flux, G.; Gear, J.; Stokke, C.; Gabina, P.M.; Bernhardt, P.; Konijnenberg, M. EANM Dosimetry Committee Series on Standard Operational Procedures: A Unified Methodology for 99mTc-MAA Pre- and 90Y Peri-Therapy Dosimetry in Liver Radioembolization with 90Y Microspheres. *EJNMMI Phys.* **2021**, *8*, 77. [CrossRef]
25. Scott, N.P.; McGowan, D.R. Optimising Quantitative 90Y PET Imaging: An Investigation into the Effects of Scan Length and Bayesian Penalised Likelihood Reconstruction. *EJNMMI Res.* **2019**, *9*, 40. [CrossRef] [PubMed]
26. Liu, C.; Alessio, A.; Pierce, L.; Thielemans, K.; Wollenweber, S.; Ganin, A.; Kinahan, P. Quiescent Period Respiratory Gating for PET/CT. *Med. Phys.* **2010**, *37*, 5037–5043. [CrossRef] [PubMed]
27. Dewaraja, Y.K.; Schipper, M.J.; Roberson, P.L.; Wilderman, S.J.; Amro, H.; Regan, D.D.; Koral, K.F.; Kaminski, M.S.; Avram, A.M. 131I-Tositumomab Radioimmunotherapy: Initial Tumor Dose-Response Results Using 3-Dimensional Dosimetry Including Radiobiologic Modeling. *J. Nucl. Med.* **2010**, *51*, 1155–1162. [CrossRef]
28. Thomas, M.A.; Pan, T. Data-Driven Gated PET/CT: Implications for Lesion Segmentation and Quantitation. *EJNMMI Phys.* **2021**, *8*, 64. [CrossRef]

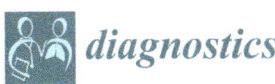

Review

Absolute Quantification in Diagnostic SPECT/CT: The Phantom Premise

Stijn De Schepper [1,2,*], Gopinath Gnanasegaran [3], John C. Dickson [4] and Tim Van den Wyngaert [1,2]

1. Department of Nuclear Medicine, Antwerp University Hospital, 2650 Edegem, Belgium; tim.vandenwyngaert@uza.be
2. Faculty of Medicine and Health Sciences (MICA—IPPON), University of Antwerp, 2610 Wilrijk, Belgium
3. Department of Nuclear Medicine, Royal Free London NHS, London NW3 2QG, UK; gopinath.gnanasegaran@nhs.net
4. Institute of Nuclear Medicine, University College of London Hospitals NHS, London NW1 2BU, UK; john.dickson2@nhs.net
* Correspondence: stijn.deschepper@uza.be

Abstract: The application of absolute quantification in SPECT/CT has seen increased interest in the context of radionuclide therapies where patient-specific dosimetry is a requirement within the European Union (EU) legislation. However, the translation of this technique to diagnostic nuclear medicine outside this setting is rather slow. Clinical research has, in some examples, already shown an association between imaging metrics and clinical diagnosis, but the applications, in general, lack proper validation because of the absence of a ground truth measurement. Meanwhile, additive manufacturing or 3D printing has seen rapid improvements, increasing its uptake in medical imaging. Three-dimensional printed phantoms have already made a significant impact on quantitative imaging, a trend that is likely to increase in the future. In this review, we summarize the data of recent literature to underpin our premise that the validation of diagnostic applications in nuclear medicine using application-specific phantoms is within reach given the current state-of-the-art in additive manufacturing or 3D printing.

Keywords: absolute quantification; SPECT/CT; phantoms; diagnostics; 3D printing

1. Introduction

From the moment radioactivity was discovered by Henri Becquerel in 1896, there was an immediate interest in quantification arising from the need to study this phenomenon. After more than a century, this interest in measuring and quantifying radioactivity is more relevant than ever within the context of SPECT/CT technology in nuclear medicine. The past two decades have seen the continuous improvement of SPECT/CT as a molecular imaging modality to a point where it can produce accurate quantitative images [1–3]. The technical advances leading to this improved accuracy have been extensively reviewed before [4,5].

Recent research on absolute quantification has primarily focused on applications related to theranostics or radionuclide therapy [6–10] and dosimetry [11–17]. Next to its use in the therapeutic setting, accurate quantification of tracer uptake could become highly relevant, providing diagnostic information beyond just the absence or presence of disease. Until now, relative quantification and comparisons against a database have dominated quantitative applications of SPECT/CT in diagnostic studies. However, while the quantitative capability of SPECT/CT as a modality is without doubt and several potential applications have already been suggested at the beginning of the previous decade [18], there is still limited use in clinical practice.

The results from a survey on the use of quantitative SPECT in the UK in 2019 show that quantitative SPECT/CT has not yet broken through in clinical practice [19]. Approximately two-thirds (67%) of responders indicated not using absolute quantification or a semiquantitative standardized uptake value (SUV). The main focus of those who do use absolute quantification is radionuclide therapy, predominantly for thyroid conditions and neuroendocrine tumors. While most respondents indicated using quantitative images only for therapy, 43% indicated having a calibration for ^{99m}Tc. When asked what the main impediment is for quantitative SPECT, 35% questioned the benefit, and 23% indicated a lack of transferability across sites and platforms. Clearly, several challenges, including clinical validation and transferability, continue to hamper the use of absolute quantification for diagnostic purposes.

Three-dimensional printing or additive manufacturing is a technique where a structure is built layer by layer, and each new layer is deposited on the previous layer [20]. Also called rapid prototyping, it was initially developed for making scale models of a prototype, which at that time were still developed by skilled craftsmen based on 2D drawings. The printers use a 3D drawing which it subdivides into the individual layers to be constructed. There is a large flexibility in methods and materials that are used for printing. Fused deposition modeling (FDM) and stereolithography (SLA) are among the most popular commercial 3D printing technologies. A wide variety of materials can be used to print, from metals like aluminum to polymers such as poly(methyl methacrylate) (PMMA). In recent years, improvements in 3D printing technology have decreased the cost while increasing the speed with which the prints are produced. This allows for efficient prototyping and iterative designs where improvements to the model are introduced with each iteration. The high quality in printing technology is reflected in the homogeneity within prints and the reproducibility of the prints. The availability of the technology combined with its reproducibility has the added benefit that phantoms can be reproduced at different sites rather than having to send a phantom from one site to the other for multicentre studies. These favorable properties have increased the interest in 3D printing for a wide variety of applications, including anthropomorphic phantoms for medical imaging [21]. In this narrative review, we summarize the available applications reported in the literature, focusing on the potential of innovative models or phantoms to improve the clinical uptake of this technology. We will show that these applications of 3D printing have already shown they can fulfill the need for application-specific anthropomorphic phantoms. These phantoms have already had a significant impact on our understanding of the physical effects that can potentially lower the accuracy of quantitative SPECT/CT imaging. It is our premise that they will further increase our understanding and allow for optimization of application-specific protocols.

2. Understanding the Need for Quantification

The concept of theranostics in nuclear medicine is well-established and increasingly successful, especially with the introduction of ^{177}Lu-based therapies [7,8,10]. Undeniably, the measurement of the absolute activity in this context is a requirement for accurate dose calculation, as these start from the number of nuclei decaying in a region of interest. Afterward, the decay energy and range of the emitted particles are used to calculate the absorbed dose. Establishing a dose-effect relationship for a given radionuclide therapy allows for a personalized therapy plan more closely resembling external beam radiotherapy. Moreover, such dosimetry calculation after radionuclide therapy has also become a legal requirement in the European Union (EU) under the Basic Safety Standard (Council Directive 2013/59/Euratom of 5 December 2013).

The use of absolute quantification in diagnostic applications is perhaps less of a requirement than in therapeutic uses. Today, uptake ratios and reference databases are routinely used, with applications in cardiac amyloidosis [22], temporomandibular joint growth [23], dopaminergic function [24], and renal function [25]. More (semi)quantitative metrics have also been popularized, of which the standardized uptake value (SUV) has been the most popular. There are several variants of SUV, but in essence, they represent a normalization of the activity in a region-of-interest by dividing the injected activity by some patient metric of distribution volume, such as body mass. There are several diagnostic applications where an increased tracer uptake is correlated with the presence or severity of the disease. Multiple authors have investigated the link between the uptake of ^{99m}Tc-labeled bone-seeking agents and whether a bone lesion is benign or malignant [26–29]. In cardiac imaging, the uptake of a ^{99m}Tc-labeled bone-seeking agent has been shown to correlate with current clinical standard quantitative measures for amyloid burden in cardiac amyloidosis, therapy response, extracellular volume as measured on NMR, and left ventricular mass index, as measured on echocardiography [30]. Together, these preliminary applications illustrate that further progress in absolute quantification in diagnostic applications can significantly increase the value of these imaging studies as a truly quantitative biomarker of disease severity, patient outcomes, or predictor of treatment response.

3. Requirements for Absolute Quantification

Accuracy and reproducibility are essential for applying absolute quantification in diagnostic medicine, which depend on technical and physical processes but also on the patient's biology and physiology. Mirroring the considerable efforts over the last decades to improve our understanding of the biological and technological factors influencing the SUV in PET imaging [31–33] and the need for standardization [34], SPECT/CT has seen similar progress, even though a number of challenges remain.

The major physical processes challenging the accuracy and reproducibility for diagnostic applications are photon attenuation and scatter and the limited spatial resolution of SPECT/CT cameras. Bone structures or metallic implants will strongly affect the image produced due to their increased density. The limited spatial resolution is caused by the collimator and the detector not being perfect systems. Many structures in the human body are very small or have an irregular shape, and depending on the application, corrections for this phenomenon need to be considered. However, while many techniques have been reported, few methods, if any, are available for routine clinical use [35].

Apart from the physical processes, the technical parameters related to image reconstruction should be optimized to guarantee sufficient accuracy and reproducibility for a given application. Different vendors use different proprietary reconstruction and correction algorithms, including, but not limited to attenuation correction [36], scatter correction [37], collimator modelling [38], and resolution modelling [35]. The parameters of these algorithms need to be validated and standardized to result in accurate and reproducible (semi)quantitative metrics.

Finally, the biokinetics of the tracer being studied can impact quantification as well. For example, variations in the clearance of activity from the background can occur (e.g., depending on renal function), and tracers may demonstrate variable washout from the target over time, influencing the estimation of uptake in a target lesion. In theory, each patient is ideally scanned multiple times to establish a time–activity curve from which the tracer kinetics can be derived, providing information on the biokinetics depending on patient biology and physiology. While some suggestions have been made for multiple time-point imaging in diagnostics [39,40], generally, only one image at a fixed time-point is available in the clinical routine. In practice, the choice of imaging time-points is usually informed by the population biokinetics of the tracer of interest [24,41–44] to minimize the biological variability and increase reproducibility [45,46].

4. From Feasibility Study to Clinical Practice

There are several lessons to be learned from the experience with PET/CT when translating feasibility studies to clinical practice. The biological variance in biokinetics and technical variance have to be well-controlled to standardize the acquisition and analysis. In SPECT, contrary to PET, only a minimum incubation period after injection is usually considered, and there is no standardization in the incubation window after injection. In bone scintigraphy, a minimum of 2 h of incubation is recommended according to the EANM guideline [42], while in the FDG PET guideline from EANM, a recommendation of imaging 55 min to 75 min post-injection is made [41]. There is currently a large variety of technology available, ranging from analog planar NaI-crystal cameras to digital circular geometry solid-state cadmium-zinc-telluride (CZT) designs. These technologies differ in sensitivity, energy resolution, spatial resolution [47,48]. Therefore, results from quantitative analysis can differ significantly, and it is difficult to translate from one technology to another.

Considerable efforts have been made to progress towards more standardization in SPECT/CT imaging. Several initiatives have attempted to extend the approach from the EARL program for FDG PET/CT [49] to SPECT/CT [11,13,47], its main advantage being the large availability of the specific phantoms within the nuclear medicine community: a cylinder with a volume of 5–7 L and the NEMA IEC phantom. First, a cross-calibration is performed using the cylinder. The cylinder is filled with a known volume of water and known activity measured in a radionuclide calibrator. The activity concentration as recovered in the SPECT/CT is compared to the known activity concentration by dividing the known volume of the cylinder and the known activity from the radionuclide calibrator measurement. The use of a large cylinder allows for a measurement without boundary interactions and related partial volume effects. Second, the NEMA IEC phantom consists of a large volume, considered as background, with spherical inserts of different sizes, considered the volumes-of-interest (VOIs). The spheres are filled with a different activity concentration than the background region. The activity concentration as recovered in the SPECT/CT is again compared to the known activity concentration. Through the partial volume effect, the activity in the spheres will deviate more for the smaller than the larger spheres. The recovery coefficients will also deviate as a function of contrast between spheres and background, as spill-in and spill-out will present differently. In general, lower contrast will result in lower recovery of the activity in the smaller spheres [50].

The translation of diagnostic SPECT/CT applications in cardiac amyloidosis or bone growth across different technologies is also hampered by a lack of validation. While it makes sense in oncological applications, such as FDG PET/CT, to use the activity recovered in a hot or cold sphere in a background volume as validation, this is not necessarily the case for applications with very different geometry. Considering the uptake of ^{99m}Tc-labeled bone-seeking agents in the myocardium, the challenges for accurate quantification are very different. The myocardium differs from a spherical shape, and there is a large volume of background activity adjacent to it. The partial volume effect (PVE) will differ when measured on cameras with different spatial resolutions or different reconstruction algorithms. Depending on the situation, there might be spill-in from the hot background into the colder VOI or spill-out from the hot VOI into the colder background affecting the results and the clinical translation.

Validation of the absolute activity concentration requires verification of the measured activity concentration. Except for the bladder, where the activity concentration in the urine can be measured afterward, such in vivo verification is most often impossible in humans [51]. Therefore, a reasonable alternative is the development of application-specific phantoms.

5. Phantoms in Nuclear Medicine

From the onset of nuclear imaging [52] and emission computed tomography [53], phantoms have been used to test image properties and imaging techniques. The quest for possible clinical applications required validation of the technology, and phantoms could provide such solid foundation. Phantoms are designed to reflect the situation under study as closely as possible, such as a cylinder with a sleeve of activity and two different-sized spherical inserts to investigate lesion contrast in brain imaging [53].

Ideally, phantoms should mimic our patients as closely as possible, a quality referred to as anthropomorphism. The most relevant properties for nuclear medicine are photon–matter interaction, and geometry and activity distribution. Fortunately, humans mostly consist of water, which is reflected in the photon attenuation coefficient of human tissue. Water and plastics, such as PMMA, which have similar attenuation coefficients, are popular materials for soft tissue applications. However, geometry is essential as patients or study populations can have very different anatomies. An obvious example is children versus adults, but also between adults in, for example, patients with very different BMI, or the density of healthy bone versus osteoporotic bone, which influences attenuation. Different pathologies and tracers can also have a very different tracer distribution in the same organ of interest. For example, a tracer for myocardial perfusion will have different kinetics and distribution than a bone-seeking agent repurposed for cardiac amyloidosis.

Several commercial phantoms are available for a human torso [54,55], spine [56], and brain [57]. These phantoms are realistic and can be used to measure the recovered activity concentration in the relevant regions. They are, however, limited to whole organ volumes, but pathology does not necessarily affect the entire organ. For example, cardiac amyloidosis deposition can be heterogeneous in the cardiac wall [58]. In that case, amyloid deposits should show as hot spots within the cardiac wall. It is immediately apparent that validation of absolute quantification for this application requires a more pathology-specific approach, and the limited number of commercially available anthropomorphic phantoms may not necessarily be appropriate for all applications. An anthropomorphic phantom has the potential to take the specific anatomical situation into account, including the depth at which the region of interest lies within the patient, but can also take almost any type of material into account. We can imagine bone structures near the region of interest or self-attenuation when bony structures are the region of interest. While water has roughly the density of soft tissue, it can be made more dense and equivalent to different types of bone by adding K_2HPO_4 to accommodate these requirements [59]. For tissue types with lower density than water, this is more difficult. The activity in the lungs is contained in water, while they are mostly filled with air. This duality presents a challenge for anthropomorphic lung phantom production, as it is difficult to reduce the density of water to that of air. A 3D-printed anthropomorphic phantom will provide with the previously mentioned exception an anatomically realistic representation, and allow for flexibility in scanning conditions and experimental designs by varying filling fluids to measure the impact of nearby material on attenuation and scatter.

Designing a phantom has long been cumbersome and expensive. Their complex shapes require a sufficient level of detail and the flexibility to adapt the phantom for a different patient or cohort while not sacrificing production speed or increasing cost. Additive manufacturing or 3D printing is a technique that can achieve this. A summary of several properties making 3D printing an attractive technique for phantom production, as well as an example of such a printed shape are shown in Figure 1 This technique has been widely applied to produce patient-specific implants and is starting to make its way into medical imaging.

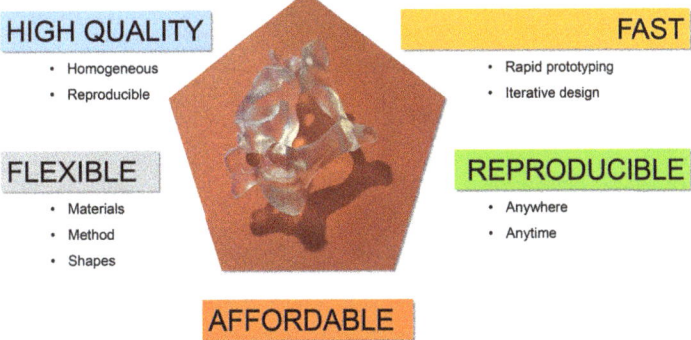

Figure 1. Summary of some properties that make 3D printing suitable for anthropomorphic phantom production. In the centre is a 3D-printed model of a cervical vertebra (C3). You can appreciate the level of detail in the processus spinosus, the processus transversus and the foramen transversarium, for example.

6. 3D-Printed Phantoms: A New Hope?

Recent technological progress has drastically lowered the cost and infrastructure needs for 3D printing, spreading its use in applied research, including nuclear medicine. In the case of phantom production, this allows more simplified development of purpose-specific phantoms. This technology makes it possible to produce almost any shape conceivable with relative ease. Several studies using 3D-printed phantoms in nuclear medicine have recently been published Table 1 for applications in the following anatomical regions: the abdomen [60–62], pancreas and kidneys [63], kidneys [64,65], brain [66–68], head and neck [69], systolic and diastolic heart [70], lungs [71], and patient-derived lesion shapes [11]. With current technology, anthropomorphic phantoms can be 3D-printed with a precision in the μm-range, well beyond the sub-millimeter resolution of CT or MRI used to develop these anatomical models.

Table 1. Summary of all articles and phantoms included in this review. SLA = stereolitography, FDM = Fused Deposition Modelling, CNR = contrast-to-noise ratio, RC = recovery coefficient, CF = calibration factors, LVEF = left ventricular ejection fraction.

Author	Region	Method	Evaluation	Isotopes
Iida et al., 2013 [66]	Brain	SLA	Visual	^{18}F, ^{99m}Tc, ^{123}I
Gear et al., 2014 [62]	Abdomen (liver, spleen, kidneys)	SLA	Visual	^{18}F, ^{99m}Tc
Gear et al., 2016 [60]	Liver, spherical inserts	FDM	Total activity	^{99m}Tc, ^{90}Y
Negus et al., 2016 [67]	Brain	FDM	Visual	^{99m}Tc
Tran-Gia et al., 2016 [64]	Kidney	FDM	CF	^{99m}Tc, ^{177}Lu, ^{131}I
Tran-Gia et al., 2018 [65]	Kidney	FDM	CF	^{177}Lu
Robinson et al., 2016 [61]	Abdomen (liver, spleen, kidney, pancreas)	FDM	CF	^{99m}Tc, ^{177}Lu
Woliner-van der Weg et al., 2016 [63]	Pancreas, kidney	FDM	Ratio	^{111}In
Alqahtani et al., 2017 [69]	Head & Neck	FDM	CNR	^{99m}Tc
Jonasson et al., 2017 [68]	Striata	FDM	RC	^{18}F
Verrecchia-Ramos et al., 2021 [70]	Heart	FDM	LVEF	^{18}F, ^{99m}Tc
Black et al., 2021 [71]	Lungs	Unknown	Not yet	N/A

As a proof-of-concept, an abdomen phantom was first developed by Gear et al. [62], including the liver, kidneys, and spherical inserts. The assessment of the phantoms included measuring concordance of the geometry with that of imaging-derived organ dimensions, which showed a maximum deviation of 7%, and a visual assessment of PET and SPECT acquisitions.

Afterwards, they created an abdomen phantom [60] for validation of quantitative imaging of ^{99m}Tc and ^{90}Y and dosimetry after liver radioembolization. The phantom included a fillable liver and lesions in a solid abdomen. The design process was discussed in detail, including considerations on attenuation, leak-tightness, and attachments. The included flowchart should provide sufficient information to reproduce a similar phantom. The 3D-printed object must match the anatomical structure as closely as possible, especially for smaller objects, to evaluate the partial volume effect accurately. For the liver, the deviation of the volume was 9.6%, even though the contours on the original MRI images were hand-drawn and were thoroughly smoothed before printing to remove pixelation. This agreement was deemed sufficient for the desired application. The X-ray properties were characterized at different photon energies for several different materials and were similar to soft tissue. The accuracy of the recovered activity was different for the lesions and liver, and very different for various isotopes on PET or SPECT. Deviations as high as 18% were observed for the liver and more than 60% for the lesions. The difference is probably caused by the partial volume effect. The authors also included the cost of their project (approximately €11,600 adjusted for inflation), demonstrating the increased affordability of 3D printers today (costing €1000–3000). At the time of writing, the phantom had undergone approximately 20 acquisition protocols, including at different sites, which illustrates the excellent durability.

Robinson et al. [61] developed an abdomen phantom to verify activity quantification in SPECT in the context of molecular radiotherapy using ^{177}Lu, including ^{99m}Tc imaging. The phantom included simplified models used in a dosimetry system common at that time (OLINDA/EXM), representing spleens and kidneys of different sizes, and also representing a pancreas and liver of the ages of 5 years, 10 years, and that of an adult (extended with a bilobar design and tumor insert). The description of the phantom properties is brief, yet information on attachments and filling ports can be useful for other projects. The prints were of similar accuracy compared to the virtual volumes as in the previous examples. They evaluated the accuracy of the quantification by estimating the calibration factor, which is the ratio of the activity recovered in the VOI over the injected activity. In the ideal measurement, this would be 1. As expected, the calibration factor decreased with decreasing organ volume. Importantly, a clear dependency of the calibration factor on organ shape could be demonstrated for ^{99m}Tc and ^{177}Lu, resulting in a reduction of the absorbed dose for the liver, spleen, and kidneys using organ-specific factors. This finding illustrates that non-spherical calibration factors from 3D-printed phantom inserts can significantly improve the accuracy of whole organ activity quantification.

The challenges of imaging pancreatic beta cells using ^{111}In-exendin, which includes high uptake in the nearby kidneys, motivated Woliner van der Weg et al. [63] to develop pancreatic and kidney phantom inserts for the NEMA IEC phantom. They compared several reconstruction algorithms and different activity concentrations in the pancreas. Visually, the images were comparable to real-life studies performed in humans and showed comparable artefacts. With this work, they could assess the need for different correction algorithms and determine the appropriate reconstruction settings most suitable for clinical use.

Tran-Gia et al. first developed a single-compartment kidney model for dosimetry [64] similar to the mathematical model from MIRD Pamphlet 19 [72] for newborns, one-year olds, five-year olds, and adults, and later, a two-compartment kidney model [65] by dividing the previous volumes into a cortex (70%) and a medulla (30%). The design and production of the single-compartment model were described in detail, including the software used and attachments. A volume assessment showed a maximum deviation of 5.8%. They compared different reconstruction algorithms and different PVC techniques to optimize imaging for ^{177}Lu radionuclide therapy. In this setup, the difference between spherical and renal recovery coefficients suggests that a more geometry-specific alternative should replace the typically applied volume-dependent lookup tables based on spherical recovery coefficients. The cost of the project was similar to that by Gear et al. [60] in the order of magnitude of €10,000.

Iida et al. [66] developed a brain phantom to simulate a static cerebral blood flow distribution in the grey matter, while including a realistic skull structure. They described the segmentation upon which the phantom was based in detail. The grey matter and skull structures were fillable with liquid. White matter was made from the polymer used by the printer. The phantom was printed in five-fold and evaluated for geometry and attenuation using CT. The volumes of all phantoms were consistently close to the original value with a maximum deviation of 2.6%. The phantom was filled with either ^{99m}Tc or ^{123}I for SPECT or ^{18}F for PET. The images were compared with a virtual image blurred using a Gaussian filter to simulate the lower resolution of SPECT and PET. The printing of hollow structures normally requires supporting pillars, yet the authors were able to forgo this requirement by reducing the temperature, speed, and pitch of the printer.

A different approach to a brain phantom was developed by Negus et al. [67] by dividing the head and brain from an MRI image into slabs. These slabs with a thickness of 4 mm are 3D-printed for attenuation purposes. A conventional inkjet printer with a cartridge with added ^{99m}Tc was used to print a greyscale image of grey matter on a sheet of paper. The appropriate paper was placed between the slabs. The phantom is shown in Figure 2. The attenuation was measured using transmission scans, and the images were visually assessed.

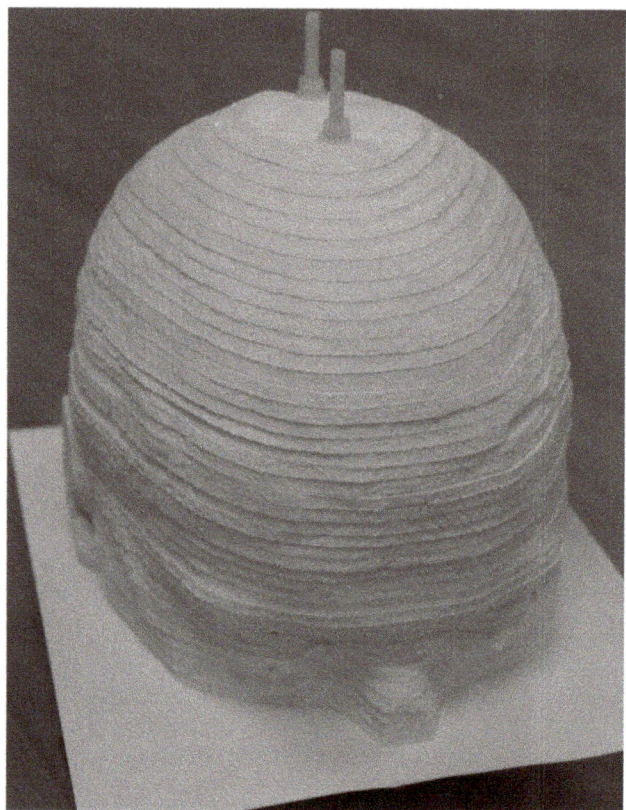

Figure 2. The brain phantom developed by Negus et al. [67] follows a different approach compared to fillable phantoms. It is a sandwich of 3D-printed slabs for attenuation and paper for activity distributions. The image was reproduced under license from the American Association of Physicists in Medicine and John Wiley & Sons, Inc. (Hoboken, NJ, USA).

The previously mentioned brain phantoms focus on grey and white matter, while imaging of the dopamine receptors also plays a significant role in neurological imaging. Jonasson et al. [68] produced a brain phantom with striatal inserts of different sizes to evaluate the influence of the size on the interpretation of PET imaging. The information on the design and production of the phantom is scarce. The background volume of the phantom and the striatum was filled with differing concentrations of ^{18}F. The recovery coefficients were compared for different reconstruction algorithms, yielding a much better recovery for all sizes of striatum using OSEM combined with the point-spread function (PSF). The PSF technique should increase the spatial resolution of the image and therefore decrease the PVE. The large increase in recovery coefficient by adding PSF to the OSEM reconstruction demonstrates this.

The head and neck region is very complex where tiny structures are densely packed, yet this region is often imaged in the context of sentinel lymph node (SLN) detection or thyroid disease. A phantom was designed and tested by Alqahtani et al. [69]; however, the analysis was aimed at assessing the imaging ability of gamma cameras for distinguishing different SLNs and the thyroid, and no evaluation of the absolute quantification was performed.

The left-ventricular ejection fraction (LVEF) is a function of the end-diastolic and end-systolic heart volume. Verrechia-Ramos et al. [70] printed the end-diastolic and end-systolic phase of the same heart based on a gated cardiac MRI, but provided little information on the design and the production process of the phantom. As the reliability of the volumes is the only important factor in determining the LVEF, no evaluation of the absolute activity measurement was done. Different isotopes and imaging modalities are used to evaluate the LVEF: MRI, planar scintigraphy (^{99m}Tc), SPECT (^{99m}Tc), and PET/CT (^{18}F). An interesting outcome was the feasibility of a very short PET/CT acquisition for a first-pass FDG scan to evaluate the LVEF.

For the validation of the accuracy of the quantification procedures in the SEL-I-METRY trial, Gregory et al. [11] developed three 3D-printed lesion inserts based on a sub-carinal node but of different sizes. The validation was performed using 123I and 131I. Little information is provided on the phantom production, nor the resulting accuracy of the quantification in the lesions.

Motion artefacts are common in molecular imaging of the thorax due to respiratory motion, and decrease the detectability and hamper quantification. Black et al. [71] developed a functional anthropomorphic lung phantom using 3D-printed molds. At the time of writing, there is no information available on the resulting images and quantification.

Recent developments attempt to improve some shortcomings of phantoms. For example, the two-compartment kidney model was complex to assemble and required the preparation of two stock solutions. Theisen et al. [73] recently presented work on a single-compartment kidney phantom. This phantom has two regions with different spatial densities by the introduction of gyroid structures. These gyroids are surfaces that limit the volume that can be filled using the stock solution. By having a denser gyroid for the medulla than for the cortex, the activity concentration will be different, even though the entire phantom is filled with the same stock solution.

There are also successful attempts at 3D-printing radioactive geometric phantoms [74–76]. The main advantage of the latter is the absence of cold walls and, when implanted with longer-lived isotopes such as ^{68}Ge (half-life = 271 days), could be used for validation in multi-center PET trials. These phantoms could play a role in quality control. However, there remains discussion on their utility as for some, this would increase the capability for diverse quality control. In contrast, according to others, they would increase the complexity while moving the difficulty in phantom preparation from the stock solution to the stock solution and the quality control of the 3D printer [77].

7. Discussion

Even though 3D printing has distinctive advantages, there is always a learning curve associated with any new technique. This learning curve could be further reduced by including more information on the design process of the phantoms and the choices made in publications. For example, Gear et al. [62] and Tran-Gia et al. [64] described the design process in more detail, including information on the attachments. This is essential information for the production of the phantom which can be used by others when designing their own phantoms. Several authors included information on wall thickness, which is useful to guarantee leak tightness. All authors included information on what printer, material, and software were used. This information all contributes to a faster uptake of the methodology in other centers. It is, however, a worrying trend that more recent publications compared to earlier work provide less information necessary for the reproduction, or to push the innovation of phantoms forward. A recommendation regarding key information to be included in future publications on 3D-printed phantoms is summarized in Table 2. It would be of considerable value if publishers and/or scientific societies would establish an online repository similar to the NIH 3D Print Exchange [78] and actively encourage making models available upon publication of research in their respective journals. The emphasis placed on data availability in the context of validation, reanalysis, and reproduction of medical research should extend to availability of phantoms.

Table 2. Examples of information which should be included in future publications of 3D-printed phantoms.

Imaging	Modality	
	Processing	
Software	Application in workflow	
3D Printer	Model	
	Material	Type
		Relevant properties
Technical	Layer thickness	
	Phantom thickness	
	Attachments	Type
		Position
	Filling method	
	Assembly	Single/multiple parts
		Assembly method
Key design choices		
Flow chart of the design process		

From the articles that mention project cost, a trend in better affordability is evident. While the price five years ago was still approximately €10,000, 3D printers are now available from as low as €1000–3000.

For anthropomorphic phantoms, it is essential that they accurately represent the anatomical image on which they are based. Therefore, verification of the geometry and the attenuation are essential. Several authors have compared the 3D-printed phantoms to the original volumes. Only small deviations from the original volumes were observed, which proves the reliability of the technique, and supports their use when reproduced given the importance of geometry on quantification. The same applies to the attenuation coefficients of the materials used. It is established that most polymers used in 3D printing have attenuation coefficients similar to soft tissue and can be used as such. Water can be made to have similar attenuation coefficients as bone by adding K_2HPO_4. It is difficult to reduce the density and attenuation coefficients of water to those of air. Therefore, anthropomorphic phantoms of the lungs are notable challenges as the activity in the lungs is present in water, while the organ mostly consists of air.

While phantoms for kidney dosimetry started as simple geometric phantoms, the complexity is still increasing with every new generation. This single-compartment phantom was improved to a two-compartment model (Figure 3). Today, even more advanced anthropomorphic phantoms and innovative designs for varying tracer concentrations within a single compartment phantom are possible. Future challenges include the 3D printing of molds for elastic anthropomorphic phantoms that can be used for dynamic imaging.

The applications of some of the discussed phantoms have already changed our view on quantitative SPECT/CT. The kidney phantom by Tran-Gia and Lassmann has been used to evaluate quantification [65], kidney dosimetry [14] using ^{177}Lu, eventually extending it to a multicentre setting [79]. The main finding of their work was that the typical volume-based approach for partial volume correction based on spherical inserts like in the IEC NEMA Body Phantom was insufficient for accurate quantification. Geometry plays an important role in the accuracy, and this should be reflected in the evaluation of specific applications. The evaluation of voxel-based dosimetry has taught us to use caution when applying this technique due to the large difference with the true measurement. This problem was improved by application of a specific partial volume correction software, indicating that quantitative imaging has to be optimised for every application. The multicentre evaluation showed a large variety in initial performance, but also the potential for harmonisation for this application.

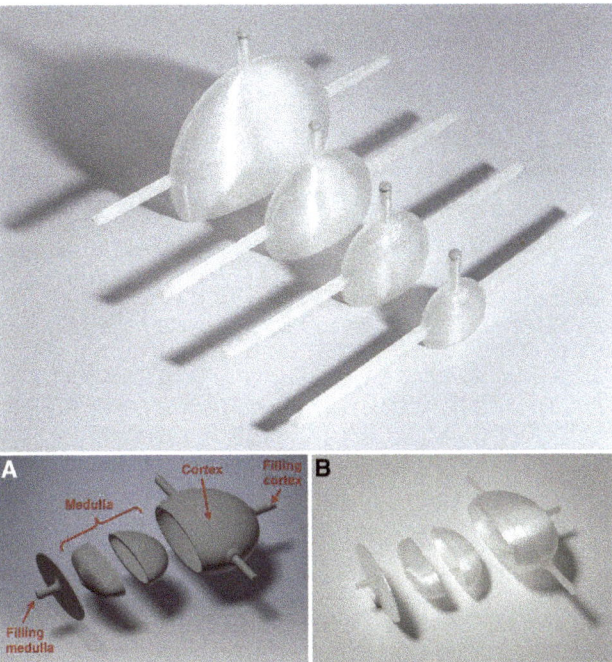

Figure 3. Three-dimensional printing allows for an iterative design process where improvements can be made for a next-generation print. The example shows the single-compartment kidney produced by Tran-Gia et al. [64] (top) and the two-compartment kidney phantom (**A**,**B**) subsequently produced by the same research group, Tran-Gia et al. [65] (bottom). This research was originally published in JNM by Tran-Gia et al. [64,65]. © SNMMI.

Until now, the major applications of 3D-printed phantoms of absolute quantification have been in the context of dosimetry. Apart from the striatal phantom, all other diagnostic applications have been evaluated visually. Yet, from these, we have learned to understand the importance of small and irregular geometries. For example, the hot spots in ^{111}In-Exendin imaging of the pancreas can result from increasing the iterations of the reconstructions and are not necessarily a result of heterogeneous uptake of the tracer. Even though there was no evaluation of the quantitative accuracy of the reconstruction, it allowed for optimization of the acquisition for visual interpretation.

8. Conclusions

Several examples have been discussed for the possible application of absolute quantification in SPECT/CT. There has, however, not been a broad uptake of these applications in diagnostic nuclear medicine so far. The establishment of absolute quantification in clinical practice depends on validation of the accuracy and reliability, and application-specific validation can benefit from anthropomorphic phantoms tailored to the application. The continued advances and availability of 3D printing allow for such application-specific phantoms to be developed at a reasonable cost and in a reasonable time with relative ease. With the current state-of-the-art, we have seen increasing possibilities and increasing complexity in the designs. These innovative designs allow for more realistic phantoms with every subsequent generation. 3D-printed phantoms have already changed our perspective on the limitations of absolute quantification while providing the possibility for further improvements. They will increase the opportunities to validate the application of absolute quantification in SPECT/CT and increase the acceptance of absolute quantification in clinical practice. This is The Phantom Premise.

Author Contributions: Conceptualization, S.D.S. and T.V.d.W.; writing: original draft preparation, S.D.S. and T.V.d.W.; review and editing, T.V.d.W., J.C.D. and G.G. All authors have read and agreed to the published version of the manuscript.

Funding: J.C.D. is part funded by the Department of Health National Institute of Health Research Biomedical Research Centre.

Institutional Review Board Statement: Not applicable.

Informed Consent Statement: Not applicable.

Conflicts of Interest: The authors declare no conflict of interest.

References

1. Bailey, D.L.; Willowson, K.P. Quantitative SPECT/CT: SPECT joins PET as a quantitative imaging modality. *Eur. J. Nucl. Med. Mol. Imaging* **2014**, *41* (Suppl. S1), S17–S25. [CrossRef]
2. Dickson, J.; Ross, J.; Voo, S. Quantitative SPECT: The time is now. *EJNMMI Phys.* **2019**, *6*, 4. [CrossRef] [PubMed]
3. Israel, O.; Pellet, O.; Biassoni, L.; De Palma, D.; Estrada-Lobato, E.; Gnanasegaran, G.; Kuwert, T.; la Fougere, C.; Mariani, G.; Massalha, S.; et al. Two decades of SPECT/CT—The coming of age of a technology: An updated review of literature evidence. *Eur. J. Nucl. Med. Mol. Imaging* **2019**, *46*, 1990–2012. [CrossRef]
4. Van den Wyngaert, T.; Elvas, F.; De Schepper, S.; Kennedy, J.A.; Israel, O. SPECT/CT: Standing on the Shoulders of Giants, It Is Time to Reach for the Sky! *J. Nucl. Med.* **2020**, *61*, 1284–1291. [CrossRef]
5. Ritt, P.; Kuwert, T. Quantitative SPECT/CT. *Recent Results Cancer Res.* **2013**, *187*, 313–330. [CrossRef] [PubMed]
6. Solnes, L.; Werner, R.; Jones, K.M.; Sadaghiani, M.S.; Bailey, C.R.; Lapa, C.; Pomper, M.G.; Rowe, S.P. Theranostics: Leveraging Molecular Imaging and Therapy to Impact Patient Management and Secure the Future of Nuclear Medicine. *J. Nucl. Med.* **2020**, *61*, 311–318. [CrossRef]
7. Hofman, M.S.; Emmett, L.; Sandhu, S.; Iravani, A.; Joshua, A.M.; Goh, J.C.; Pattison, D.A.; Tan, T.H.; Kirkwood, I.D.; Ng, S.; et al. [(177)Lu]Lu-PSMA-617 versus cabazitaxel in patients with metastatic castration-resistant prostate cancer (TheraP): A randomised, open-label, phase 2 trial. *Lancet* **2021**, *397*, 797–804. [CrossRef]
8. Strosberg, J.; El-Haddad, G.; Wolin, E.; Hendifar, A.; Yao, J.; Chasen, B.; Mittra, E.; Kunz, P.L.; Kulke, M.H.; Jacene, H.; et al. Phase 3 Trial of (177)Lu-Dotatate for Midgut Neuroendocrine Tumors. *N. Engl. J. Med.* **2017**, *376*, 125–135. [CrossRef]
9. Konik, A.; O'Donoghue, J.A.; Wahl, R.L.; Graham, M.M.; Van den Abbeele, A.D. Theranostics: The Role of Quantitative Nuclear Medicine Imaging. *Semin. Radiat. Oncol.* **2021**, *31*, 28–36. [CrossRef] [PubMed]
10. Sartor, O.; de Bono, J.; Chi, K.N.; Fizazi, K.; Herrmann, K.; Rahbar, K.; Tagawa, S.T.; Nordquist, L.T.; Vaishampayan, N.; El-Haddad, G.; et al. Lutetium-177-PSMA-617 for Metastatic Castration-Resistant Prostate Cancer. *N. Engl. J. Med.* **2021**, *385*, 1091–1103. [CrossRef] [PubMed]
11. Gregory, R.A.; Murray, I.; Gear, J.; Leek, F.; Chittenden, S.; Fenwick, A.; Wevrett, J.; Scuffham, J.; Tipping, J.; Murby, B.; et al. Standardised quantitative radioiodine SPECT/CT Imaging for multicentre dosimetry trials in molecular radiotherapy. *Phys. Med. Biol.* **2019**, *64*, 245013. [CrossRef]
12. Kennedy, J.A.; Lugassi, R.; Gill, R.; Keidar, Z. Digital Solid-State SPECT/CT Quantitation of Absolute (177)Lu Radiotracer Concentration: In Vivo and In Vitro Validation. *J. Nucl. Med.* **2020**, *61*, 1381–1387. [CrossRef]
13. Peters, S.M.B.; Meyer Viol, S.L.; van der Werf, N.R.; de Jong, N.; van Velden, F.H.P.; Meeuwis, A.; Konijnenberg, M.W.; Gotthardt, M.; de Jong, H.; Segbers, M. Variability in lutetium-177 SPECT quantification between different state-of-the-art SPECT/CT systems. *EJNMMI Phys.* **2020**, *7*, 9. [CrossRef]
14. Tran-Gia, J.; Salas-Ramirez, M.; Lassmann, M. What You See Is Not What You Get—On the Accuracy of Voxel-Based Dosimetry in Molecular Radiotherapy. *J. Nucl. Med.* **2019**, *61*, 1178–1186. [CrossRef] [PubMed]
15. Wang, J.; Zang, J.; Wang, H.; Liu, Q.; Li, F.; Lin, Y.; Huo, L.; Jacobson, O.; Niu, G.; Fan, X.; et al. Pretherapeutic 68Ga-PSMA-617 PET May Indicate the Dosimetry of 177Lu-PSMA-617 and 177Lu-EB-PSMA-617 in Main Organs and Tumor Lesions. *Clin. Nucl. Med.* **2019**, *44*, 431–438. [CrossRef] [PubMed]
16. Willowson, K.P.; Tapner, M.; Team, Q.I.; Bailey, D.L. A multicentre comparison of quantitative (90)Y PET/CT for dosimetric purposes after radioembolization with resin microspheres: The QUEST Phantom Study. *Eur. J. Nucl. Med. Mol. Imaging* **2015**, *42*, 1202–1222. [CrossRef] [PubMed]
17. Rosar, F.; Schon, N.; Bohnenberger, H.; Bartholoma, M.; Stemler, T.; Maus, S.; Khreish, F.; Ezziddin, S.; Schaefer-Schuler, A. Comparison of different methods for post-therapeutic dosimetry in [(177)Lu]Lu-PSMA-617 radioligand therapy. *EJNMMI Phys.* **2021**, *8*, 40. [CrossRef]
18. Bailey, D.L.; Willowson, K.P. An evidence-based review of quantitative SPECT imaging and potential clinical applications. *J. Nucl. Med.* **2013**, *54*, 83–89. [CrossRef] [PubMed]
19. Dickson, J.C. Quantitative SPECT: A survey of current practice in the UK Nuclear Medicine Community. *Nucl. Med. Commun.* **2019**, *40*, 986–994. [CrossRef] [PubMed]
20. Pham, D.T.; Gault, R.S. A comparison of rapid prototyping technologies. *Int. J. Mach. Tools Manuf.* **1998**, *38*, 1257–1287. [CrossRef]

21. Filippou, V.; Tsoumpas, C. Recent advances on the development of phantoms using 3D printing for imaging with CT, MRI, PET, SPECT, and ultrasound. *Med. Phys.* **2018**, *45*, e740–e760. [CrossRef] [PubMed]
22. Masri, A.; Bukhari, S.; Eisele, Y.S.; Soman, P. Molecular Imaging of Cardiac Amyloidosis. *J. Nucl. Med.* **2020**, *61*, 965–970. [CrossRef]
23. Saridin, C.P.; Raijmakers, P.G.; Al Shamma, S.; Tuinzing, D.B.; Becking, A.G. Comparison of different analytical methods used for analyzing SPECT scans of patients with unilateral condylar hyperactivity. *Int. J. Oral Maxillofac. Surg.* **2009**, *38*, 942–946. [CrossRef] [PubMed]
24. Morbelli, S.; Esposito, G.; Arbizu, J.; Barthel, H.; Boellaard, R.; Bohnen, N.I.; Brooks, D.J.; Darcourt, J.; Dickson, J.C.; Douglas, D.; et al. EANM practice guideline/SNMMI procedure standard for dopaminergic imaging in Parkinsonian syndromes 1.0. *Eur. J. Nucl. Med. Mol. Imaging* **2020**, *47*, 1885–1912. [CrossRef] [PubMed]
25. Blaufox, M.D.; De Palma, D.; Taylor, A.; Szabo, Z.; Prigent, A.; Samal, M.; Li, Y.; Santos, A.; Testanera, G.; Tulchinsky, M. The SNMMI and EANM practice guideline for renal scintigraphy in adults. *Eur. J. Nucl. Med. Mol. Imaging* **2018**, *45*, 2218–2228. [CrossRef]
26. Qi, N.; Meng, Q.; You, Z.; Chen, H.; Shou, Y.; Zhao, J. Standardized uptake values of (99m)Tc-MDP in normal vertebrae assessed using quantitative SPECT/CT for differentiation diagnosis of benign and malignant bone lesions. *BMC Med. Imaging* **2021**, *21*, 39. [CrossRef]
27. Mohd Rohani, M.F.; Mat Nawi, N.; Shamim, S.E.; Wan Sohaimi, W.F.; Wan Zainon, W.M.N.; Musarudin, M.; Said, M.A.; Hashim, H. Maximum standardized uptake value from quantitative bone single-photon emission computed tomography/computed tomography in differentiating metastatic and degenerative joint disease of the spine in prostate cancer patients. *Ann. Nucl. Med.* **2020**, *34*, 39–48. [CrossRef]
28. Tabotta, F.; Jreige, M.; Schaefer, N.; Becce, F.; Prior, J.O.; Nicod Lalonde, M. Quantitative bone SPECT/CT: High specificity for identification of prostate cancer bone metastases. *BMC Musculoskelet Disord.* **2019**, *20*, 619. [CrossRef]
29. Zhang, Y.; Li, B.; Yu, H.; Song, J.; Zhou, Y.; Shi, H. The value of skeletal standardized uptake values obtained by quantitative single-photon emission computed tomography-computed tomography in differential diagnosis of bone metastases. *Nucl. Med. Commun.* **2021**, *42*, 63–67. [CrossRef]
30. Dorbala, S.; Park, M.A.; Cuddy, S.; Singh, V.; Sullivan, K.; Kim, S.; Falk, R.H.; Taqueti, V.; Skali, H.; Blankstein, R.; et al. Absolute Quantitation of Cardiac (99m)Tc-pyrophosphate Using Cadmium Zinc Telluride-based SPECT/CT. *J. Nucl. Med.* **2021**, *62*, 716–722. [CrossRef]
31. Huang, S.C. Anatomy of SUV. Standardized uptake value. *Nucl. Med. Biol.* **2000**, *27*, 643–646. [CrossRef]
32. Boellaard, R.; Krak, N.C.; Hoekstra, O.S.; Lammertsma, A.A. Effects of noise, image resolution, and ROI definition on the accuracy of standard uptake values: A simulation study. *J. Nucl. Med.* **2004**, *45*, 1519–1527. [PubMed]
33. Adams, M.C.; Turkington, T.G.; Wilson, J.M.; Wong, T.Z. A systematic review of the factors affecting accuracy of SUV measurements. *AJR Am. J. Roentgenol.* **2010**, *195*, 310–320. [CrossRef]
34. Kaalep, A.; Sera, T.; Rijnsdorp, S.; Yaqub, M.; Talsma, A.; Lodge, M.A.; Boellaard, R. Feasibility of state of the art PET/CT systems performance harmonisation. *Eur. J. Nucl. Med. Mol. Imaging* **2018**, *45*, 1344–1361. [CrossRef] [PubMed]
35. Erlandsson, K.; Buvat, I.; Pretorius, P.H.; Thomas, B.A.; Hutton, B.F. A review of partial volume correction techniques for emission tomography and their applications in neurology, cardiology and oncology. *Phys. Med. Biol.* **2012**, *57*, R119–R159. [CrossRef]
36. O'Connor M, K.; Kemp, B.; Anstett, F.; Christian, P.; Ficaro, E.P.; Frey, E.; Jacobs, M.; Kritzman, J.N.; Pooley, R.A.; Wilk, M. A multicenter evaluation of commercial attenuation compensation techniques in cardiac SPECT using phantom models. *J. Nucl. Cardiol.* **2002**, *9*, 361–376. [CrossRef] [PubMed]
37. Hutton, B.F.; Buvat, I.; Beekman, F.J. Review and current status of SPECT scatter correction. *Phys. Med. Biol.* **2011**, *56*, R85–R112. [CrossRef]
38. Sohlberg, A.O.; Kajaste, M.T. Fast Monte Carlo-simulator with full collimator and detector response modelling for SPECT. *Ann. Nucl. Med.* **2012**, *26*, 92–98. [CrossRef]
39. Cheng, G.; Torigian, D.A.; Zhuang, H.; Alavi, A. When should we recommend use of dual time-point and delayed time-point imaging techniques in FDG PET? *Eur. J. Nucl. Med. Mol. Imaging* **2013**, *40*, 779–787. [CrossRef]
40. Lin, Y.Y.; Chen, J.H.; Ding, H.J.; Liang, J.A.; Yeh, J.J.; Kao, C.H. Potential value of dual-time-point (1)(8)F-FDG PET compared with initial single-time-point imaging in differentiating malignant from benign pulmonary nodules: A systematic review and meta-analysis. *Nucl. Med. Commun.* **2012**, *33*, 1011–1018. [CrossRef]
41. Boellaard, R.; Delgado-Bolton, R.; Oyen, W.J.; Giammarile, F.; Tatsch, K.; Eschner, W.; Verzijlbergen, F.J.; Barrington, S.F.; Pike, L.C.; Weber, W.A.; et al. FDG PET/CT: EANM procedure guidelines for tumour imaging: Version 2.0. *Eur. J. Nucl. Med. Mol. Imaging* **2015**, *42*, 328–354. [CrossRef]
42. Van den Wyngaert, T.; Strobel, K.; Kampen, W.U.; Kuwert, T.; van der Bruggen, W.; Mohan, H.K.; Gnanasegaran, G.; Delgado-Bolton, R.; Weber, W.A.; Beheshti, M.; et al. The EANM practice guidelines for bone scintigraphy. *Eur. J. Nucl. Med. Mol. Imaging* **2016**, *43*, 1723–1738. [CrossRef] [PubMed]
43. Kapucu, O.L.; Nobili, F.; Varrone, A.; Booij, J.; Vander Borght, T.; Nagren, K.; Darcourt, J.; Tatsch, K.; Van Laere, K.J. EANM procedure guideline for brain perfusion SPECT using 99mTc-labelled radiopharmaceuticals, version 2. *Eur. J. Nucl. Med. Mol. Imaging* **2009**, *36*, 2093–2102. [CrossRef]

44. Bartel, T.B.; Kuruva, M.; Gnanasegaran, G.; Beheshti, M.; Cohen, E.J.; Weissman, A.F.; Yarbrough, T.L. SNMMI Procedure Standard for Bone Scintigraphy 4.0. *J. Nucl. Med. Technol.* **2018**, *46*, 398–404.
45. Ackerhalt, R.E.; Blau, M.; Bakshi, S.; Sondel, J.A. A comparative study of three 99mTc-labeled phosphorus compounds and 18F-fluoride for skeletal imaging. *J. Nucl. Med.* **1974**, *15*, 1153–1157.
46. Phelps, M.E.; Huang, S.C.; Hoffman, E.J.; Selin, C.; Sokoloff, L.; Kuhl, D.E. Tomographic measurement of local cerebral glucose metabolic rate in humans with (F-18)2-fluoro-2-deoxy-D-glucose: Validation of method. *Ann. Neurol.* **1979**, *6*, 371–388. [CrossRef] [PubMed]
47. Peters, S.M.B.; van der Werf, N.R.; Segbers, M.; van Velden, F.H.P.; Wierts, R.; Blokland, K.; Konijnenberg, M.W.; Lazarenko, S.V.; Visser, E.P.; Gotthardt, M. Towards standardization of absolute SPECT/CT quantification: A multi-center and multi-vendor phantom study. *EJNMMI Phys.* **2019**, *6*, 29. [CrossRef]
48. Hutton, B.F.; Erlandsson, K.; Thielemans, K. Advances in clinical molecular imaging instrumentation. *Clin. Transl. Imaging* **2018**, *6*, 31–45. [CrossRef]
49. EANM. EARL. Available online: https://earl.eanm.org/ (accessed on 12 October 2021).
50. Zhang, R.; Wang, M.; Zhou, Y.; Wang, S.; Shen, Y.; Li, N.; Wang, P.; Tan, J.; Meng, Z.; Jia, Q. Impacts of acquisition and reconstruction parameters on the absolute technetium quantification of the cadmium-zinc-telluride-based SPECT/CT system: A phantom study. *EJNMMI Phys.* **2021**, *8*, 66. [CrossRef]
51. Kennedy, J.A.; Reizberg, I.; Lugassi, R.; Himmelman, S.; Keidar, Z. Absolute radiotracer concentration measurement using whole-body solid-state SPECT/CT technology: In vivo/in vitro validation. *Med. Biol. Eng. Comput.* **2019**, *57*, 1581–1590. [CrossRef] [PubMed]
52. Kuhl, D.E.; Edwards, R.Q. Image Separation Radioisotope Scanning. *Radiology* **1963**, *80*, 653–662. [CrossRef]
53. Jaszczak, R.J.; Murphy, P.H.; Huard, D.; Burdine, J.A. Radionuclide emission computed tomography of the head with 99mCc and a scintillation camera. *J. Nucl. Med.* **1977**, *18*, 373–380.
54. Ismail, F.S.; Mansor, S. Impact of Resolution Recovery in Quantitative (99m)Tc SPECT/CT Cardiac Phantom Studies. *J. Med. Imaging Radiat. Sci.* **2019**, *50*, 449–453. [CrossRef] [PubMed]
55. Blaire, T.; Bailliez, A.; Ben Bouallegue, F.; Bellevre, D.; Agostini, D.; Manrique, A. First assessment of simultaneous dual isotope ((123)I/(99m)Tc) cardiac SPECT on two different CZT cameras: A phantom study. *J. Nucl. Cardiol.* **2018**, *25*, 1692–1704. [CrossRef] [PubMed]
56. Fukami, M.; Matsutomo, N.; Yamamoto, T. Optimization of Number of Iterations as a Reconstruction Parameter in Bone SPECT Imaging Using a Novel Thoracic Spine Phantom. *J. Nucl. Med. Technol.* **2021**, *49*, 143–149. [CrossRef]
57. Rakvongthai, Y.; Fahey, F.; Borvorntanajanya, K.; Tepmongkol, S.; Vutrapongwatana, U.; Zukotynski, K.; El Fakhri, G.; Ouyang, J. Joint reconstruction of Ictal/inter-ictal SPECT data for improved epileptic foci localization. *Med. Phys.* **2017**, *44*, 1437–1444. [CrossRef]
58. Syed, I.S.; Glockner, J.F.; Feng, D.; Araoz, P.A.; Martinez, M.W.; Edwards, W.D.; Gertz, M.A.; Dispenzieri, A.; Oh, J.K.; Bellavia, D.; et al. Role of cardiac magnetic resonance imaging in the detection of cardiac amyloidosis. *JACC Cardiovasc. Imaging* **2010**, *3*, 155–164. [CrossRef]
59. de Dreuille, O.; Strijckmans, V.; Ameida, P.; Loc'h, C.; Bendriem, B. Bone equivalent liquid solution to assess accuracy of transmission measurements in SPECT and PET. *IEEE Trans. Nucl. Sci.* **1997**, *44*, 1186–1190. [CrossRef]
60. Gear, J.I.; Cummings, C.; Craig, A.J.; Divoli, A.; Long, C.D.; Tapner, M.; Flux, G.D. Abdo-Man: A 3D-printed anthropomorphic phantom for validating quantitative SIRT. *EJNMMI Phys.* **2016**, *3*, 17. [CrossRef]
61. Robinson, A.P.; Tipping, J.; Cullen, D.M.; Hamilton, D.; Brown, R.; Flynn, A.; Oldfield, C.; Page, E.; Price, E.; Smith, A.; et al. Organ-specific SPECT activity calibration using 3D-printed phantoms for molecular radiotherapy dosimetry. *EJNMMI Phys.* **2016**, *3*, 12. [CrossRef]
62. Gear, J.I.; Long, C.; Rushforth, D.; Chittenden, S.J.; Cummings, C.; Flux, G.D. Development of patient-specific molecular imaging phantoms using a 3D printer. *Med. Phys.* **2014**, *41*, 082502. [CrossRef]
63. Woliner-van der Weg, W.; Deden, L.N.; Meeuwis, A.P.; Koenrades, M.; Peeters, L.H.; Kuipers, H.; Laanstra, G.J.; Gotthardt, M.; Slump, C.H.; Visser, E.P. A 3D-printed anatomical pancreas and kidney phantom for optimizing SPECT/CT reconstruction settings in beta cell imaging using (111)In-exendin. *EJNMMI Phys.* **2016**, *3*, 29. [CrossRef] [PubMed]
64. Tran-Gia, J.; Schlogl, S.; Lassmann, M. Design and Fabrication of Kidney Phantoms for Internal Radiation Dosimetry Using 3D Printing Technology. *J. Nucl. Med.* **2016**, *57*, 1998–2005. [CrossRef] [PubMed]
65. Tran-Gia, J.; Lassmann, M. Optimizing Image Quantification for (177)Lu SPECT/CT Based on a 3D Printed 2-Compartment Kidney Phantom. *J. Nucl. Med.* **2018**, *59*, 616–624. [CrossRef] [PubMed]
66. Iida, H.; Hori, Y.; Ishida, K.; Imabayashi, E.; Matsuda, H.; Takahashi, M.; Maruno, H.; Yamamoto, A.; Koshino, K.; Enmi, J.; et al. Three-dimensional brain phantom containing bone and grey matter structures with a realistic head contour. *Ann. Nucl. Med.* **2013**, *27*, 25–36. [CrossRef]
67. Negus, I.S.; Holmes, R.B.; Jordan, K.C.; Nash, D.A.; Thorne, G.C.; Saunders, M. Technical Note: Development of a 3D-printed subresolution sandwich phantom for validation of brain SPECT analysis. *Med. Phys.* **2016**, *43*, 5020. [CrossRef]
68. Jonasson, L.S.; Axelsson, J.; Riklund, K.; Boraxbekk, C.J. Simulating effects of brain atrophy in longitudinal PET imaging with an anthropomorphic brain phantom. *Phys. Med. Biol.* **2017**, *62*, 5213–5227. [CrossRef]

69. Alqahtani, M.S.; Lees, J.E.; Bugby, S.L.; Samara-Ratna, P.; Ng, A.H.; Perkins, A.C. Design and implementation of a prototype head and neck phantom for the performance evaluation of gamma imaging systems. *EJNMMI Phys.* **2017**, *4*, 19. [CrossRef]
70. Verrecchia-Ramos, E.; Morel, O.; Retif, P.; Ben Mahmoud, S. Innovative procedure for measuring left ventricular ejection fraction from (18)F-FDG first-pass ultra-sensitive digital PET/CT images: Evaluation with an anthropomorphic heart phantom. *EJNMMI Phys.* **2021**, *8*, 42. [CrossRef]
71. Black, D.G.; Yazdi, Y.O.; Wong, J.; Fedrigo, R.; Uribe, C.; Kadrmas, D.J.; Rahmim, A.; Klyuzhin, I.S. Design of an anthropomorphic PET phantom with elastic lungs and respiration modeling. *Med. Phys.* **2021**, *48*, 4205–4217. [CrossRef]
72. Bouchet, L.G.; Bolch, W.E.; Blanco, H.P.; Wessels, B.W.; Siegel, J.A.; Rajon, D.A.; Clairand, I.; Sgouros, G. MIRD Pamphlet No 19: Absorbed fractions and radionuclide S values for six age-dependent multiregion models of the kidney. *J. Nucl. Med.* **2003**, *44*, 1113–1147.
73. Afanasenka, K.; Vaitkienė, D.; Kulakienė, I.; Šedienė, S.; Šimeliūnaitė, I. European Association of Nuclear Medicine October 20–23, 2021 Virtual. *Eur. J. Nucl. Med. Mol. Imaging* **2021**, *48*, 1–648. [CrossRef]
74. Gear, J.I.; Cummings, C.; Sullivan, J.; Cooper-Rayner, N.; Downs, P.; Murray, I.; Flux, G.D. Radioactive 3D printing for the production of molecular imaging phantoms. *Phys. Med. Biol.* **2020**, *65*, 175019. [CrossRef]
75. Lappchen, T.; Meier, L.P.; Furstner, M.; Prenosil, G.A.; Krause, T.; Rominger, A.; Klaeser, B.; Hentschel, M. 3D printing of radioactive phantoms for nuclear medicine imaging. *EJNMMI Phys.* **2020**, *7*, 22. [CrossRef] [PubMed]
76. Gillett, D.; Marsden, D.; Ballout, S.; Attili, B.; Bird, N.; Heard, S.; Gurnell, M.; Mendichovszky, I.A.; Aloj, L. 3D printing (18)F radioactive phantoms for PET imaging. *EJNMMI Phys.* **2021**, *8*, 38. [CrossRef] [PubMed]
77. Ehler, E.; Craft, D.; Rong, Y. 3D printing technology will eventually eliminate the need of purchasing commercial phantoms for clinical medical physics QA procedures. *J. Appl. Clin. Med. Phys.* **2018**, *19*, 8–12. [CrossRef] [PubMed]
78. NIH. NIH 3D Print Exchange. Available online: https://3dprint.nih.gov/ (accessed on 12 October 2021).
79. Tran-Gia, J.; Denis-Bacelar, A.M.; Ferreira, K.M.; Robinson, A.P.; Calvert, N.; Fenwick, A.J.; Finocchiaro, D.; Fioroni, F.; Grassi, E.; Heetun, W.; et al. A multicentre and multi-national evaluation of the accuracy of quantitative Lu-177 SPECT/CT imaging performed within the MRTDosimetry project. *EJNMMI Phys.* **2021**, *8*, 55. [CrossRef] [PubMed]

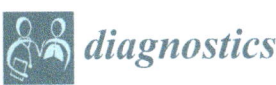

Article

Diagnostic Performance of [¹⁸F]FDG PET in Staging Grade 1–2, Estrogen Receptor Positive Breast Cancer

Ramsha Iqbal [1,*], Lemonitsa H. Mammatas [2], Tuba Aras [1], Wouter V. Vogel [3], Tim van de Brug [4], Daniela E. Oprea-Lager [5], Henk M. W. Verheul [6], Otto S. Hoekstra [5], Ronald Boellaard [5] and Catharina W. Menke-van der Houven van Oordt [1,*]

1. Department of Medical Oncology, Cancer Center Amsterdam, Amsterdam UMC, Vrije Universiteit Amsterdam, 1081 HV Amsterdam, The Netherlands; t.aras@student.vu.nl
2. Department of Medical Oncology, Reinier de Graaf Gasthuis, 2625 AD Delft, The Netherlands; l.mammatas@rdgg.nl
3. Department of Nuclear Medicine and Department of Radiation Oncology, The Netherlands Cancer Institute—Antoni van Leeuwenhoek, 1066 CX Amsterdam, The Netherlands; w.vogel@nki.nl
4. Department of Epidemiology and Data Science, Amsterdam Public Health Research Institute, Amsterdam UMC, Vrije Universiteit Amsterdam, 1081 HV Amsterdam, The Netherlands; t.vandebrug@amsterdamumc.nl
5. Department of Radiology and Nuclear Medicine, Cancer Center Amsterdam, Amsterdam UMC, Vrije Universiteit Amsterdam, 1081 HV Amsterdam, The Netherlands; d.oprea-lager@amsterdamumc.nl (D.E.O.-L.); os.hoekstra@amsterdamumc.nl (O.S.H.); r.boellaard@amsterdamumc.nl (R.B.)
6. Department of Medical Oncology, Radboud University Medical Center, 6525 GA Nijmegen, The Netherlands; Henk.Verheul@radboudumc.nl
* Correspondence: r.iqbal@amsterdamumc.nl (R.I.); c.menke@amsterdamumc.nl (C.W.M.-v.d.H.v.O.)

Abstract: Positron emission tomography using [¹⁸F]fluorodeoxyglucose (FDG PET) potentially underperforms for staging of patients with grade 1–2 estrogen receptor positive (ER+) breast cancer. The aim of this study was to retrospectively investigate the diagnostic accuracy of FDG PET in this patient population. Suspect tumor lesions detected on conventional imaging and FDG PET were confirmed with pathology or follow up. PET-positive lesions were (semi)quantified with standardized uptake values (SUV) and these were correlated with various pathological features, including the histological subtype. Pre-operative imaging detected 155 pathologically verified lesions (in 74 patients). A total of 115/155 (74.2%) lesions identified on FDG PET were classified as true positive, i.e., malignant (in 67 patients) and 17/155 (10.8%) lesions as false positive, i.e., benign (in 9 patients); 7/155 (4.5%) as false negative (in 7 patients) and 16/155 (10.3%) as true negative (in 14 patients). FDG PET incorrectly staged 16/70 (22.9%) patients. The FDG uptake correlated with histological subtype, showing higher uptake in ductal carcinoma, compared to lobular carcinoma ($p < 0.05$). Conclusion: Within this study, FDG PET inadequately staged 22.9% of grade 1–2, ER + BC cases. Incorrect staging can lead to inappropriate treatment choices, potentially affecting survival and quality of life. Prospective studies investigating novel radiotracers are urgently needed.

Keywords: positron emission tomography (PET); [¹⁸F]FDG; breast cancer; estrogen receptor; staging

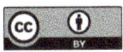

1. Introduction

Breast cancer (BC) is the most frequently diagnosed malignancy among women worldwide [1]. In the Netherlands, 16,000 women are newly diagnosed with BC annually, most of whom have stage I (40.4%) or stage II (32.6%) disease, whereas 9.6% patients have stage III and 4.6% stage IV [2]. For stage IIB/III (advanced T-stage disease often with nodal involvement) or locoregional recurrent disease, curative treatment generally consists of surgery, radiotherapy and (neoadjuvant or adjuvant) systemic therapy (i.e., chemo-, endocrine and targeted therapy) [3]. In the case of metastatic disease without curative options, burdensome locoregional as well as systemic therapy should be avoided in order to maintain quality of life. On the other hand, identification of oligometastatic disease may improve the chance of (prolonged disease free) survival by including these sites in the local therapy plan [4]. Therefore, accurate pre-operative staging is essential to identify locoregionally affected lymph nodes and (distant) metastases, as it will affect treatment choices.

The initial work-up for BC includes physical examination, mammography, ultrasound and magnetic resonance imaging (MRI) of the breast and axilla, to assess the extent of locoregional disease [3]. Standard staging procedures detect (distant) metastases in approximately 7% and 8–21% of clinical stage IIB and III patients, respectively, and in 33% of those presenting with locoregional recurrences [5–7]. Furthermore, 10–25% will develop recurrences within 2 years, suggesting, at least in part, missed (occult) metastases at presentation [8]. According to (inter)national guidelines, staging is often performed with 2-[^{18}F]fluoro-2-deoxy-D-glucose (FDG) positron emission tomography accompanied by a low-dose CT scan for attenuation correction (FDG PET) [3,9,10]. In addition to this, a diagnostic computed tomography (CT) scan of the thorax and abdomen is often performed [3,9]. For primary staging of clinical stage II/III BC, the sensitivity and specificity of FDG PET to identify lymph node involvement and distant metastases is 63–100% and 98–100%, respectively [5,11], and in recurrent disease, it is 90% and 81%, respectively [12].

However, FDG uptake of BC can be quite variable, due to various underlying biological features [11–18]. FDG uptake is often lower in lobular BC (vs. ductal BC) [15,16,18,19], in low-intermediate grade (vs. high grade) [12–18] tumors and in ER-positive tumors, compared to triple negative tumors (ER-/PR-/HER2-) [11,13,15–17,20–23]. Alternatively, triple negative BC (ER-/PR-/HER2-), a more aggressive phenotype, shows higher FDG uptake than ER+/PR+ and HER2- BC [20]. Thus, these biological factors can affect the FDG avidity of lesions potentially limiting the accuracy of FDG PET/CT for the staging of grade 1–2 ER+ BC [16].

Although there are data that FDG uptake (usually expressed as standard uptake value (SUV)) is lower in low grade ER+ BC than in other types of BC and that staging might be suboptimal [24,25], no study has specifically investigated the extent to which this affects the staging of BC. Therefore, the primary aim of this study was to retrospectively investigate the diagnostic performance of FDG PET in staging patients with grade 1–2 ER + BC. The secondary aims were to study whether the level of tracer uptake in the primary tumor was associated with the accuracy of staging, and to investigate which histopathological features might predict the accuracy of FDG PET.

2. Materials and Methods

2.1. Patient Population

In this retrospective study, we included women ≥18 years with histologically proven ER+, grade 1–2, clinical stage IIB/III or locoregional recurrent BC, treated at the Amsterdam UMC (VUmc) and The Netherlands Cancer Institute-Antoni van Leeuwenhoek (NKI-AvL) in the Netherlands between 2008–2016 and 2014–2015, respectively. All patients underwent FDG PET/CT for staging and had their follow-up visits for at least 18 months. Patients with other malignancies in the last five years prior to diagnosis of (recurrent) BC were excluded.

Prior to inclusion, patients provided written informed consent, except when it was not possible to approach them for consent, due to various reasons (e.g., death or no contact details available). The study was approved by the local Medical Ethics Committee of the VUmc (No. 2017.382).

2.2. Imaging Procedures

According to the standard of care, patients underwent mammography, ultrasound and MRI of the breast and axilla for locoregional staging. Patients at VUmc underwent an additional diagnostic CT scan of the thorax/abdomen and at both centers bone scans were performed if indicated (i.e., 'conventional imaging'). FDG PET scans were performed using

Gemini TF-64 or Ingenuity TF-64 PET/CT scanner at VUmc and Gemini TF-16 or Gemini TF-Big Bore 16 (Philips Medical Systems, Cleveland, Ohio, United States of America) at AvL, according to the guidelines of the European Association of Nuclear Medicine (EANM) [26]. Patients were administered 3.5 MBq/kg FDG at VUmc, and 190–240 MBq (according to the body mass index) at AvL [26]. All patients underwent a low-dose CT scan for attenuation correction, followed by the PET scan (skull vertex to mid-thigh) at 60 min post-injection, with 2 min per bed position.

2.3. Histopathology

According to standard of care, the biopsy of the primary tumor was used to evaluate the histological subtype, grade (according to the Bloom–Richardson grading system), ER, PR, HER2 expression and mitotic activity. Compliant with Dutch guidelines ER-/PR-positivity on immunohistochemistry (IHC) was established if $\geq 10\%$ of cell nuclei were immunoreactive, and HER2 was classified positive with 3+ or 2+ and amplified [3]. Mitotic activity was defined as the number of mitoses per 2 mm^2. Suspect locoregional or distant lesions visible on conventional imaging and/or FDG PET that were decisive for therapy choices were verified by core needle biopsy and/or fine-needle aspiration cytology.

The pathological reports of lymph node resection were classified as follows: in the case of the presence of malignant cells, pathologically verified malignant lymph node; in the case of fibrosis compatible with complete response after neo-adjuvant therapy, pathologically verified malignant lymph node before neo-adjuvant treatment; and in the case of no malignant cells or fibrosis by cytology and/or histology, benign lymph node.

2.4. Patient-Based Analysis

The patient-based outcomes consisted of determining the stage of disease at baseline and at the end of follow-up. The stage of disease was determined at clinical presentation together with conventional imaging and subsequently by FDG PET together with pathological confirmation.

2.5. Lesional Analysis: Qualitative and Semi-Quantitative FDG PET Readings

Conventional imaging was performed ≤ 5 weeks before or after FDG PET. Clinically relevant lesions suspicious for malignancy on any imaging modality were included in this analysis, with a maximum of 5 largest lesions per tissue type in the case of distant metastases. The included lesions were either pathologically confirmed as benign or malignant (group A) or, in the case of absent/inconclusive pathology, verified by additional imaging and/or follow up for 18 months after primary diagnosis (group B). Based on these data, we classified lesions as true positives (=malignant lesions suspect on FDG PET), true negatives (=benign lesions not suspect on FDG PET), false positives (=benign lesions suspect on FDG PET) and false negatives (=malignant lesions not suspect on FDG PET). In the case of multiple axillary lymph nodes on FDG PET, only those which were pathologically proven to be malignant were included in group A.

Quantitative analysis was performed, using in-house developed software (version 04092018, Accurate tool, R. Boellaard, Amsterdam, The Netherlands) [27]. This analysis only included lesions visible on FDG PET. Volumes of interest (VOIs) were semi-automatically defined using 50% thresholds of peak standardized uptake values (SUV$_{peak}$) adapted for local background[26] and verified by radiologists. For each VOI, we determined the SUV$_{max}$, SUV$_{mean}$, SUV$_{peak}$ and total lesion glycolysis (TLG). In addition, for primary breast lesions, VOIs were manually defined on the low-dose CT scans to calculate anatomical volumes. The correlation between these FDG PET parameters and various histopathological features of the primary tumor was assessed to investigate whether histopathological features predicted the accuracy of the FDG PET.

2.6. Clinical Implications on Treatment Plan

We investigated the impact of incorrect lesion identification by FDG PET. The pathological outcome of the surgically resected axillary lymph nodes was retrospectively compared to lymph nodes identified on FDG PET, excluding patients that had progressive disease during neo-adjuvant therapy. We postulated that without progression, any additional pathologically verified malignant node in the resection specimen, compared to baseline FDG PET, should be classified as false negative on FDG PET. In the case that this would lead to stage migration of the N-stage, from N1 to N2, such patients would require an axillary lymph node dissection, according to current guidelines instead of sentinel node/marked node resection [3].

Similarly, the number of distant metastases is relevant for the treatment plan. In the case of oligometastatic disease (<4 lesions), local treatment with curative intent can be considered, whereas in the case of extensive disease (≥ 4 distant metastases) a palliative option will prevail. We compared the distant lesions on FDG PET to the number of distant metastases confirmed through pathological verification and/or additional imaging at baseline and during the follow-up period.

2.7. Statistical Analysis

Statistical analysis was performed, using SPSS Statistics 22.0 (IBM Corp.). Accuracy was measured at the patient and lesional levels, separately for groups A and B. The difference between FDG PET parameters (SUV_{max}, SUV_{peak}, SUV_{mean} and TLG) across the different categories in the two groups (true positives, false positives and false negatives, group A and B) was assessed using the Kruskal–Wallis test. The association between the tracer uptake in the primary tumor and accuracy of staging was assessed by using the Mann–Whitney U test. The association between histopathological features of the primary tumor and accuracy of staging was assessed by using a chi-square test or a Mann–Whitney U test. The association between semi-quantitative FDG PET parameters and histopathological features of the primary tumor was investigated, using a mixed model analysis with an intercept on patient level. Results were considered significant for a p-value of <0.05.

3. Results

3.1. Patients

Seventy-four patients (37 from each center) with a median age of 49 years (range: 28–94) were included. Most patients presented with clinical stage IIB (48.6%) or III (47.3%) BC (Table 1). FDG PET/CT was performed after primary surgery in four patients, and prior to surgery ($n = 6$) or systemic treatment ($n = 58$ neo-adjuvant and $n = 6$ palliative) in the remaining 70 patients.

Table 1. Patient characteristics.

	N (%) or Median (Range)
Age at diagnosis (y)	49 (28–94)
Clinical stage at presentation	
IIB	36 (48.6)
III	35 (47.3)
Locoregional recurrence	3 (4.1)
Histological subtype *	
Ductal	57 (77.0)
Lobular	17 (22.7)
Micropapillary	1 (1.3)
Grade	
1	7 (9.5)
2	67 (91.5)

Table 1. Cont.

	N (%) or Median (Range)
ER receptor	
Positive	74 (100.0)
PR receptor	
Negative	13 (17.6)
Positive	61 (82.4)
HER2neu receptor	
Negative	65 (87.8)
Positive	9 (12.2)
Treatment received	
Neo-adjuvant therapy (after FDG PET imaging)	
yes	58 (78.4)
- chemotherapy	- 53 (91.4)
- endocrine therapy	- 5 (8.6)
no **	16 (21.6)
Surgery	
- yes	65 (87.8)
- before FDG PET imaging	- 4 (6.2)
- after FDG PET imaging	- 61 (93.8)
- no	9 (12.2)
Adjuvant therapy	
- yes	69 (93.2)
- no	2 (2.7)
- unknown	3 (4.1)

* One patient with multifocal BC presented with 2 lesions in the breast, each having a different histological subtype. ** These patients directly underwent surgery before ($n = 4$) or after the FDG PET scan ($n = 6$) or received endocrine treatment for metastatic disease ($n = 5$) or locoregional recurrence ($n = 1$) after FDG PET imaging.

3.2. Patient-Based Analysis

In 67% (47/70), the FDG PET stage was identical to the clinical stage at baseline and in 10% (7/70), FDG PET correctly upstaged patients (Table 2). However, of the remaining 16 patients, 3 were incorrectly downstaged and 13 were incorrectly upstaged. Four patients underwent staging with FDG PET after surgery, as they had stage IIB or III disease post-surgery: one of these patients had an additional suspect breast lesion on FDG PET, and subsequent mastectomy showed multifocal breast cancer.

Table 2. FDG PET staged 16/70 patients incorrectly compared to final baseline stage. Patients who received FDG PET imaging prior to surgery or who did not receive surgical treatment are included ($n = 70$). The table indicates the number of patients with their corresponding stage. (A) Staging based on clinical assessment, pathology and conventional imaging performed at baseline. (B) Staging based on FDG PET imaging. (C) Final stage determined after FDG PET imaging, additional imaging and/or biopsy/cytology of new identified suspect lesions.

(A) Clinical Stage	(B) [18F]FDG PET Stage	(C) Final Stage Baseline			
		Local Recurrence	IIB	III	IV
Local recurrence	Local recurrence	2	0	0	0
	IIB	0	0	0	0
	III	0	0	0	0
	IV	0	0	0	1

Table 2. Cont.

(A) Clinical Stage	(B) [18F]FDG PET Stage	(C) Final Stage Baseline			
		Local Recurrence	IIB	III	IV
IIB	Local recurrence/stage I/IIA	0	0	0	0
	IIB	0	21	0	0
	III	0	3	0	0
	IV	0	4	0	1
	No lesions visible on scan	0	1	0	0
III	Local recurrence/stage I/IIA	0	0	0	0
	IIB	0	0	2	0
	III	0	0	24	0
	IV	0	0	6	5

■ : Correctly identified by FDG PET, ■ : Incorrectly downstaged by FDG PET, ■ : Correctly upstaged by FDG PET, ■ : Incorrectly upstaged by FDG PET.

At the end of follow-up (after 18 months), 81.4% were disease-free (Table S1). Of 67 patients who were diagnosed with locoregional disease at baseline, 3 developed metastases during follow-up. One patient had stage III by FDG PET at baseline; during follow-up, multiple bone metastases were diagnosed after 12 months. The second patient had multiple FDG-avid mediastinal lymph nodes, which were classified as reactive lymph nodes (no biopsy/cytology performed), and 17 months later, she developed pathologically proven liver metastases (without growing mediastinal nodes). The third patient had enhanced uptake in parasternal and paratracheal lymph nodes (no biopsy/cytology performed), which was interpreted at baseline as reactive lymph nodes probably due to esophagitis; 9 months later she presented with mastitis carcinomatosa, growing parasternal lymph nodes and liver metastases.

3.3. Lesional Analysis

In group A, 155 lesions were pathologically verified prior to neo-adjuvant therapy and primary surgical treatment (breast: 86, locoregional lymph nodes: 58, distant: 11; Table S2A). Visual analysis of FDG PET correctly classified 115/155 (74.2%) lesions as malignant, and 16/155 (10.3%) as benign. FDG PET incorrectly categorized 24/155 (15.5%) lesions: 7/155 (4.5%) lesions in 7 patients were malignant but showed no uptake, whereas 17/155 (11.0%) lesions in 9 patients (5 with 1 lesion, 2 with 2 lesions, and 2 with 4 lesions) were benign but showed enhanced uptake (Figure 1). On this pathologically confirmed lesional basis, FDG PET had a sensitivity and specificity of 94.3% and 48.4%, respectively.

Group B consisted of 112 lesions (Table S2B). FDG PET classified 61/112 (54.5%) and 8/112 (7.2%) lesions as true positives and true negatives, respectively. Forty-three (43/112, 38.4%) lesions were classified incorrectly: 12/112 (10.8%) malignant lesions showed no uptake, whereas 31/112 (27.7%) lesions showed enhanced uptake reported as suspect but were benign. On this, with imaging/follow up confirmed lesional basis, FDG PET had a sensitivity and specificity of 83.6% and 20.5%, respectively.

Results of groups A and B taken together (Table S2C) yielded a sensitivity and specificity of 90.3% (95% CI 85.3–93.7%) and 33.3% (23.5–44.8%), respectively. Misclassification by FDG PET mostly involved axillary lymph nodes and bone tissue, respectively (Table S3).

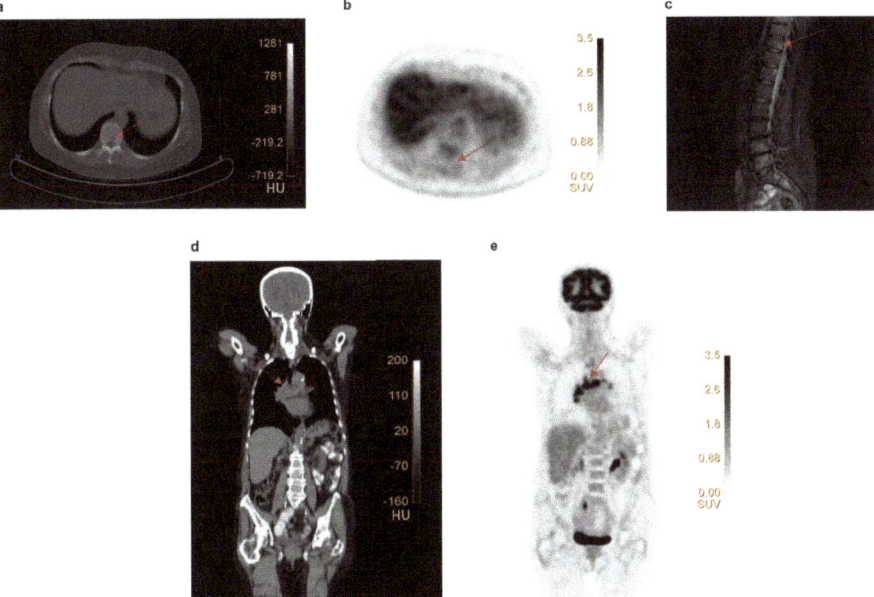

Figure 1. Examples of false negative and false positive lesions on FDG PET. (a–c) Patient with primary ER+ breast cancer with faint uptake in the primary tumor (SUV$_{max}$ 2.3). Low-dose CT (**a**) revealed a lytic lesion in the 10th thoracic vertebra (Th10) without enhanced FDG uptake (**b**). An MRI scan (**c**) revealed multiple vertebral metastases (Th4, Th11, Th12, L4, L5), including the one at Th10. This lesion was classified as false negative on FDG PET. (**d–e**) Patient with multiple mediastinal FDG avid, suspect lymph nodes. Coronal section of a low-dose CT-scan (**d**) and FDG PET scan (**e**). Endobronchial ultrasound–guided biopsy of 3 mediastinal lymph nodes showed reactive cells. These lesions were, therefore, classified as false positive on FDG PET.

A similar lesion-based analysis was performed for conventional imaging, including the diagnostic CT scan (Table S4), showing high sensitivity and low-moderate specificity rates of 95.9% and 15.2% and 80.8% and 66.7% for groups A and B, respectively. Outcomes of conventional and FDG PET imaging were also combined together for group A (Table S5), showing that conventional imaging alone identified 23 additional suspect lesions of which 7 were malignant. FDG PET alone identified 10 other suspect lesions of which 5 were malignant.

Quantification of visually identified lesions on FDG PET did not improve discrimination between true and false positives lesions (Figure 2, Table S6 and Figures S1–S3), in either group (A and B).

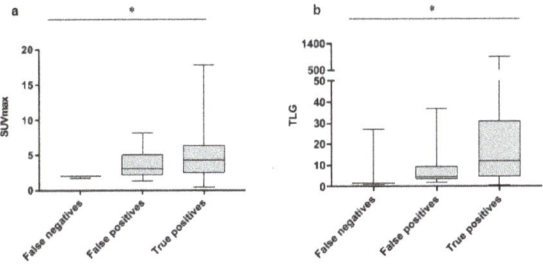

Figure 2. *Cont.*

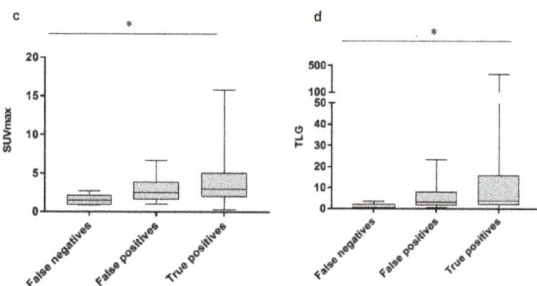

Figure 2. SUV_{max} and TLG show no significant differences between false and true positive lesions. Lesions were classified into 3 groups, i.e. false negatives, false positives and true positives; lesions have been verified with pathology (**a,b**) or additional imaging and/or follow-up (**c,d**). Similar results have been obtained for SUV_{peak} and SUV_{mean} (Supplementary Figures S1 and S2). * $p < 0.05$.

3.4. Correlation between FDG PET Parameters and Histopathology

FDG uptake in the primary tumor was not associated with the accuracy of FDG PET staging ($p = 0.67$). Ductal carcinoma had a higher SUV_{peak} and SUV_{mean} than lobular carcinoma ($p < 0.05$), and HER2+ tumors had a significantly higher TLG compared to HER2- tumors ($p < 0.05$) (Table S7). The % ER positivity correlated with TLG ($p < 0.05$)

3.5. Implications for the Plan

In summary, in 22/74 (29.8%) patients, the treatment plan based solely on FDG PET imaging would have been incorrect. In total, 65/74 (87.8%) patients underwent surgical resection, and in 34/65 patients (52.3%), surgery included also axillary lymph node dissection. No patient on neo-adjuvant therapy had progressive disease during treatment. Pathological analysis of axillary specimens classified 143 of 346 lymph nodes as malignant, whereas 203 were benign (Table S8). Since it is impossible to match each lymph node in the pathology specimen with their location on imaging, we compared the numbers of suspicious nodes on FDG PET with malignant nodes in the specimen. 83/143 (58.0%) malignant lymph nodes in 16 patients were classified as false negatives on FDG PET. In 7 patients, diagnosed with N1-stage disease on FDG PET, axillary lymph node dissection showed N2-disease (Table S9). In 2 patients with one malignant node on FDG PET, 1 or 2 additional nodes were identified when the axillary lymph node dissection was performed. Additionally, FDG PET falsely identified N3 disease (infraclavicular lymph node) in one patient, whereas in one case, N3 disease (intramammary lymph node) was missed. In the remaining patients, FDG PET showed the same number or fewer affected lymph nodes than the resection specimen, the latter most likely due to the effect of the neo-adjuvant systemic treatment. As the neo-adjuvant treatment affects the lesion size, no correlation between FDG PET positivity and the size of the lymph node metastasis could be made.

Metastatic disease was missed by FDG PET in two patients: one patient had multiple bone metastases and the other patient had a lung metastasis. In eight other patients, false positive lesions were identified in the liver, thyroid, bone and lymph nodes located in the neck, mediastinum and inguinal region (Table S3).

4. Discussion

To our knowledge, this is the first study assessing the diagnostic performance of FDG PET in patients with stage IIB/III or LRR, grade 1–2, ER+ breast cancer. In this study, the sensitivity of FDG PET for disease staging was 77.1%. Previous studies have reported a sensitivity of up to 100% for primary breast cancer [15,28] and 81–97% for restaging of LRR [15], for all types of breast cancer combined. In a meta-analysis performed by Han et al. [29], it could be seen that FDG PET outcomes led to changes in staging in 25% of patients. In addition, various studies have shown that FDG PET outcomes affected the treatment plan in 6.5–18% of patients with primary breast cancer [11,15,29]. These data reinforce the importance of additional imaging modalities next to the conventional imaging to obtain the correct stage, which is essential for an adequate treatment plan. In our case, the treatment plan was correctly adapted by FDG PET in 7/70 (10%) patients, but in 16/70 (23%) patients FDG PET would have led to an incorrect treatment plan (Table 2). Thus, our results support the hypothesis that FDG PET is insufficient for (re)staging of grade 1-2 ER+ breast cancer.

4.1. TNM Lesion Detection

When looking into more detail to detection of individual lesions, this study shows that the sensitivity and specificity of FDG PET for lesion detection (pre-operatively) was 94.3% and 48.8% (group A)/83.6% and 20.5% (group B), respectively in patients with grade 1–2, ER+ BC. Differentiation of lesion detection based on the type of lesion (i.e., primary breast lesions, locoregional lymph nodes and distant metastases), showed that FDG PET accurately detects primary breast tumors (83/87 (95.4%). Our data are in line with a prospective study that showed similar detection rate of BC lesions when comparing FDG PET/CT with MRI (95% vs. 100%, p = 1.0) [30]. However, compared to other conventional imaging techniques, such as MRI, it is known that FDG PET has less sensitivity and less accuracy for determining the size of the tumor and to assess the presence of multifocal disease [15]. For locoregional lymph nodes, previous studies have shown that micrometastases are suboptimally detected with FDG PET (CT) [31,32]. However, in current clinical practice, it is essential to identify all affected nodes before neo-adjuvant treatment, as only extensively affected axillary lymph nodes (i.e., $\geq$N2-disease/'bulky' disease) remaining after neo-adjuvant systemic treatment will, in general, require axillary lymph node dissection. In the case of N1-disease (1–$\leq$ 3 affected lymph nodes) at diagnosis and response to neo-adjuvant treatment, resection of the sentinel node(s) and marked node is deemed sufficient when followed by locoregional radiotherapy [3]. In our study, 26/96 (27.1%) axillary lymph nodes were incorrectly identified: 3.1% of the axillary lymph nodes were identified as false negatives and 24.0% as false positive nodes (Table S3). These incorrect identified nodes could potentially change the N-stage and eventually the locoregional treatment, making it even more important that these nodes are correctly identified.

In the case of distant metastases, FDG PET(CT) is known to have a high yield as shown in inflammatory and stage II/III BC [6,15,33–35]. In this study, distant metastases were identified in 7/70 patients (10%), which is at the lower end of what would be expected from the literature for stages IIB/III/LRR [5–7]. In 4 patients, FDG PET confirmed the suspicion of metastases as seen on conventional imaging, and in 3 patients, metastatic lesions were correctly identified on FDG PET alone. However, FDG PET also missed lung and bone metastases in 7 patients. Distant metastases were mainly located in extra-axillary lymph nodes, the lungs and bone. FDG PET lacks sensitivity for the detection of (small) lung nodules (due to partial volume effect and respiratory movement) and identifies osteoblastic lesions suboptimally (often showing low or no FDG uptake in these lesions) [15,36]. In our study, most of the lung lesions were small (range: 4–11 mm) and therefore correct identification of these might have been hampered by the partial volume effect; however, the low grade, ER+ breast cancer subtype might also have played a role. Most of the bone lesions included in this study were osteolytic and also for these lesions, applied that the specified low grade, ER+ breast cancer subtype might have affected its identification on PET.

4.2. Association between FDG PET Parameters and Histopathology

Quantification of FDG uptake only showed a trend for higher SUV_{max} and TLG values in malignant (true positive) lesions, compared to false positives and false negatives. However, no specific threshold for malignancy could be determined, as was described in other studies [37,38]. The histological subtype, however, correlates with FDG uptake, with ductal BC having higher FDG uptake, compared to lobular BC. This is in accordance with other studies and can probably be explained by a lower tumor cell density, a low level of GLUT1 expression, diffuse infiltration of surrounding tissue and a decreased proliferation rate in lobular BC, eventually resulting in lower FDG uptake [17,19,20].

We did not observe a difference in FDG uptake between grade 1 and grade 2 tumors. In the literature, it is known that grade 3 tumors have significantly higher FDG uptake than grade 1–2 tumors, but no information is available regarding the correlation between FDG uptake and grade 1 and 2 tumors, separately [12–18]. Regarding the receptor status, we found that the % ER positivity and HER2 status correlated with TLG. No correlations could be found between the PR status and FDG uptake. Previous studies are somewhat contradictory about this: a few studies have shown that there is no correlation between the hormone receptor status (positive or negative) and FDG uptake [14,39], whereas others have shown that FDG uptake is affected by hormone receptor status [13,15–17,20–22]. These studies do not take the expression levels of ER and PR, separately and in combination, into account, which may be essential to identify the relation with FDG uptake. For HER2, no correlation could be found between its status (positive/negative) and FDG SUV, which is consistent with other studies [16,17,22]. However, the HER2 status did correlate with TLG, but we could not confirm this from other studies, as they did not include TLG in their analyses.

We did not find a correlation between the FDG uptake and the mitotic activity index (mean ± standard deviation: 3.1 (±4.1); range: 0–19), probably as we only included tumors, which are expected to be less metabolically active than other subtypes of breast cancer. Studies including more metabolically active tumors, identified by a higher Ki-67 expression, have reported higher FDG uptake [17,40].

4.3. Limitations

Due to the retrospective set-up of this study not all clinical, imaging, and pathology data were available for all patients. We had access to all the FDG PET scans, but the scans of other imaging modalities were not always present. In those cases, the available report of the radiologist was used to compare lesions on the different imaging modalities. Furthermore, of the 267 lesions investigated, 155/267 lesions were pathologically verified (reference method), whereas for 112/267 lesions, only additional imaging and/or follow-up data were available, which precludes a definitive diagnosis regarding these lesions. However, our separate analyses for both groups yielded results in a similar range, supporting the chosen approach. For the visual analysis, we also included all axillary lymph nodes, benign or malignant, as verified according to the pathology report. However, in the case of multiple avid lymph nodes on the FDG PET scan, it can be difficult to match the exact lymph node that was pathologically proven benign or malignant to the correct lesion on the scan. In that case, it was assumed that the lesion that is most avid on the scan is also most likely the one of which biopsy or cytology is performed, and this lesion could also be quantified. Of the remaining lesions, only the number of affected lymph nodes were taken into account in the analysis.

4.4. Scientific Implications

Imaging with FDG PET for patients with grade 1–2, ER + BC can potentially lead to incorrect staging. In the search for alternative methods to improve staging, imaging based on the ER, which is independent of metabolic activity, might be of interest. Several clinical studies have shown that 16α-[^{18}F]-fluoro-17β-estradiol ([^{18}F]FES) PET/CT has overall high sensitivity (82–84%) and specificity (93–98%) rates [41], making it an interesting ER-targeting PET tracer to compare with FDG for the staging of patients with grade 1–2, ER + BC.

5. Conclusions

The data presented in this study show that FDG PET imaging inadequately staged 22.9% of grade 1–2, ER+ BC cases. This can lead to incorrect staging and subsequently to inappropriate treatment choices, potentially affecting survival and quality of life. Prospective studies investigating novel radiotracers are urgently needed to improve the current imaging staging procedures.

Supplementary Materials: The following are available online at https://www.mdpi.com/2075-4418/11/11/1954/s1. Please see 'Supplemental data'.

Author Contributions: Conceptualization: R.I., C.W.M.-v.d.H.v.O.; methodology: R.I., L.H.M., C.W.M.-v.d.H.v.O.; data acquisition: R.I., L.H.M., W.V.V., C.W.M.-v.d.H.v.O.; data analysis: R.I., T.A., T.v.d.B.; data interpretation and revision: R.I., L.H.M., T.A., W.V.V., T.v.d.B., D.E.O.-L., H.M.W.V., O.S.H., R.B., C.W.M.-v.d.H.v.O.; writing—original draft preparation: R.I.; supervision: H.M.W.V., O.S.H., R.B., C.W.M.-v.d.H.v.O. All authors have read and agreed to the published version of the manuscript.

Funding: This research was financially supported by the Cancer Center Amsterdam.

Institutional Review Board Statement: The study was conducted according to the guidelines of the Declaration of Helsinki, and approved by the Institutional Review Board (or Ethics Committee) of the Amsterdam UMC—location VUmc (protocol number: 2017.382; date of approval: 23 February 2018).

Informed Consent Statement: Informed consent was obtained from subjects involved in the study except when it was not possible to approach them for consent due to various reasons (e.g., death or no contact details available).

Data Availability Statement: The data supporting the conclusions of this article are included within the article.

Acknowledgments: The authors would like to thank the patients for participating in this study and the members of the associated departments of the VUmc and NKI-AvL for tracer production and data acquisition.

Conflicts of Interest: The authors declare no conflict of interest.

References

1. Bray, F.; Ferlay, J.; Soerjomataram, I.; Siegel, R.L.; Torre, L.A.; Jemal, A. Global cancer statistics 2018: GLOBOCAN estimates of incidence and mortality worldwide for 36 cancers in 185 countries. *CA Cancer J. Clin.* **2018**, *68*, 394–424. [CrossRef]
2. Vondeling, G.T.; Menezes, G.L.; Dvortsin, E.P.; Jansman, F.G.A.; Konings, I.R.; Postma, M.J.; Rozenbaum, M.H. Burden of early, advanced and metastatic breast cancer in The Netherlands. *BMC Cancer* **2018**, *18*, 262. [CrossRef]
3. Breast Cancer Dutch Guideline. Available online: https://richtlijnendatabase.nl/richtlijn/borstkanker/algemeen.html (accessed on 11 October 2020).
4. Kwapisz, D. Oligometastatic breast cancer. *Breast Cancer* **2019**, *26*, 138–146. [CrossRef] [PubMed]
5. Brennan, M.E.; Houssami, N. Evaluation of the evidence on staging imaging for detection of asymptomatic distant metastases in newly diagnosed breast cancer. *Breast* **2012**, *21*, 112–123. [CrossRef]
6. Segaert, I.; Mottaghy, F.; Ceyssens, S.; De Wever, W.; Stroobants, S.; Van Ongeval, C.; Van Limbergen, E.; Wildiers, H.; Paridaens, R.; Vergote, I.; et al. Additional Value of PET-CT in Staging of Clinical Stage IIB and III Breast Cancer. *Breast J.* **2010**, *16*, 617–624. [CrossRef]
7. Elfgen, C.; Schmid, S.M.; Tausch, C.J.; Montagna, G.; Güth, U. Radiological Staging for Distant Metastases in Breast Cancer Patients with Confirmed Local and/or Locoregional Recurrence: How Useful are Current Guideline Recommendations? *Ann. Surg. Oncol.* **2019**, *26*, 3455–3461. [CrossRef]
8. Early Breast Cancer Trialists' Collaborative Group; McGale, P.; Correa, C.; Cutter, D.; Duane, F.; Ewertz, M.; Gray, R.; Mannu, G.; Peto, R.; Whelan, T.; et al. Effect of radiotherapy after mastectomy and axillary surgery on 10-year recurrence and 20-year breast cancer mortality: Meta-analysis of individual patient data for 8135 women in 22 randomised trials. *Lancet* **2014**, *383*, 2127–2135. [PubMed]
9. Cardoso, F.; Kyriakides, S.; Ohno, S.; Penault-Llorca, F.; Poortmans, P.; Rubio, I.T.; Zackrisson, S.; Senkus, E. Early breast cancer: ESMO Clinical Practice Guidelines for diagnosis, treatment and follow-up. *Ann. Oncol.* **2019**, *30*, 1194–1220. [CrossRef]
10. National Comprehensive Cancer Network. Breast Cancer (Version 8.2021). Available online: https://www.nccn.org/professionals/physician_gls/pdf/breast.pdf (accessed on 11 October 2021).
11. Groheux, D.; Cochet, A.; Humbert, O.; Alberini, J.-L.; Hindié, E.; Mankoff, D. 18F-FDG PET/CT for Staging and Restaging of Breast Cancer. *J. Nucl. Med.* **2016**, *57*, 17S–26S. [CrossRef] [PubMed]
12. Xiao, Y.; Wang, L.; Jiang, X.; She, W.; He, L.; Hu, G. Diagnostic efficacy of 18F-FDG-PET or PET/CT in breast cancer with suspected recurrence: A systematic review and meta-analysis. *Nucl. Med. Commun.* **2016**, *37*, 1180–1188. [CrossRef]

13. Gil-Rendo, A.; Martínez-Regueira, F.; Zornoza, G.; Garcia-Velloso, M.J.; Beorlegui, C.; Rodriguez-Spiteri, N. Association between [18F]fluorodeoxyglucose uptake and prognostic parameters in breast cancer. *J. Br. Surg.* **2009**, *96*, 166–170. [CrossRef]
14. Crippa, F.; Seregni, E.; Agresti, R.; Chiesa, C.; Pascali, C.; Bogni, A.; Decise, D.; De Sanctis, V.; Greco, M.; Daidone, M.G.; et al. Association between [18F]fluorodeoxyglucose uptake and postoperative histopathology, hormone receptor status, thymidine labelling index and p53 in primary breast cancer: A preliminary observation. *Eur. J. Nucl. Med. Mol. Imaging* **1998**, *25*, 1429–1434. [CrossRef] [PubMed]
15. Groheux, D.; Espie, M.; Giachetti, S.; Hindie, E. Performance of FDG PET/CT in the clinical management of breast cancer. *Radiology* **2013**, *266*, 388–405. [CrossRef]
16. Groheux, D.; Giacchetti, S.; Moretti, J.-L.; Porcher, R.; Espié, M.; Lehmann-Che, J.; De Roquancourt, A.; Hamy, A.-S.; Cuvier, C.; Vercellino, L.; et al. Correlation of high 18F-FDG uptake to clinical, pathological and biological prognostic factors in breast cancer. *Eur. J. Nucl. Med. Mol. Imaging* **2011**, *38*, 426–435. [CrossRef] [PubMed]
17. Jung, N.Y.; Kim, S.H.; Choi, B.B.; Sung, M.S. Associations between the standardized uptake value of 18F-FDG PET/CT and the prognostic factors of invasive lobular carcinoma: In comparison with invasive ductal carcinoma. *World J. Surg. Oncol.* **2015**, *13*, 113. [CrossRef]
18. Kumar, R.; Chauhan, A.; Zhuang, H.; Chandra, P.; Schnall, M.; Alavi, A. Clinicopathologic factors associated with false negative FDG–PET in primary breast cancer. *Breast Cancer Res. Treat.* **2006**, *98*, 267–274. [CrossRef] [PubMed]
19. Bos, R.; Van der Hoeven, J.J.; Van der Wall, E.; Van der Groep, P.; Van Diest, P.J.; Comans, E.F.; Semenza, G.L.; Hoekstra, O.S.; Lammertsma, A.A.; Molthoff, C.F.M. Biologic correlates of (18)fluorodeoxyglucose uptake in human breast cancer measured by positron emission tomography. *J. Clin. Oncol.* **2002**, *20*, 379–387. [CrossRef] [PubMed]
20. Basu, S.; Chen, W.; Tchou, J.; Mavi, A.; Cermik, T.; Czerniecki, B.; Schnall, M.; Alavi, A. Comparison of triple-negative and estrogen receptor-positive/progesterone receptor-positive/HER2-negative breast carcinoma using quantitative fluorine-18 fluorodeoxyglucose/positron emission tomography imaging parameters: A potentially useful method for disease characterization. *Cancer* **2008**, *112*, 995–1000.
21. Mavi, A.; Cermik, T.F.; Urhan, M.; Puskulcu, H.; Basu, S.; Jian, Q.Y.; Zhuang, H.; Czerniecki, B.; Alavi, A. The effects of estrogen, progesterone, and C-erbB-2 receptor states on 18F-FDG uptake of primary breast cancer lesions. *J. Nucl. Med.* **2007**, *48*, 1266–1272. [CrossRef]
22. Osborne, J.R.; Port, E.; Gonen, M.; Doane, A.; Yeung, H.; Gerald, W.; Cook, J.B.; Larson, S. 18F-FDG PET of locally invasive breast cancer and association of estrogen receptor status with standardized uptake value: Microarray and immunohistochemical analysis. *J. Nucl. Med.* **2010**, *51*, 543–550. [CrossRef]
23. Weigelt, B.; Geyer, F.C.; Reis-Filho, J.S. Histological types of breast cancer: How special are they? *Mol. Oncol.* **2010**, *4*, 192–208. [CrossRef]
24. Lemarignier, C.; Martineau, A.; Teixeira, L.; Vercellino, L.; Espié, M.; Merlet, P.; Groheux, D. Correlation between tumour characteristics, SUV measurements, metabolic tumour volume, TLG and textural features assessed with 18F-FDG PET in a large cohort of oestrogen receptor-positive breast cancer patients. *Eur. J. Nucl. Med. Mol. Imaging* **2017**, *44*, 1145–1154. [CrossRef]
25. Groheux, D.; Martineau, A.; Teixeira, L.; Espié, M.; De Cremoux, P.; Bertheau, P.; Merlet, P.; Lemarignier, C. 18FDG-PET/CT for predicting the outcome in ER+/HER2- breast cancer patients: Comparison of clinicopathological parameters and PET image-derived indices including tumor texture analysis. *Breast Cancer Res.* **2017**, *19*, 3. [CrossRef]
26. Boellaard, R.; Delgado-Bolton, R.; Oyen, W.J.G.; Giammarile, F.; Tatsch, K.; Eschner, W.; Verzijlbergen, F.J.; Barrington, S.F.; Pike, L.C.; Weber, W.A.; et al. FDG PET/CT: EANM procedure guidelines for tumour imaging: Version 2.0. *Eur. J. Nucl. Med. Mol. Imaging* **2015**, *42*, 328–354. [CrossRef]
27. Boellaard, R. Quantitative oncology molecular analysis suite: ACCURATE. *J. Nucl. Med.* **2018**, *59*, 1753.
28. Vogsen, M.; Jensen, J.D.; Christensen, I.Y.; Gerke, O.; Jylling, A.M.B.; Larsen, L.B.; Braad, P.-E.; Søe, K.L.; Bille, C.; Ewertz, M.; et al. FDG-PET/CT in high-risk primary breast cancer—a prospective study of stage migration and clinical impact. *Breast Cancer Res. Treat.* **2021**, *185*, 145–153. [CrossRef] [PubMed]
29. Han, S.; Choi, J.Y. Impact of 18F-FDG PET, PET/CT, and PET/MRI on staging and management as an initial staging modality in breast cancer: A systematic review and meta-analysis. *Clin. Nucl. Med.* **2021**, *46*, 271–282. [CrossRef]
30. Heusner, T.A.; Kuemmel, S.; Umutlu, L.; Koeninger, A.; Freudenberg, L.S.; Hauth, E.A.; Kimmig, K.R.; Forsting, M.; Bockisch, A.; Antoch, G. Breast Cancer Staging in a Single Session: Whole-Body PET/CT Mammography. *J. Nucl. Med.* **2008**, *49*, 1215–1222. [CrossRef] [PubMed]
31. Fuster, D.; Duch, J.; Paredes, P.; Velasco, M.; Muñoz, M.; Santamaría, G.; Fontanillas, M.; Pons, F. Preoperative Staging of Large Primary Breast Cancer with [18F]Fluorodeoxyglucose Positron Emission Tomography/Computed Tomography Compared with Conventional Imaging Procedures. *J. Clin. Oncol.* **2008**, *26*, 4746–4751. [CrossRef]
32. Veronesi, U.; De Cicco, C.; Galimberti, V.; Fernandez, J.; Rotmensz, N.; Viale, G.; Spano, G.; Luini, A.; Intra, M.; Berrettini, A.; et al. A comparative study on the value of FDG-PET and sentinel node biopsy to identify occult axillary metastases. *Ann. Oncol.* **2007**, *18*, 473–478. [CrossRef] [PubMed]
33. Alberini, J.-L.; Lerebours, F.; Wartski, M.; Fourme, E.; Le Stanc, E.; Gontier, E.; Madar, O.; Cherel, P.; Pecking, A.P. 18F-fluorodeoxyglucose positron emission tomography/computed tomography (FDG-PET/CT) imaging in the staging and prognosis of inflammatory breast cancer. *Cancer* **2009**, *115*, 5038–5047. [CrossRef] [PubMed]

34. Carkaci, S.; Macapinlac, H.A.; Cristofanilli, M.; Mawlawi, O.; Rohren, E.; Angulo, A.M.G.; Dawood, S.; Resetkova, E.; Le-Petross, H.T.; Yang, W.-T. Retrospective Study of 18F-FDG PET/CT in the Diagnosis of Inflammatory Breast Cancer: Preliminary Data. *J. Nucl. Med.* **2009**, *50*, 231–238. [CrossRef]
35. van der Hoeven, J.J.; Krak, N.C.; Hoekstra, O.S.; Comans, E.F.; Boom, R.P.; Van Geldere, D.; van der Wall, E.; Buter, J.; Pinedo, H.M.; Teule, G.J.J.; et al. 18F-2-fluoro-2-deoxy-d-glucose positron emission tomography in staging of locally advanced breast cancer. *J. Clin. Oncol.* **2004**, *22*, 1253–1259. [CrossRef]
36. Cook, G.J.; Azad, G.K.; Goh, V. Imaging Bone Metastases in Breast Cancer: Staging and Response Assessment. *J. Nucl. Med.* **2016**, *57*, 27S–33S. [CrossRef]
37. Shin, K.M.; Kim, H.J.; Jung, S.J.; Lim, H.S.; Lee, S.W.; Cho, S.H.; Jang, Y.-J.; Lee, H.J.; Kim, G.C.; Jung, J.H.; et al. Incidental Breast Lesions Identified by18F-FDG PET/CT: Which Clinical Variables Differentiate between Benign and Malignant Breast Lesions? *J. Breast Cancer* **2015**, *18*, 73–79. [CrossRef]
38. Pencharz, D.; Nathan, M.; Wagner, T.L. Evidence based management of incidental focal uptake of fluorodeoxyglucose on PET-CT. *Br. J. Radiol.* **2017**, *91*, 20170774. [CrossRef]
39. Avril, N.; Menzel, M.; Dose, J.; Schelling, M.; Weber, W.; Jänicke, F.; Nathrath, W.; Schwaiger, M. Glucose metabolism of breast cancer assessed by 18F-FDG PET: Histologic and immunohistochemical tissue analysis. *J. Nucl. Med.* **2001**, *42*, 9–16. [PubMed]
40. Buck, A.; Schirrmeister, H.; Kühn, T.; Shen, C.; Kalker, T.; Kotzerke, J.; Dankerl, A.; Glatting, G.; Reske, S.; Mattfeldt, T. FDG uptake in breast cancer: Correlation with biological and clinical prognostic parameters. *Eur. J. Nucl. Med. Mol. Imaging* **2002**, *29*, 1317–1323. [CrossRef] [PubMed]
41. Kurland, B.F.; Wiggins, J.R.; Coche, A.; Fontan, C.; Bouvet, Y.; Webner, P.; Divgi, C.; Linden, H.M. Whole-body characterization of estrogen receptor status in metastatic breast cancer with 16α-18F-fluoro-17β-estradiol positron emission tomography: Meta-analysis and recommendations for integration into clinical applications. *Oncologist* **2020**, *25*, 835–844. [CrossRef] [PubMed]

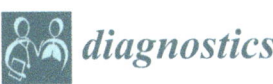

Article

Evaluation of Quantitative Ga-68 PSMA PET/CT Repeatability of Recurrent Prostate Cancer Lesions Using Both OSEM and Bayesian Penalized Likelihood Reconstruction Algorithms

Mark J. Roef [1,*], Sjoerd Rijnsdorp [2], Christel Brouwer [1], Dirk N. Wyndaele [1] and Albert J. Arends [2]

1. Department of Nuclear Medicine, Catharina Hospital Eindhoven, Michelangelolaan 2, 5623 EJ Eindhoven, The Netherlands; christel.brouwer@catharinaziekenhuis.nl (C.B.); dirk.wyndaele@catharinaziekenhuis.nl (D.N.W.)
2. Department of Medical Physics, Catharina Hospital Eindhoven, Michelangelolaan 2, 5623 EJ Eindhoven, The Netherlands; srijnsdorp@outlook.com (S.R.); bertjan.arends@catharinaziekenhuis.nl (A.J.A.)
* Correspondence: mark.roef@catharinaziekenhuis.nl; Tel.: +31-40-239-9111; Fax: +31-40-2398600

Abstract: Rationale: To formally determine the repeatability of Ga-68 PSMA lesion uptake in both relapsing and metastatic tumor. In addition, it was hypothesized that the BPL algorithm Q. Clear has the ability to lower SUV signal variability in the small lesions typically encountered in Ga-68 PSMA PET imaging of prostate cancer. Methods: Patients with biochemical recurrence of prostate cancer were prospectively enrolled in this single center pilot test-retest study and underwent two Ga-68 PSMA PET/CT scans within 7.9 days on average. Lesions were classified as suspected local recurrence, lymph node metastases or bone metastases. Two datasets were generated: one standard PSF + OSEM and one with PSF + BPL reconstruction algorithm. For tumor lesions, SUVmax was determined. Repeatability was formally assessed using Bland–Altman analysis for both BPL and standard reconstruction. Results: A total number of 65 PSMA-positive tumor lesions were found in 23 patients (range 1 to 12 lesions a patient). Overall repeatability in the 65 lesions was $-1.5\% \pm 22.7\%$ (SD) on standard reconstructions and $-2.1\% \pm 29.1\%$ (SD) on BPL reconstructions. Ga-68 PSMA SUVmax had upper and lower limits of agreement of +42.9% and −45.9% for standard reconstructions and +55.0% and −59.1% for BPL reconstructions, respectively (NS). Tumor SUVmax repeatability was dependent on lesion area, with smaller lesions exhibiting poorer repeatability on both standard and BPL reconstructions (F-test, $p < 0.0001$). Conclusion: A minimum response of 50% seems appropriate in this clinical situation. This is more than the recommended 30% for other radiotracers and clinical situations (PERCIST response criteria). BPL does not seem to lower signal variability in these cases.

Keywords: repeatability; Ga-68 PSMA PET/CT; Bayesian penalized likelihood reconstruction; prostate cancer

Citation: Roef, M.J.; Rijnsdorp, S.; Brouwer, C.; Wyndaele, D.N.; Arends, A.J. Evaluation of Quantitative Ga-68 PSMA PET/CT Repeatability of Recurrent Prostate Cancer Lesions Using Both OSEM and Bayesian Penalized Likelihood Reconstruction Algorithms. *Diagnostics* **2021**, *11*, 1100. https://doi.org/10.3390/diagnostics11061100

Academic Editor: Lioe-Fee de Geus-Oei

Received: 8 April 2021
Accepted: 12 June 2021
Published: 16 June 2021

Publisher's Note: MDPI stays neutral with regard to jurisdictional claims in published maps and institutional affiliations.

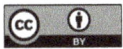

Copyright: © 2021 by the authors. Licensee MDPI, Basel, Switzerland. This article is an open access article distributed under the terms and conditions of the Creative Commons Attribution (CC BY) license (https://creativecommons.org/licenses/by/4.0/).

1. Introduction

In western Europe, United States and Canada, prostate cancer has the highest incidence of all cancers in men, with a global incidence estimated at over 1.6 million in 2015 [1]. Nearly half of the patients will experience a relapse during their lifespan, either locally in the prostate (bed) and/or in lymph node or bone metastases [2]. Biochemical relapse (BCR) is defined as a PSA relapse after initial treatment, with different definitions for BCR after radical prostatectomy or radiotherapy (i.e., external beam radiotherapy or brachytherapy) [3]. Management strategies in BCR are focused on early detection of disease, with patients with low volume disease having the best prognosis [4]. Patients with low volume disease may have only a few lesions of small size that make them qualify for focal therapy, e.g., stereotactic body radiotherapy (SBRT), with the intent of postponing systemic therapy [5]. Focal therapy can thus be directed against either local relapses or against metastases (metastasis directed therapy, MDT). PSMA PET/CT is a widely accepted imaging modality in BCR, showing lesions with high contrast to their background [6]. Using PSMA PET/CT for monitoring of focal therapy to these lesions is generally less well accepted but promising [7].

A standardized quantitative approach still needs to be developed, however.

It is known that uptake measurements of radiolabeled tracers with PET in vivo suffer from many inaccuracies, as demonstrated by experience with FDG [8], and that this requires evaluation and standardization prior to application as response parameter [9]. This probably applies equally to PSMA-PET expression. Before quantification of PSMA, expression can be used as a surrogate biological parameter to identify response to treatment, and before we can design sufficiently powered response evaluation studies, we need to know the characteristics of the measurement technique. An important factor that is currently less known is the normal day-to-day variability in Ga-68 PSMA expression of tumor, i.e., repeatability.

The main aim of this pilot study is to formally determine the repeatability of Ga-68 PSMA in both relapsing and metastatic tumor, with focus on small lesions. In small lesions, partial volume effects become increasingly relevant. Partial volume effects start to play a role when lesion size falls below 2 to 3 times the spatial resolution of the PET system defined by its full width at half maximum (FWHM), and are expected to increase signal variability [10,11].

The spatial resolution that can be achieved in PET imaging is limited by physical characteristics such as positron range and noncollinearity of annihilation photons depends furthermore on scanner properties such as detector size and geometry, acquisition parameters and on the reconstruction method applied.

For 18F-fluordeoxyglucose (FDG), Rogasch et al. have demonstrated that the Bayesian penalized likelihood (BPL) reconstruction algorithm called Q.Clear (GE Healthcare, Milwaukee, WI, USA) can yield consistently improved reconstructed spatial resolution at high and medium signal to background ratios, compared to OSEM +PSF + TOF and OSEM + TOF [12].

Q.Clear is an iterative reconstruction algorithm that runs to full convergence by controlling the noise introducing a relative difference noise penalty [13,14]. The noise control term is a function of the signal values in neighboring voxels and is controlled by a unitless penalization factor (the beta value), which is the only user-input variable set in the algorithm [14]. In solitary pulmonary nodules (SPNs), BPL is claimed to improve lesion visibility, when compared to OSEM [15,16]. We hypothesized that in small prostate cancer lesions, which also may comprise of only 2 or 3 voxels, the noise penalty of the BPL algorithm would improve uptake quantification to the voxel level, thus lowering signal variability. This is the second aim of our study.

2. Materials and Methods

2.1. Patients

Thirty patients with biochemical recurrence of prostate cancer scheduled for routine clinical Ga-68PSMA PET/CT were prospectively enrolled in this pilot study (NL52809.100. 16/R16.058/Ga-68 PSMA test-retest study) between January 2018 and July 2019. Their scans were screened for evaluable PSMA-positive tumor lesions by two board certified nuclear physicians (MJR and CB). Seven patients had no evaluable tumor lesions and were excluded from the study. The remaining twenty-three had their second (retest) scan within on average 7.9 days (range 6 to 23) of their initial (test) scan and were evaluated for measurements in assigned tumor lesions. Only one patient had a relatively long interval of 23 days between test and retest due to logistical issues, where the next highest value was 10 days. Tumor lesions were classified as suspected local recurrence, lymph node metastases or bone metastases. Both baseline scans were performed before any treatment had begun. The study was approved by the local institutional ethics review board, and all patients had given written approval before any scanning was done (NL52809.100.16/R16.058/Ga-68 PSMA test-retest study, date of approval 22 March 2017).

PET images were acquired on a PET/CT scanner (GE Healthcare Discovery 710), with a 2.5 min acquisition per bed position, on average 58 (range 55 to 69) min after injection of on average 1.4 (range 0.9 to 1.7) MBq/kg dose of Ga-68 PSMA. Two datasets were reconstructed: one standard ordered subset expectation maximization (OSEM) reconstruction including both time-of-flight (TOF) and point spread function (PSF) modelling and a second one using the Bayesian penalized likelihood (BPL) algorithm, called Q.Clear [17]. For the OSEM reconstruction, 2 iterations and 24 subsets were used. BPL reconstruction also included TOF and PSF. BPL (including TOF and PSF) is subsequently referred to as BPL, same as for OSEM. A matrix size of 256 × 256 was used, resulting in voxels of 2.73 × 2.73 × 3.27 mm^3. With respect to filtering, a 6.4 mm Gaussian filter and 1:4:1 filter in axial direction were applied. Both used low dose CT for attenuation correction. For the BPL algorithm, a beta value of 600 was used. This value was found optimal in a Ga-68 PSMA phantom study using spheres of 5–37 mm diameter (this special issue).

2.2. PET and CT Analysis

For both the test and the retest datasets, the PET and low-dose CT images were processed independently. Imaging reading was performed using dedicated software for PET/CT imaging (Philips IntelliSpace Portal 9.0, Eindhoven, The Netherlands).

In PET, tumor lesion size was measured in the axial plane using a fixed PET windowing upper level (UL) of 10 used for stretching of the greyscale. Both long and short axis were measured; lesion area was calculated according to the simple formula for round and oval lesions: A = π × half long axis × half short axis. Within this area, the pixel with the highest standardized uptake value is designated the SUVmax (injected dose/kg body weight). Thus SUVmax was measured in all tumor lesions. The small size of most of the lesions did not allow for measurement of other meaningful SUVs such as SUVpeak that need lesions of at least 1 cm^3. Low dose CT was used to check for appropriateness of the lesion area measured in PET if possible (i.e., with the exception of some bone metastases not visible on CT).

2.3. Statistical Analysis

The repeatability of SUVmax in tumor lesions was assessed with Bland–Altman analysis by reporting the mean (bias) and limits of agreement (defined as mean ± 1.96 SD) of the differences between the two measurements of individual lesions. Bland–Altman analysis was preferred over intra class correlation coefficients on the basis of previous recommendations [18,19]. Assessment of signal variability between lesion areas and SUVmax was assessed with F-testing.

For the comparison of the two reconstruction techniques a paired t-test was used, i.e., BPL versus standard OSEM.

3. Results

A total number of 65 PSMA-positive tumor lesions were found in 23 patients (range 1 to 12 lesions), see Table 1 for patient characteristics. In addition, in 7 patients no lesions were found, and therefore, these were excluded. In theory, a perfect test–retest will result in identical values for the test and the retest. In daily practice, however, measurements of a lesions SUVmax in repeated acquisitions will yield results normally distributed around the true value. In tumor lesions showing an increased SUVmax from test to retest, the average increase was 16.8% ± 10.6% (SD) on standard OSEM reconstructions (33 lesions) and 22.1% ± 18.6% (SD) on BPL reconstructions (30 lesions). In tumor lesions showing a decreased SUVmax from test to retest, these values were −21.0% ± 15.2% (SD) on standard OSEM reconstructions (32 lesions) and −23.2% ± 19.7% (SD) on BPL reconstructions (35 lesions), respectively. Overall repeatability in 65 lesions was −1.5% ± 22.7% (SD) on standard OSEM reconstructions and −2.1% ± 29.1% (SD) on BPL reconstructions. The small difference between both reconstructions was not statistically significant.

Table 1. Patient characteristics.

Pat no.	Age	PSA	Gleason Score	Activity Test Scan (MBq/kg)	Activity Retest Scan (MBq/kg)	Time Test Scan (min)	Time Re-Test Scan (min)	Total Number of Lesions	Prostate Bed	Lymph Node Metastases	Bone	Initial Therapy	Year of Therapy
1	83	2.4	7	1.2	1.4	60	65	3	-	3	-	LND +EBRT	2009
2	71	4.1	8	1.2	1.5	58	58	1	-	-	1	RALP +LND	2017
3	75	4.5	7	1.4	1.5	57	60	1	-	-	1	RALP	2009
4	73	8.4	6	1.3	1.6	57	57	6	-	3	3	AS+BT +LND	2012
5	69	0.7	7	1.3	0.9	55	56	2	-	2	-	RALP +ELND	2015
6	78	16.0	6	1.5	1.4	55	56	3	1	2	-	BT	2011
7	84	9.0	6	1.5	1.5	58	58	4	1	3	-	BT	2012
8	80	0.7	8	1.3	1.5	57	57	2	1	-	1	RALP +LND	2008
9	62	3.9	6	1.5	1.6	60	55	1	1	-	-	BT	2013
10	77	3.0	7	0.9	0.9	69	72	1	-	1	-	RALP +ELND	2010
11	71	3.5	7	1.3	1.5	55	56	1	1	-	-	BT	2014
12	67	5.7	-	1.3	1.1	55	55	3	1	1	1	BT	2007
13	78	1.7	8	1.4	1.4	61	56	1	-	1	-	BT	2016
14	75	2.8	6	1.4	1.4	55	55	3	-	3	-	BT	2009
15	74	2.0	7	1.5	1.5	59	62	1	-	1	-	RP+LND +EBRT	2009
16	77	1.2	7	1.0	1.5	55	55	3	-	3	-	RALP	2009
17	72	2.5	7	1.7	1.6	55	55	12	-	-	12	RALP +ELND	2018
18	73	2.8	7	1.7	1.4	58	58	1	-	-	1	BT	2007
19	78	5.4	6	1.5	1.4	57	55	3	-	3	-	RALP +LND	2008
20	77	3.7	8	1.5	1.3	55	55	4	2	2	-	EBRT +HT	2009
21	69	5.2	6	1.4	1.3	59	59	1	1	-	-	EBRT	2012
22	68	0.6	7	1.3	1.5	60	60	3	-	3	-	RALP +LND	2015
23	78	7.0	7	0.9	1.5	55	58	5	-	5	-	EBRT	2017

AS = active surveillance, BT = brachytherapy, EBRT = external beam radiotherapy, ELND = extended lymph node dissection, HT = hormonal therapy, LND = lymph node dissection, RP = radical prostatectomy (open procedure), RALP = robot assisted radical prostatectomy.

As shown in Figure 1A, overall repeatability of SUVmax had upper and lower limits of agreement of +42.9% and −45.9% for standard OSEM reconstructions and +55.0% and −59.1% for BPL reconstructions, respectively. For suspected local recurrence, SUVmax had a repeatability of −5.0% ± 14.4%, with upper and lower limits of agreement of +23.2% and −33.1% for standard OSEM reconstructions. For BPL reconstructions, SUVmax repeatability was −9.5% ± 16.8%, with upper and lower limits at +23.5% and −42.5%. See Figure 1B. For suspected lymph node metastases, SUVmax repeatability was −4.5% ± 22.8% for standard OSEM reconstructions, with upper and lower limits of +40.1% and −49.1%. For BPL reconstructions, SUVmax repeatability was −3.3% ± 30.6%, with upper and lower limits at +56.6% and −63.2%. See Figure 1C. For suspected bone metastases, SUVmax had a repeatability of +4.4% ± 26.1%, with upper and lower limits of agreement of +55.7% and −46.8% for standard OSEM reconstructions. For BPL reconstructions, SUVmax repeatability was +2.7% ± 32.8%, with upper and lower limits at +67.0% and −61.6%. See

Figure 1D. None of the differences between standard OSEM and BPL reconstructions were statistically significant.

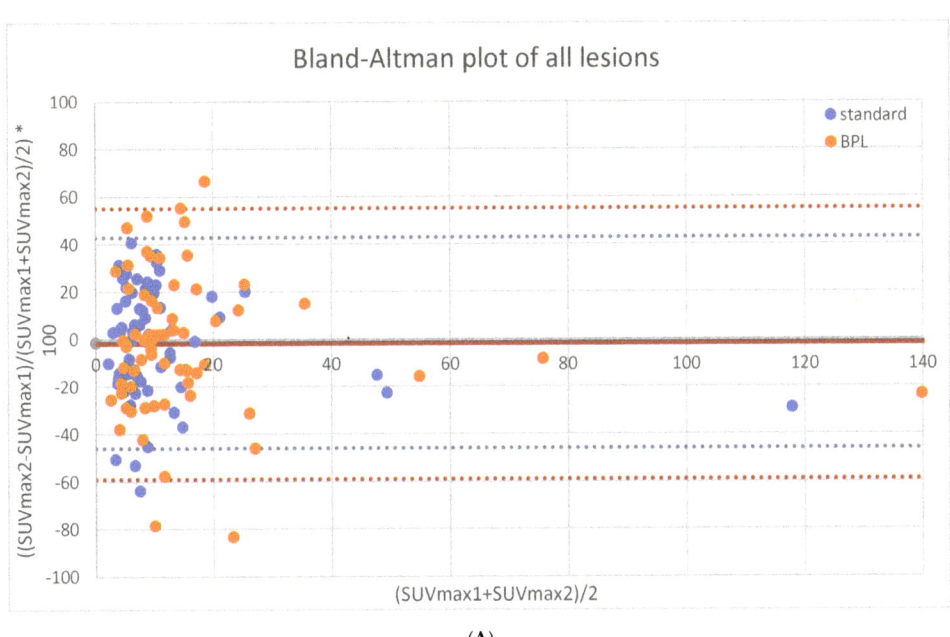

(A)

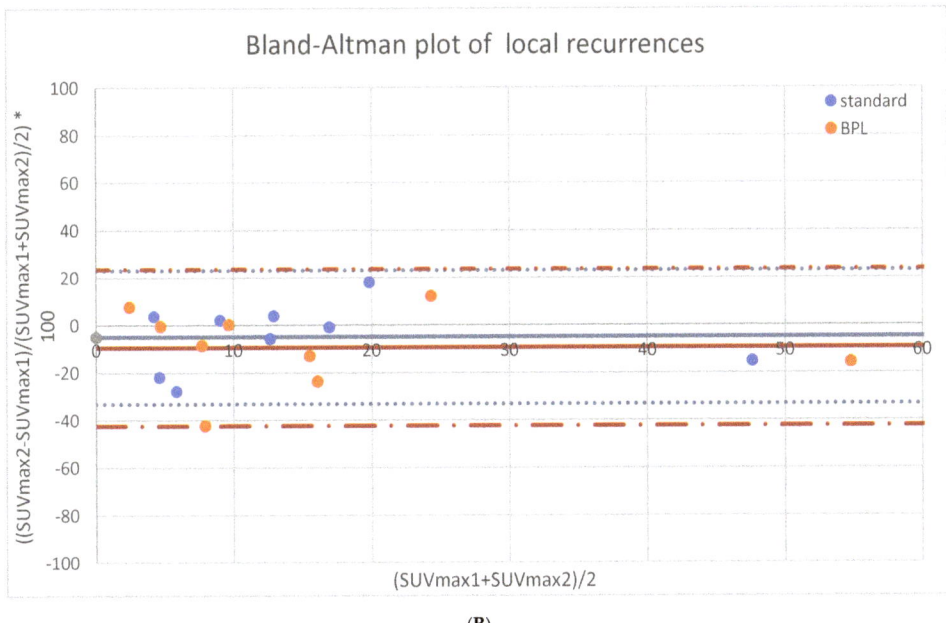

(B)

Figure 1. *Cont.*

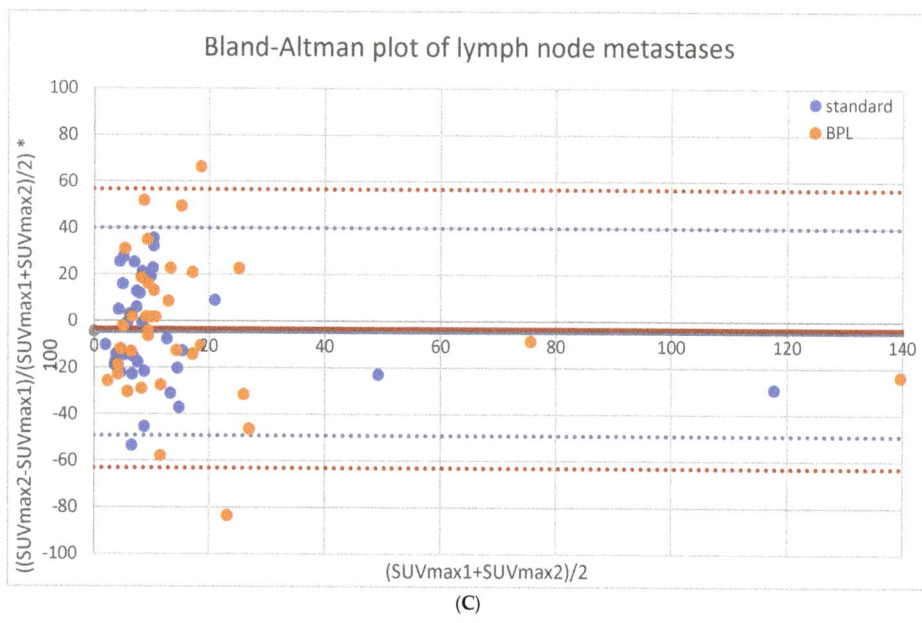

(C)

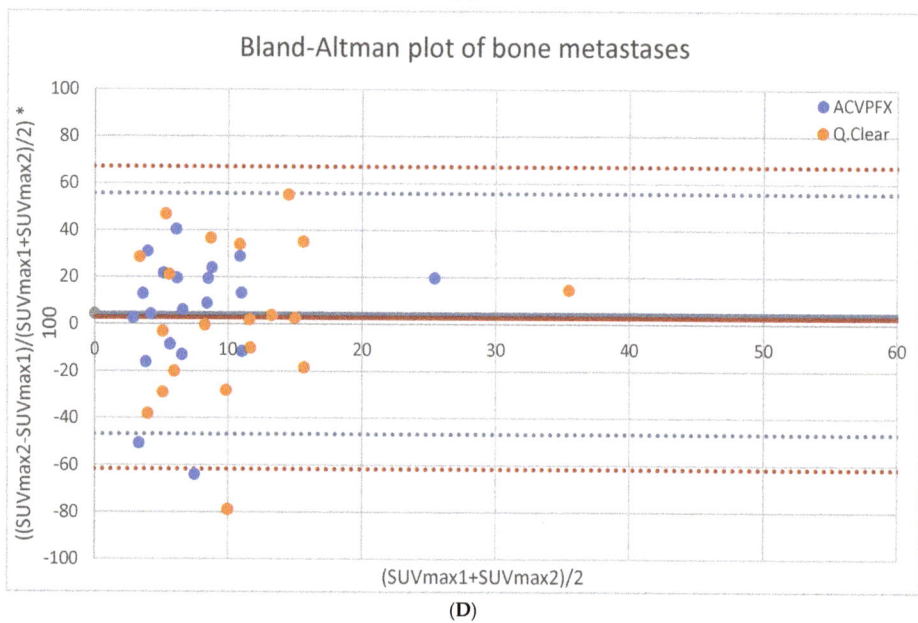

(D)

Figure 1. Repeatability results of SUVmax for both reconstructions in all lesions (65 lesions, (**A**)), local recurrences (9 lesions, (**B**)), lymph node metastases (36 lesions, (**C**)) and bone metastases (20 lesions, (**D**)).

Tumor SUVmax repeatability was dependent on lesion area, with smaller lesions exhibiting poorer repeatability on both standard OSEM and BPL reconstructions (F-test, $p < 0.0001$). See Figure 2A,B.

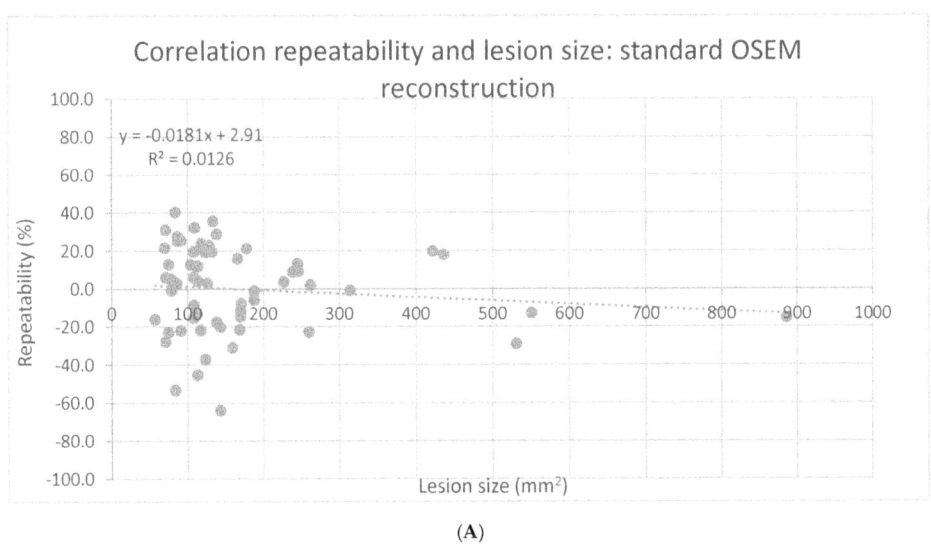

(A)

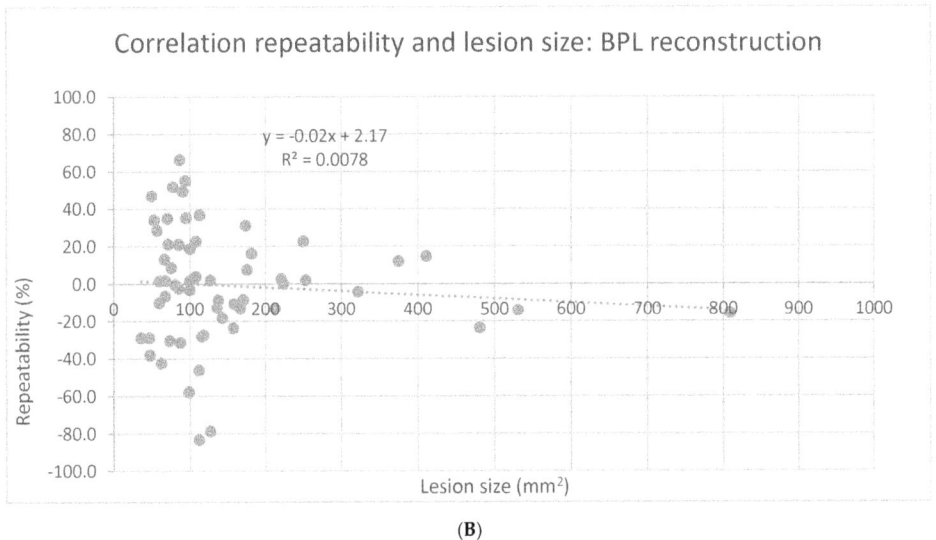

(B)

Figure 2. Correlation between SUVmax repeatability and lesion size for standard OSEM (**A**) and BPL reconstruction (**B**).

Tumor absolute SUVmax was higher in BPL reconstructions than in standard OSEM reconstructions for all lesions (data not shown). The relative increase in measured SUVmax in the BPL reconstructions (as compared to standard OSEM reconstruction) was dependent on lesion size. Smaller lesions (lesion area < 200 mm^2) showed a significant larger increase of SUVmax as compared to larger lesions (lesion area > 200 mm^2): 44.3% ± 4.6% versus 25.5% ± 42.2% for the test scans (p = 0.004) and 43.5% ± 3.9% versus 18.6% ± 3.1% for the retest scans (p < 0.001), respectively. See Table 2.

Table 2. BPL SUVmax increase (relative to standard reconstruction) for smaller and larger lesions.

	Test BPL Relative Increase of Suvmax (%)	SEM	Retest BPL Relative Increase of SUVmax (%)	SEM
lesions < 200 mm^2	44.3	4.6	43.5	3.9
lesions $\geq$ 200 mm^2	25.5	4.2	18.6	3.1
2-sided t-test	$p = 0.004$		$p < 0.001$	

4. Discussion

In this prospective test–retest study, we formally report the repeatability of Ga-68 PSMA in both relapsing and metastatic tumor. The main finding of this study is the relatively high day-to-day variability of tumor SUVmax with repeatability levels of agreement varying between +43% and −46% for all lesions taken together. For local recurrences, values vary between +23% and −33%; for the smaller lymph node and bone metastases, values are +40% to −49% and +56% to −47%, respectively. In addition to this, we show a significant correlation between lesion size and SUVmax repeatability levels of agreement.

With respect to our second aim, no significant differences in repeatability between standard OSEM reconstruction and BPL reconstruction could be shown in this pilot study. There was a small but not significant difference in favor of the standard OSEM reconstruction. However, BPL reconstructions resulted in significantly higher SUVmax of tumor lesions as compared to standard OSEM reconstructions, with significantly higher relative increases in smaller lesions.

Pollard et al. reported on the repeatability of Ga-68 PSMA-HBED-CC (PSMA-11) SUVmax in relapsing prostate cancer [20]. Repeatability levels of agreement were given for lymph node and bone metastases only and were lower than in our study: 30–40% versus 40–60%. Moreover, for other radiotracers like F-18 DCFPyL, F-18 FDG and F-18 FLT, values in the 30–40% range were reported for SUVmax [21,22]. A possible explanation for the higher day-to-day variability in our study is the relative high number of small lesions. Our study hints at a negative correlation between lesion SUVmax variability and lesion size (Figure 2A). We believe the patient cohort of this pilot study to be representative for patients with relapsing prostate cancer showing relatively small tumor lesions in lymph nodes and bones. Pollard et al. did not find any relationship between lesion size and SUVmax variability [20]. A possible explanation for this is that they only reported on relationships within classes, i.e., within typically smaller lymph node and bone metastases, where we report on all lesions including the larger relapses of the primary tumor in the prostate bed. Olde Heuvel et al. also reported on larger tumors in the setting of primary staging of prostate cancer and found smaller day-to-day variability [23].

A larger day-to-day variability may have implications for lesion-specific response in treatment monitoring. With respect to treatment response monitoring using F-18 FDG, Wahl et al. proposed a minimum of 30% SUVmax decrease for a true response in their PERCIST response criteria [24]. Although the PERCIST criteria have not been validated for Ga-68 PSMA PET yet, we think that a minimum of 30% response is probably not appropriate for the majority of the relatively small lesions that are typically found in (early) relapsing prostate cancer. Our study shows that a minimum response of 50% might be more appropriate in these cases, when using Ga-68 PSMA. Being deferred from a single center single vendor study, an even more conservative approach might be warranted when multiple centers and/or vendors are involved.

When confronted with the relatively small tumor lesions in patients with (early) relapsing prostate cancer, partial volume effects have to be anticipated. This will be particularly the case when quantifying tracer expression in small lesions using tracers with high tumor-to-background ratios like Ga-68 PSMA but is not always appreciated [25,26]. For example, in a report on the effects of androgen deprivation therapy on Ga-68 PSMA

SUVmax in primary prostate cancer, lymph node and bone metastases as recent as April 2020, possible impact of partial volume effects was not discussed at all [27].

The possible importance of partial volume effects can be illustrated by the BPL versus standard reconstructions, as applied in our study. Two factors that contribute to the partial volume effect (spill-in and spill-out) are the finite spatial resolution of the imaging system (involving scanner hardware, acquisition parameters and reconstruction method) and image sampling on a discrete voxel grid imperfectly matching the actual contours of tracer distribution [12]. Impact of partial volume effects is strongly dependent on lesion size and is coming into play when lesion size falls below 2 to 3 times the resolution of the system, i.e., below 10 to 15 mm for an average PET/CT scanner system [10]. With respect to tracer SUVmax measurements, partial volume effect will generally result in lower SUVmax values. As SUVmean is usually defined as the average SUV in a 3D isocontour at a certain threshold set as a percentage of the SUVmax [28]. In standard OSEM reconstruction, the number of iterations is very limited, to prevent the emergence of excessive noise [13]. The Bayesian penalized likelihood (BPL) reconstruction algorithm called Q.Clear allows for improved spatial resolution because of its convergence, applying a noise penalty at the voxel level during image reconstruction [14]. The resulting higher uptake/expression values in small lesions (compared to standard reconstruction) have been reported for several radiotracers, including F-18 PSMA-1007 in prostate cancer patients [29]. In the latter study, SUVmax with BPL reconstruction has been compared to standard OSEM reconstruction, stratified for lesion size. A significant reported increase in SUVmax with BPL reconstruction for lesions smaller than 10 mm diameter only was reported. In our study, we confirm these findings for the ^{68}Ga-PSMA tracer, including the relationship with lesion size (Table 2), thus highlighting the importance of partial volume effects and its correction.

We hypothesized that the BPL reconstruction algorithm Q.Clear has the ability to lower signal variability in the small lesions typically encountered in early relapse or early metastatic disease of prostate cancer. Our study did not confirm our hypothesis. On the contrary, signal variability tended to be higher with BPL reconstruction compared to standard reconstruction (although not significant). A possible explanation for this could be the 'overshoot' reported with BPL reconstruction for small spheres at high sphere-to-background ratios in a phantom study using F-18 FDG [30]. The high sphere-to-background ratios in this study may correspond to the high tumor-to-background ratios typically encountered in Ga-68 PSMA avid prostate cancer lesions.

Limitations. This single site study has several limitations. For a formal test–retest study, there is a relatively wide range in administered activity (0.9–1.7 MBq/kg) and time from injection to acquisition (55–69 min). However, in most patients, the activity was administered within reasonable limits with respect to dose and equilibration time, thus reflecting daily practice. Especially, with regard to relatively short-lived radiopharmaceuticals like Ga-68, exact dosing can be cumbersome. For example, timely administration of the radiopharmaceutical was hampered by the pending results of the quality control just prior to injection in some patients. The assignment of tumor lesions was only done by two experienced image readers, and inter-observer variability was not assessed. This was considered acceptable because the exact nature of the lesions was less important in light of the general aim of the study, i.e., assessment of signal variability. The same holds for the fact that for the majority of the lesions there has been no confirmation by histopathology. Moreover, potential detrimental effects of patient motion cannot be ruled out. This may be especially relevant because most lesions were small.

With respect to the comparison of the BPL and standard OSEM reconstructions, the image reading was not blinded. This was deemed acceptable because the visual appearance of both reconstructions is different, precluding true blinded image reading.

No significant difference was found between BPL and standard OSEM reconstruction signal variability, probably because the study was underpowered. Being a pilot study, the results can be used for power calculations for a possible future study.

5. Conclusions

The main finding of this study is the relatively high day-to-day variability of tumor SUVmax with repeatability levels of agreement varying between +43% and −46% for all lesions taken together. Small lesions tend to have larger day-to-day variability of tumor SUVmax when compared to larger lesions. With respect to response monitoring, minimum response of 50% for Ga-68 PSMA PET might be more appropriate.

With respect to our second aim no significant differences in repeatability between standard OSEM reconstruction and BPL reconstruction could be shown in this pilot study. There was a small but not significant difference in favor of the standard reconstruction, however. These results do not support the use of BPL with respect to our hypothesis that it might lower signal variability.

Author Contributions: M.J.R. was the leading contributor to study design, data analysis and interpretation as well as to writing the manuscript. S.R. and A.J.A. were major contributors to study design and to writing the manuscript. C.B. and D.N.W. were major contributors to data analysis and interpretation. All authors have read and agreed to the published version of the manuscript.

Funding: The study was funded by General Electrics Health Care (investigator-sponsored research support for principal investigator Mark J. Roef). The study was investigator driven. General Electrics Health Care played no role in study design, data analysis or in writing the manuscript.

Institutional Review Board Statement: The study was conducted according to the guidelines of the Declaration of Helsinki and approved by the local institutional ethics review board (NL52809.100.16/R16.058/Ga-68 PSMA test–retest study, 27 March 2017).

Informed Consent Statement: Informed consent was obtained from all subjects involved in the study.

Data Availability Statement: The data presented in this study are available on request from the corresponding author.

Acknowledgments: First: we thank all the patients who agreed to participate in the study. Furthermore, we want to thank our PET/CT team for their excellent support. We would also like to thank Marcel van 't Veer for his statistical help.

Conflicts of Interest: The authors declare no conflict of interest. The sponsors had no role in the design, execution, interpretation or writing of the study.

References

1. Global Burden of Disease Cancer Collaboration. Global, Regional, and National Cancer Incidence, Mortality, Years of Life Lost, Years Lived with Disability, and Disability-Adjusted Life-years for 32 Cancer Groups, 1990 to 2015A Systematic Analysis for the Global Burden of Disease Study. *JAMA Oncol.* **2017**, *3*, 524–548. [CrossRef]
2. Mottet, N.; Bellmunt, J.; Bolla, M.; Briers, E.; Cumberbatch, M.G.; De Santis, M.; Fossati, N.; Gross, T.; Henry, A.M.; Joniau, S.; et al. EAU—ESTRO—SIOG Guidelines on Prostate Cancer. Part 1: Screening, Diagnosis, and Local Treatment with Curative Intent. *Eur. Urol.* **2017**, *71*, 618–629. [CrossRef]
3. Moul, J.W. Prostate specific antigen only progression of prostate cancer. *J. Urol.* **2000**, *163*, 1632–1642. [CrossRef]
4. Artibani, W.; Porcaro, A.B.; De Marco, V.; Cerruto, M.A.; Siracusano, S. Management of Biochemical Recurrence after Primary Curative Treatment for Prostate Cancer: A Review. *Urol. Int.* **2018**, *100*, 251–262. [CrossRef] [PubMed]
5. Battaglia, A.; De Meerleer, G.; Tosco, L.; Moris, L.; Van den Broeck, T.; Devos, G.; Everaerts, W.; Joniau, S. Novel Insights into the Management of Oligometastatic Prostate Cancer: A Comprehensive Review. *Eur. Urol. Oncol.* **2019**, *2*, 174–188. [CrossRef] [PubMed]
6. Inubushi, M.; Miura, H.; Kuji, I.; Ito, K.; Minamimoto, R. Current status of radioligand therapy and positron-emission tomography with prostate-specific membrane antigen. *Ann. Nucl. Med.* **2020**, *34*, 879–883. [CrossRef] [PubMed]
7. Miura, N.; Pradere, B.; Mori, K.; Mostafaei, H.; Quhal, F.; Misrai, V.; D'Andrea, D.; Albisinni, S.; Papalia, R.; Saika, T.; et al. Metastasis-directed therapy and prostate-targeted therapy in oligometastatic prostate cancer: A systematic review. *Minerva Urol. Nefrol.* **2020**, *72*, 531–542. [CrossRef]
8. de Langen, A.J.; Vincent, A.; Velasquez, L.M.; Van Tinteren, H.; Boellaard, R.; Shankar, L.K.; Boers, M.; Smit, E.F.; Stroobants, S.; Weber, W.A.; et al. Repeatability of 18F-FDG uptake measurements in tumors: A metaanalysis. *J. Nucl. Med.* **2012**, *53*, 701–708. [CrossRef]

9. Aide, N.; Lasnon, C.; Veit-Haibach, P.; Sera, T.; Sattler, B.; Boellaard, R. EANM/EARL harmonization strategies in PET quantification: From daily practice to multicentre oncological studies. *Eur. J. Nucl. Med. Mol. Imaging* 2017, *44* (Suppl. 1), 17–31. [CrossRef]
10. Hoffman, E.J.; Huang, S.-C.; Phelps, M.E. Quantitation in positron emission computed tomography: 1. Effect of object size. *J. Comput. Assist. Tomogr.* 1979, *3*, 299–308. [CrossRef]
11. Kessler, R.M.; Ellis, J.R.; Eden, M. Analysis of emission tomographic scan data: Limitations imposed by resoulution and background. *J. Comput. Assist. Tomogr.* 1984, *8*, 514–522. [CrossRef] [PubMed]
12. Rogasch, J.M.; Suleiman, S.; Hofheinz, F.; Bluemel, S.; Lukas, M.; Amthauer, H.; Furth, C. Reconstructed spatial resolution and contrast recovery with Bayesian penalized likelihood reconstruction (Q.Clear) for FDG-PET compared to time-of-flight (TOF) with point spread function (PSF). *EJNMMI Phys.* 2020, *7*, 2. [CrossRef]
13. Jaskowiak, C.J.; Bianco, J.A.; Perlman, S.B.; Fine, J.P. Influence of reconstruction iterations on 18F-FDG PET/CT standardized uptake values. *J. Nucl. Med.* 2005, *46*, 424–428.
14. Teoh, E.J.; McGowan, D.R.; Macpherson, R.E.; Bradley, K.M.; Gleeson, F.V. Phantom and Clinical Evaluation of the Bayesian Penalized Likelihood Reconstruction Algorithm Q.Clear on an LYSO PET/CT System. *J. Nucl. Med.* 2015, *56*, 1447–1452. [CrossRef] [PubMed]
15. Teoh, E.J.; McGowan, D.R.; Bradley, K.M.; Belcher, E.; Black, E.; Gleeson, F.V. Novel penalised likelihood reconstruction of PET in the assessment of histologically verified small pulmonary nodules. *Eur. Radiol.* 2016, *26*, 576–584. [CrossRef]
16. Howard, B.A.; Morgan, R.; Thorpe, M.P.; Turkington, T.G.; Oldan, J.; James, O.G.; Borges-Neto, S. Comparison of Bayesian penalized likelihood reconstruction versus OS-EM for cahracterization of small pulmonary nodules in oncologic PET/CT. *Ann. Nucl. Med.* 2017, *31*, 623–628. [CrossRef]
17. Te Riet, J.; Rijnsdorp, S.; Roef, M.J.; Arends, A.J. Evaluation of a Bayesian penalized likelihood reconstruction algorithm for low-counts clinical 18F-FDG PET/CT. *EJNMMI Phys.* 2019, *6*, 32. [CrossRef]
18. Zaki, R.; Bulgiba, A.; Ismail, R.; Ismail, N.A. Statistical methods used to test for agreement of medical instruments measuring continuous variables in method comparison studies: A systematic review. *PLoS ONE* 2012, *7*, e37908. [CrossRef] [PubMed]
19. Lodge, M.A. Repeatability of SUV in Oncologic 18 F-FDG PET. *J. Nucl. Med.* 2017, *58*, 523–532. [CrossRef]
20. Pollard, J.H.; Raman, C.; Zakharia, Y.; Tracy, C.R.; Nepple, K.G.; Ginader, T.; Breheny, P.; Sunderland, J.J. Quantitative test-retest measurement of ^{68}Ga-PSMA-HBED-CC (PSMA-11) in tumor and normal tissue. *J. Nucl. Med.* 2020, *61*, 1145–1152. [CrossRef]
21. Jansen, B.H.E.; Cysouw, M.C.F.; Vis, A.N.; Van Moorselaar, R.J.A.; Voortman, J.; Bodar, Y.J.L.; Schober, P.R.; Hendrikse, N.H.; Hoekstra, O.S.; Boellaard, R.; et al. Repeatability of Quantitative ^{18}F-DCFPyL PET/CT Measurements in Metastatic Prostate Cancer. *J. Nucl. Med.* 2020, *61*, 1320–1325. [CrossRef]
22. Hatt, M.; Cheze-Le Rest, C.; Aboagye, E.O.; Kenny, L.M.; Rosso, L.; Turkheimer, F.E.; Albarghach, N.M.; Metges, J.P.; Pradier, O.; Visvikis, D. Reproducibility of 18F-FDG and 3′-deoxy-3′-18F-fluorothymidine PET Tumor Volume Measurements. *J. Nucl. Med.* 2010, *51*, 1368–1376. [CrossRef]
23. Olde Heuvel, J.; de Wit-van der Veen, B.J.; Donswijk, M.L.; Slump, C.H.; Stokkel, M.P.M. Day-to-day variability of [^{68}Ga]Ga-PSMA-11 accumulation in primary prostate cancer: Effects on tracer uptake and visual interpretation. *EJNMMI Res.* 2020, *10*, 132. [CrossRef] [PubMed]
24. Wahl, R.L.; Jacene, H.; Kasamon, Y.; Lodge, M.A. From RECIST to PERCIST: Evolving Considerations for PET Response Criteria in Solid Tumors. *J. Nucl. Med.* 2009, *50* (Suppl. 1), 122S–150S. [CrossRef] [PubMed]
25. Afshar-Oromieh, A.; Malcher, A.; Eder, M.; Eisenhut, M.; Linhart, H.G.; Hadaschik, B.A.; Holland-Letz, T.; Giesel, F.L.; Kratochwil, C.; Haufe, S.; et al. PET imaging with a [68Ga]gallium-labelled PSMA ligand for the diagnosis of prostate cancer: Biodistribution in humans and first evaluation of tumour lesions. *Eur. J. Nucl. Med. Mol. Imaging* 2013, *40*, 486–495. [CrossRef]
26. Berliner, C.; Tienken, M.; Frenzel, T.; Kobayashi, Y.; Helberg, A.; Kirchner, U.; Klutmann, S.; Beyersdorff, D.; Budäus, L.; Wester, H.J.; et al. Detection rate of PET/CT in patients with biochemical relapse of prostate cancer using [68Ga]PSMA I&T and comparison with published data of [68Ga]PSMA HBED-CC. *Eur. J. Nucl. Med. Mol. Imaging* 2017, *44*, 670–677.
27. Ettala, O.; Malaspina, S.; Tuokkola, T.; Luoto, P.; Löyttyniemi, E.; Boström, P.J.; Kemppainen, J. Prospective Study on the Effect of Short-Term Androgen Deprivation Therapy on PSMA Uptake Evaluated With ^{68}Ga-PSMA-11 PET/MRI in Men With treatment-naïve Prostate Cancer. *Eur. J. Nucl. Med. Mol. Imaging* 2020, *47*, 665–673. [CrossRef] [PubMed]
28. Boellaard, R.; O'Doherty, M.J.; Weber, W.A.; Mottaghy, F.M.; Lonsdale, M.N.; Stroobants, S.G.; Oyen, W.J.; Kotzerke, J.; Hoekstra, O.S.; Pruim, J.; et al. FDG PET and PET/CT: EANM procedure guidelines for tumour PET imaging version 1.0. *Eur. J. Nucl. Med. Mol. Imaging* 2010, *37*, 181–200. [CrossRef]
29. Witkowska-Patena, E.; Budzyńska, A.; Giżewska, A.; Dziuk, M.; Walęcka-Mazur, A. Ordered Subset Expectation Maximisation vs Bayesian Penalised Likelihood Reconstruction Algorithm in 18F-PSMA-1007 PET/CT. *Ann. Nucl. Med.* 2020, *34*, 192–199. [CrossRef]
30. Yamaguchi, S.; Wagatsuma, K.; Miwa, K.; Ishii, K.; Inoue, K.; Fukushi, M. Bayesian Penalized-Likelihood Reconstruction Algorithm Suppresses Edge Artifacts in PET Reconstruction Based on Point-Spread-Function. *Phys. Med.* 2018, *47*, 73–79. [CrossRef]

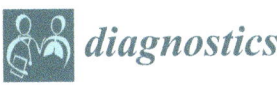

Article

Prognostic Value of Combing Primary Tumor and Nodal Glycolytic–Volumetric Parameters of ^{18}F-FDG PET in Patients with Non-Small Cell Lung Cancer and Regional Lymph Node Metastasis

Yu-Hung Chen [1,2], Sung-Chao Chu [2,3], Ling-Yi Wang [4], Tso-Fu Wang [2,3], Kun-Han Lue [5], Chih-Bin Lin [2,6], Bee-Song Chang [7], Dai-Wei Liu [2,8], Shu-Hsin Liu [1,5] and Sheng-Chieh Chan [1,2,*]

[1] Department of Nuclear Medicine, Hualien Tzu Chi Hospital, Buddhist Tzu Chi Medical Foundation, Hualien 97002, Taiwan; jedimasterchen@hotmail.com (Y.-H.C.); kaopectin@yahoo.com.tw (S.-H.L.)
[2] School of Medicine, College of Medicine, Tzu Chi University, Hualien 97002, Taiwan; oldguy-chu1129@umail.hinet.net (S.-C.C.); tfwang@tzuchi.com.tw (T.-F.W.); ferlin@tzuchi.com.tw (C.-B.L.); dwliu5177@yahoo.com.tw (D.-W.L.)
[3] Department of Hematology and Oncology, Hualien Tzu Chi Hospital, Buddhist Tzu Chi Medical Foundation, Hualien 97002, Taiwan
[4] Epidemiology and Biostatistics Consulting Center, Department of Medical Research, Hualien Tzu Chi Hospital, Buddhist Tzu Chi Medical Foundation and Department of Pharmacy, School of Medicine, Tzu Chi University, Hualien 97002, Taiwan; wangly1212@gmail.com
[5] Department of Medical Imaging and Radiological Sciences, Tzu Chi University of Science and Technology, Hualien 97005, Taiwan; john.lue@protonmail.com
[6] Department of Internal Medicine, Hualien Tzu Chi Hospital, Buddhist Tzu Chi Medical Foundation, Hualien 97002, Taiwan
[7] Department of Cardiothoracic Surgery, Hualien Tzu Chi Hospital, Buddhist Tzu Chi Medical Foundation, Hualien 97002, Taiwan; rr122336@gmail.com
[8] Department of Radiation Oncology, Hualien Tzu Chi Hospital, Buddhist Tzu Chi Medical Foundation, Hualien 97002, Taiwan
* Correspondence: williamsm.tw@gmail.com; Tel.: +886-3-856-1825

Abstract: We investigated whether the combination of primary tumor and nodal ^{18}F-FDG PET parameters predict survival outcomes in patients with nodal metastatic non-small cell lung cancer (NSCLC) without distant metastasis. We retrospectively extracted pre-treatment ^{18}F-FDG PET parameters from 89 nodal-positive NSCLC patients (stage IIB–IIIC). The Cox proportional hazard model was used to identify independent prognosticators of overall survival (OS) and progression-free survival (PFS). We devised survival stratification models based on the independent prognosticators and compared the model to the American Joint Committee on Cancer (AJCC) staging system using Harrell's concordance index (c-index). Our results demonstrated that total TLG (the combination of primary tumor and nodal total lesion glycolysis) and age were independent risk factors for unfavorable OS ($p < 0.001$ and $p = 0.001$) and PFS (both $p < 0.001$), while the Eastern Cooperative Oncology Group scale independently predicted poor OS ($p = 0.022$). Our models based on the independent prognosticators outperformed the AJCC staging system (c-index = 0.732 versus 0.544 for OS and c-index = 0.672 versus 0.521 for PFS, both $p < 0.001$). Our results indicate that incorporating total TLG with clinical factors may refine risk stratification in nodal metastatic NSCLC patients and may facilitate tailored therapeutic strategies in this patient group.

Keywords: ^{18}F-FDG; PET; non-small cell lung cancer; prognosis; glycolytic; volumetric

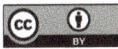

1. Introduction

The incidence of lung cancer is the highest among all types of cancers, with lung cancer being the leading cause of cancer mortality worldwide [1–3]. Non-small cell lung cancer (NSCLC) accounts for 85% of all lung cancer cases [4–6]. In patients with NSCLC without distant metastasis, regional lymph node metastasis is common; 13.0% to 40.3% of these cases develop nodal metastases despite early primary tumor status [7]. With current therapeutic advances, regional nodal metastasis without distant spreading can be curatively treated by definitive concurrent chemoradiotherapy (CCRT), radiotherapy, or surgery. However, the treatment response and survival outcome of NSCLC cases with regional nodal metastasis are quite heterogeneous. The 5 year overall survival (OS) rates range from 9% to 60% [8–11]. Furthermore, the nodal classification in the eighth edition of the American Joint Committee on Cancer (AJCC) may be inadequate for prognostic stratification of NSCLC cases with regional lymph node metastasis [11–13]. Therefore, a more reliable prognosticator is imperative in this patient group to guide more sophisticated risk-adapted treatment strategies.

^{18}F-fluorodeoxyglucose (^{18}F-FDG) positron emission tomography (PET) is highly sensitive for detecting the disease extent of NSCLC, and this imaging modality has become the standard-of-care tool for staging and re-staging patients with NSCLC [14]. Because ^{18}F-FDG PET provides a way of featuring the glycolytic activity of the tumor, it is also able to represent the tumor viability and can be used to assess the treatment response [15]. Furthermore, the glycolytic activity in tumors is associated with vicious signaling pathways [16,17]. Several ^{18}F-FDG PET semiquantitative parameters have been developed to quantify the glycolytic activity and metabolic volume of tumors, including standardized uptake value (SUV) and volumetric parameters such as the metabolic tumor volume (MTV) and total lesion glycolysis (TLG). Higher metabolic activity and larger metabolic burdens are associated with worse survival outcomes; thus, many studies have focused on the use of ^{18}F-FDG PET-derived semiquantitative parameters as prognostic biomarkers to predict survival outcomes in patients with NSCLC [15,18–21]. In addition, the semiquantitative ^{18}F-FDG PET parameters can not only be derived from the primary tumor but can also be measured from the metastatic nodes, as the genotypes and the consequent phenotypes may not be the same in the metastatic lesions and primary tumors [22,23]. To date, most studies for nodal metastatic NSCLC have evaluated the ^{18}F-FDG PET parameters from the primary tumor and metastatic lesions separately; studies combining ^{18}F-FDG PET parameters from both metastatic nodes and primary tumor in nodal metastatic NSCLC are limited [21].

Therefore, the objective of this study was to investigate the feasibility of combining ^{18}F-FDG PET parameters from primary tumors with regional metastatic nodes to assess the survival outcomes in patients with nodal-positive NSCLC without distant metastasis.

2. Materials and Methods

2.1. Patient Population

This retrospective study was conducted in accordance with the Declaration of Helsinki and the protocol was approved by the local Institutional Review Board and Ethics Committee at our hospital (IRB109-235-B). Due to the retrospective nature of this study, the requirement of informed consent for this study was waived. We retrospectively enrolled patients with a new diagnosis of NSCLC from January 2010 to September 2019. The diagnoses of NSCLC in all study patients were established using histopathology. Serial examinations were performed in all study participants for lung cancer staging and treatment planning at the time of the initial diagnosis. The examinations included contrast-enhanced computed tomography (CT) of the chest to the upper abdomen, ^{18}F-FDG PET/CT, gadolinium-enhanced MRI of the brain, and pulmonary function tests. For lesions in the images that were indicative of malignancy, image-guided biopsies were collected whenever possible. If biopsies were not feasible or if the biopsy result was negative, the patient was closely monitored with imaging. Patients were re-staging according to the eighth edition of the AJCC staging manual [13]. We only included patients with a clinically positive regional nodal metastatic disease (patients with an N1 to N3 classification were included) and without evidence of distant metastasis at the time of the initial diagnosis. Patients' daily living performance at the initial diagnosis was assessed using the Eastern Cooperative Oncology Group scale (ECOG) [24]. Patients included in this study received curative surgery (resection of the primary tumor and mediastinal lymph node dissection) with or without neoadjuvant CCRT, definitive CCRT, or definitive radiotherapy as the initial treatment. The radiotherapy dose was 2 Gy/fraction daily up to a targeted dose of 60 to 66 Gy. A cisplatin-based chemotherapeutic regimen was administered if CCRT was chosen as the initial treatment [25,26]. Patients receiving only systemic chemotherapy or target therapy were excluded. The choice of first-line treatment was based on the decision of the attending physician. The findings of all examinations in each individual and the pre-treatment staging were discussed and determined at a multidisciplinary lung cancer conference convened by our thoracic oncology research team.

2.2. Imaging Protocol and Analysis of ^{18}F-FDG PET Scan

All study participants fasted for at least 4 h before ^{18}F-FDG injection (400 MBq) and had blood glucose levels no greater than 200 mg/dL. The ^{18}F-FDG PET/CT scans were performed 45 to 60 min after radiotracer administration using a GE Discovery ST scanner (GE Healthcare, Milwaukee, WI, USA). The PET/CT system was equipped with a PET unit containing 10,080 bismuth germanate crystals in 24 rings and a 16-detector row transmission CT unit. CT scans were performed first for attenuation correction without administration of contrast medium. The voltage and current of the tube were 120 kV and 120 mA, respectively. The pitch of the CT was 1.75 and sampling of CT images was done in the helical mode with a helical thickness of 3.75 mm. Immediately after the transmission CT, PET images were acquired from the midthigh to the vertex in a static 3-dimensional mode. The scanning time was three min for each table position (15 cm for each table position, with a 3 cm overlap for every contiguous frame). PET images were reconstructed with an ordered-subset expectation maximization algorithm (2 iterations, 21 subsets, and a 2.14 mm full width at half maximum Gaussian post-filter). The imaging matrix size, pixel size, and slice thickness for the reconstructed PET images were 128 × 128, 5.47 × 5.47, and 3.27 mm, respectively.

The platform used for display and semiquantitative analysis of ^{18}F-FDG PET/CT images was a PMOD 4.0 system (PMOD Technologies Ltd., Zurich, Switzerland). An experienced nuclear medicine physician interpreted the ^{18}F-FDG PET images. For image quantification, the experienced nuclear medicine physician identified and placed the volume-of-interest (VOI) on the primary tumor and the regional metastatic nodes on the ^{18}F-FDG PET/CT image. The VOIs were placed and segmented separately for the primary tumor and the metastatic nodes. The SUV of ^{18}F-FDG PET was calculated and normalized to each patient's body weight as follows:

$$SUV = \frac{(decay - corrected\ activity\ (kBq)\ per\ milliliter\ of\ tissue\ volume)}{(injected\ 18F - FDG\ activity\ (kBq)/body\ weight\ in\ g)}$$

The ^{18}F-FDG lesions were segmented using a 41% threshold of the maximum standard uptake value method [27]. The segmented volumes were used to define the MTV. The PMOD 4.0 software automatically generated the mean SUV within the MTV. The TLG was then calculated as TLV = mean SUV × MTV. The VOI and segmentation results were confirmed by another expert nuclear medicine physician. We recorded the SUV_{max} and TLG values of the primary tumors (described as primary tumor SUV_{max} and primary tumor TLG) and the regional metastatic nodes (nodal SUV_{max} and nodal TLG). Furthermore, we calculated the nodal to primary tumor SUV_{max} ratio (NTSUVR), the nodal to primary tumor TLG ratio (NTTLGR), the product of the primary tumor and nodal SUV_{max} (TNSUVproduct), and the sum of the primary tumor and nodal TLG (total TLG) based on the following formulas:

$$\text{NTSUVR} = \frac{(\text{nodal SUVmax})}{(\text{primary tumor SUVmax})}$$

$$\text{NTTLGR} = \frac{(\text{nodal TLG})}{(\text{primary tumor TLG})}$$

$$\text{TNSUVproduct} = (\text{primary tumor SUVmax}) \times (\text{nodal SUVmax})$$

$$\text{total TLG} = \text{primary tumor TLG} + \text{nodal TLG}$$

The procedure used for image feature extraction is outlined in Figure 1.

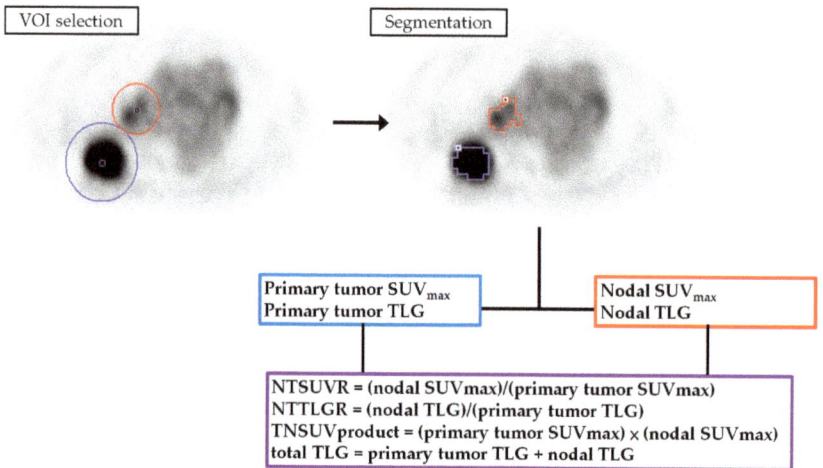

Figure 1. The method used for feature extraction from ^{18}F-FDG PET. VOI, volume-of-interest; SUV, standardized uptake value; TLG, total lesion glycolysis; NTSUVR, nodal to primary tumor SUV$_{max}$ ratio; NTTLGR, nodal to primary tumor TLG ratio; TNSUVproduct, product of primary tumor and nodal SUV$_{max}$.

2.3. Follow-Up of Study Participants

After diagnosis, we followed patients with weekly outpatient clinic visits during treatment, at 3-month intervals after initial curative treatment, at 6-month intervals for 2 years, and annually thereafter. When signs of disease recurrence or progression emerged, contrast-enhanced CT, gadolinium-enhanced MRI of the brain, or ^{18}F-FDG PET/CT were performed. Biopsies were taken for suspicious lesions whenever possible. New bloody effusion or positive fluid cytology was considered as recurrence or disease progression.

2.4. Data Analysis

We followed all study participants until death or March 2021 (whichever occurred first). Patient demographics were expressed as frequencies (percentage), means (standard deviation), or medians (interquartile range). The primary endpoints were OS and progression-free survival (PFS). The OS was defined as the date of cancer diagnosis to the date of death or censored at the date of the last follow-up for surviving patients. PFS was calculated from the date of treatment initiation to the date of disease progression (e.g., growth of a residual tumor or development of new metastatic lesion), the date of disease recurrence after complete remission, the date of death, or censoring at the date of the last follow-up. Continuous variables were selected and the optimal cut-off values for each continuous variable were determined using receiver-operating characteristic (ROC) curve analyses. Only variables that were statistically significant predictors of death in the ROC curve analyses were selected for the survival analysis. Cut-off values with the highest summation of sensitivity and specificity were selected as the optimal cut-offs for each continuous variable [28–30]. The variable selection and optimal cut-off determinations are summarized in the Supplementary Table S1. The continuous variables adjusted in the survival analysis were age, primary tumor SUV_{max}, primary tumor TLG, nodal SUV_{max}, nodal TLG, total TLG, and TNSUVproduct, and their optimal cut-off values were 75.5, 8.05, 42.5, 2.94, 18.3, 81, and 27, respectively. We used univariate and multivariate Cox regression analyses to study the association of the study variables with survival outcomes. First, we tested the effects of each variable on OS and PFS using univariate analyses. Then, the statistically significant variables from the univariate analysis were incorporated into the multivariate analysis to identify independent predictors of survival. We expressed the results of the survival analysis as hazard ratios (HR) and 95% confidence intervals. Statistical analyses were performed using SPSS software (version 20.0; SPSS Inc., Chicago, IL, USA).

The results of the multivariate Cox regression analysis were used to model the OS and PFS. The patient survival hazard was calculated by multiplying the HRs of the existing independent risk factors. For example, if a patient had three independent risk factors (HR1–HR3), the total hazard for this patient was calculated as HR1 × HR2 × HR3. If a patient had no risk factors, then the total hazard was the baseline hazard. If a patient had risk factors 1 and 3, then the risk of having shorter survival compared to no risk factor was HR1 × HR3.

2.5. Survival Model Validation and Comparison

The results of the multivariate Cox regression survival analysis were validated using the bootstrapping method. The validation process was performed with 1000 bootstrap samples. The results of bootstrapping validation were expressed as β, bias-corrected accelerated 95% confidence intervals, standard errors, and *p*-values. The validation process was executed using SPSS software (version 20.0; SPSS Inc., Chicago, IL, USA). The performance of our Cox regression models was assessed and compared with the AJCC staging system using Harrell's concordance index (c-index) and Kaplan–Meier curves (log-rank test) [19,31]. Different c-indices were compared using the "compareC" package installed on the R open-source statistical software version 3.4.2 (R Foundation, Vienna, Austria). A two-tailed *p*-value of <0.05 was considered statistically significant.

3. Results

3.1. Patient Characteristics

Eighty-nine patients were eligible for analysis, whose baseline characteristics are summarized in Table 1. In total, 15 (16.9%), 53 (59.6%), and 21 (23.6%) patients were clinically classified as N1, N2, and N3 status, respectively. Thirty-seven (41.6%) patients received curative surgery or neoadjuvant CCRT and surgery as the initial treatment. Fifty-two (58.4%) patients received definitive CCRT or definitive radiotherapy. The median (interquartile range, IQR) time from the ^{18}F-FDG PET/CT to initiation of treatment was 14 (12) days. The median follow-up period was 25.4 months (range, 1.7–130.2 months) for all patients and 48.7 months (range, 10.0–130.2 months) for the 34 surviving patients. Sixty (67.4%) patients experienced recurrence or disease progression after or during the initial treatment; 32 of these patients had locoregional recurrence or progression only and 15 patients developed distant metastases without locoregional failure. The remaining 13 patients had both locoregional failure and distant metastasis. By the time of the last follow-up, 55 (61.8%) patients died. The 5-year OS and PFS rates were 33.4% and 24.7%, respectively.

Table 1. Baseline characteristics for patients in this study ($n = 89$).

Characteristics	Value
Age, years, mean ± SD	67 ± 11.4
Sex, n (%)	
Male	59 (66.3)
Female	30 (33.7)
Histology	
Adenocarcinoma	43 (48.3)
Squamous cell carcinoma	45 (50.6)
NSCLC—otherwise specified	1 (1.1)
T classification, n (%) [a]	
T1b	2 (2.2)
T1c	16 (18.0)
T2a	10 (11.2)
T2b	11 (12.3)
T3	25 (28.1)
T4	25 (28.1)
N classification, n (%) [a]	
N1	15 (16.9)
N2	53 (59.6)
N3	21 (23.6)
Overall stage, n (%) [a]	
Stage IIB	12 (13.5)
Stage IIIA	23 (25.8)
Stage IIIB	41 (46.1)
Stage IIIC	13 (14.6)
ECOG, n (%)	
0	20 (22.5)
1	59 (66.3)
2	9 (10.1)
3	1 (1.1)
Initial treatment, n (%)	
Surgery	30 (33.7)
Neoadjuvant CCRT and surgery	7 (7.9)
Definitive CCRT	33 (37.0)
Definitive Radiotherapy	19 (21.4)
Time from ^{18}F-FDG PET to initial treatment, d, median (IQR)	14 (12)
Quantitative analysis of ^{18}F-FDG PET, mean ± SD	
Primary tumor SUV_{max}	11.3 ± 5.22
Primary tumor TLG	292.1 ± 420.86
Nodal SUVmax	7.0 ± 4.96
NTSUVR	0.68 ± 0.415
Nodal TLG	67.4 ± 161.46
NTTLGR	0.79 ± 2.023
total TLG	359.6 ± 489.10
TNSUVproduct	89.7 ± 89.74

NSCLC, non-small cell lung cancer; ECOG, Eastern Cooperative Oncology Group; CCRT, concurrent chemoradiotherapy; SD, standard deviation; IQR, interquartile range; SUV, standardized uptake value; TLG, total lesion glycolysis; NTSUVR, nodal to primary tumor SUV_{max} ratio; NTTLGR, nodal to primary tumor TLG ratio; TNSUVproduct, product of primary tumor and nodal SUV_{max}. [a] Staging according to 8th edition of American Joint Committee on Cancer manual.

3.2. Univariate and Multivariate Survival Analyses

Our ROC curve analysis identified six semiquantitative ^{18}F-FDG PET parameters that were associated with patient death. These parameters were included in the survival analysis (Supplementary Table S1), including the primary tumor SUV_{max}, primary tumor TLG, nodal SUV_{max}, nodal TLG, total TLG, and TNSUVproduct. The median OS and median PFS were 31.5 months (range, 1.7–130.2 months) and 15.1 months (range, 0.2–126.8 months), respectively. The results of the univariate and multivariate Cox regression analyses are outlined in Table 2. The univariate analysis of OS showed that age > 75.5 year-old, squamous cell pathology, T2–T4 disease, ECOG status > 0, never received surgery, only received radiotherapy, primary tumor SUV_{max} > 8.05, primary tumor TLG > 42.5, nodal SUV_{max} > 2.94, nodal TLG > 18.3, total TLG > 81, and TNSUVproduct > 27 were associated with shorter OS. The univariate Cox regression analysis for PFS showed that age >75.5 year-old, never received surgery, only received radiotherapy, primary tumor SUV_{max} > 8.05, primary tumor TLG > 42.5, total TLG > 81, and NSUVproduct > 27 were predictive of shorter time to progression. The statistically significant variables in the univariate analysis were fitted into multivariate Cox regression models. Age > 75.5 year-old, ECOG status > 0, and total TLG > 81 independently predicted unfavorable OS, whereas age > 75.5 year-old and total TLG > 81 were independent risk factors for shorter PFS.

Table 2. Univariate and multivariate analyses for survival prognostic factors.

Variable	No.	OS Univariate HR (95% CI)	p-Value	OS Multivariate HR (95% CI)	p-Value	PFS Univariate HR (95% CI)	p-Value	PFS Multivariate HR (95% CI)	p-Value
Age			<0.001		0.001		0.001		<0.001
>75.5	24	2.8 (1.6–4.9)		2.6 (1.5–4.6)		2.5 (1.5–4.2)		2.7 (1.6–4.7)	
≤75.5	65	Reference		Reference		Reference		Reference	
Histopathology			0.012		0.126		0.175		NA
Squamous cell	45	2.0 (1.2–3.5)				1.4 (0.9–2.3)			
Others	44	Reference				Reference			
At least T2 disease			0.045		0.590		0.053		NA
Yes	71	2.3 (1.0–5.0)				2.0 (1.0–3.9)			
No	18	Reference				Reference			
N3 disease			0.303		NA		0.408		NA
Yes	21	1.4 (0.8–2.5)				1.3 (0.7–2.2)			
No	68	Reference				Reference			
Staging			0.257		NA		0.169		NA
Stage III	77	1.6 (0.7–3.8)				1.7 (0.8–3.8)			
Stage II	12	Reference				Reference			
ECOG status			0.007		0.022		0.084		NA
ECOG > 0	69	4.1 (1.5–11.4)		3.3 (1.2–9.4)		1.8 (0.9–3.6)			
ECOG = 0	20	Reference		Reference		Reference			
Received surgery [a]			0.001		0.240		0.030		0.938
Absence	52	2.6 (1.5–4.7)				1.8 (1.1–2.9)			
Presence	37	Reference				Reference			
Radiotherapy only [b]			<0.001		0.338		0.002		0.642
Yes	19	3.2 (1.8–5.6)				2.4 (1.4–4.2)			
No	70	Reference				Reference			
Primary tumor SUV_{max}			<0.001		0.135		<0.001		0.238
>8.05	62	4.9 (2.2–10.9)				3.0 (1.6–5.6)			
≤8.05	27	Reference				Reference			
Primary tumor TLG			0.001		0.873		0.024		0.064
>42.5	63	3.7 (1.7–8.3)				2.0 (1.1–3.6)			
≤42.5	26	Reference				Reference			
Nodal SUVmax			0.012		0.114		0.204		NA
>2.94	70	3.0 (1.3–6.9)				1.5 (0.8–2.8)			
≤2.94	19	Reference				Reference			
Nodal TLG			0.014		0.454		0.104		NA
>18.3	40	2.0 (1.1–3.3)				1.5 (0.9–2.4)			
≤18.3	49	Reference				Reference			
total TLG			<0.001		<0.001		0.001		<0.001
>81	63	5.2 (2.2–12.2)		5.1 (2.2–12.0)		3.0 (1.6–5.7)		3.3 (1.7–6.2)	
≤81	26	Reference		Reference		Reference		Reference	
TNSUVproduct			<0.001		0.164		0.011		0.481
>27	67	5.3 (2.1–13.3)				2.3 (1.2–4.3)			
≤27	22	Reference				Reference			

OS, overall survival; PFS, progression-free survival; HR, hazard ratio; CI, confidence interval; ECOG, Eastern Cooperative Oncology Group; SUV, standardized uptake value; TLG, total lesion glycolysis; TNSUVproduct, product of primary tumor and nodal SUV_{max}; NA, not applicable. [a] Received curative surgery or neoadjuvant chemoradiation followed by curative surgery. [b] Only received radiotherapy as the initial treatment.

3.3. Survival Model Construction and Validation

The independent risk factors were used to develop prediction models for OS (age > 75.5 years, ECOG > 0, and total TLG > 81) and PFS (age > 75.5 years and total TLG > 81). The construction of our survival models is demonstrated in the Supplementary Figure S1. The risk for each patient was calculated by multiplying the hazard ratio of each risk factor. In the OS model, the HRs for age > 75.5 years, ECOG > 0, and total TLG > 81 were 2.6, 3.3, and 5.1, respectively; in the PFS model, the HRs for age > 75.5 years and total TLG > 81 were 2.7 and 3.3, respectively (Table 2). If a patient had all three independent risk factors for OS, the total hazard of poor OS for this patient was 43.8 (2.6 × 3.3 × 5.1). If a patient had no risk factor, then the total hazard was the baseline hazard. If a patient was > 75.5 years and had a total TLG > 81, then the risks of having a shorter OS and poor PFS compared to no risk factor would be 13.3 (2.6 × 5.1) and 8.9 (2.7 × 3.3), respectively. The resulting hazards ranged from 1 to 43.8 for the OS model and 1 to 8.9 for the PFS model. Patients with similar 5 year survival outcomes in the Kaplan–Meier curve analysis were re-stratified into one risk group. Finally, we obtained three separate risk categories (HR < 3, HR = 3–10, and HR > 10 for the OS model; HR < 3, HR = 3–5, and HR > 5 for the PFS model).

The bootstrap method was used to validate our survival analysis results. Supplementary Table S2 presents the results of the bootstrap validation. The β estimate of each independent prognosticator was statistically significant in predicting OS and PFS.

3.4. Model Performance and Comparison to AJCC Staging System

The Cox regression models in our study significantly stratified patients into different survival risk groups (Figure 2). The c-indices of our Cox regression model for OS and PFS were 0.732 and 0.672, respectively. The Cox regression model developed in our study cohort significantly outperformed the AJCC staging system. In addition, our models (combining the independent clinical prognosticators with total TLG) showed the highest c-indices compared with other models using the combination of independent clinical risk factors with primary tumor TLG or nodal TLG (Table 3).

Table 3. A Comparison of the c-indices between the traditional cancer staging system and our models.

Model	c-Index for OS	p-Value [d]	c-Index for PFS	p-Value [d]
AJCC staging system [a]	0.544	NA	0.521	NA
Our Cox regression model	0.732	<0.001	0.672	<0.001
Model with primary tumor TLG [b]	0.696	0.002	0.639	0.012
Model with nodal TLG [c]	0.708	0.001	0.632	0.010

NA, not applicable; AJCC, American Joint Committee on Cancer; TLG, total lesion glycolysis. [a] Staging according to 8th edition of AJCC manual. [b] Model constructed from the independent clinical risk factors and primary tumor TLG. [c] Model constructed from the independent clinical risk factors and nodal TLG. [d] In comparison with AJCC staging system.

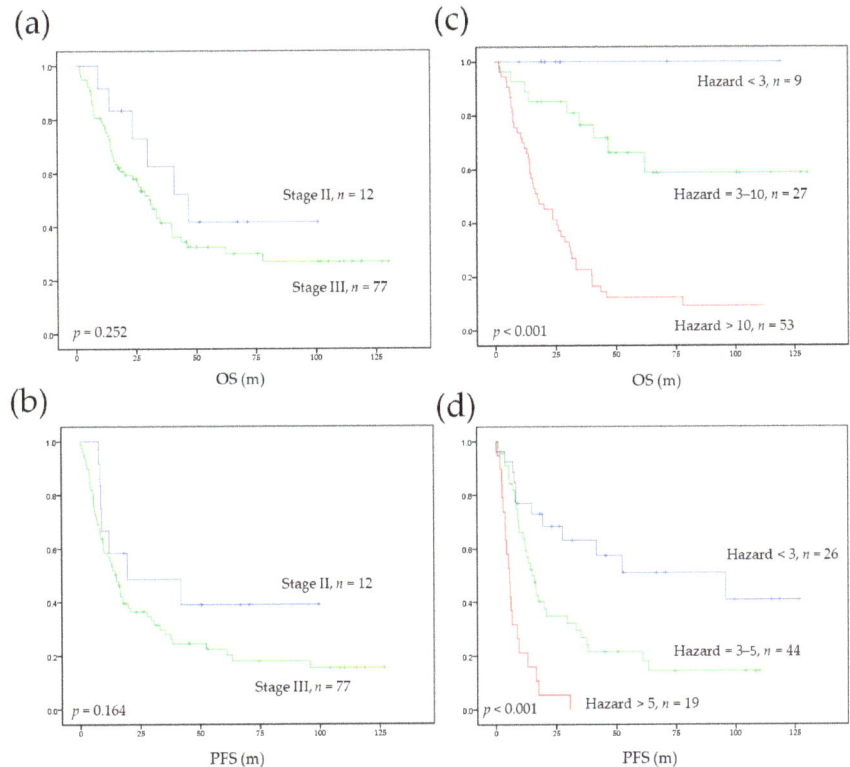

Figure 2. The Kaplan–Meier curves for OS and PFS in patients with nodal metastatic NSCLC without distant metastasis. Survival was stratified according to the eighth edition of the AJCC system (**a**,**b**) and our survival prediction model (**c**,**d**). OS, overall survival; PFS, progression-free survival; AJCC, American Joint Committee on Cancer.

3.5. Model Performance in Subgroups of Different Initial Treatments

We also applied our survival prediction models to subgroups according to different initial treatments (curative surgery or definitive CCRT). Our models significantly stratified patients into different survival risks independent of the initial treatment strategy (Figure 3). The c-indices of our models were compared to the AJCC staging system in the subgroups. Our models significantly outperformed the AJCC staging system, except the c-index for PFS in patients who received initial curative surgery, which only showed a statistical trend (Table 4).

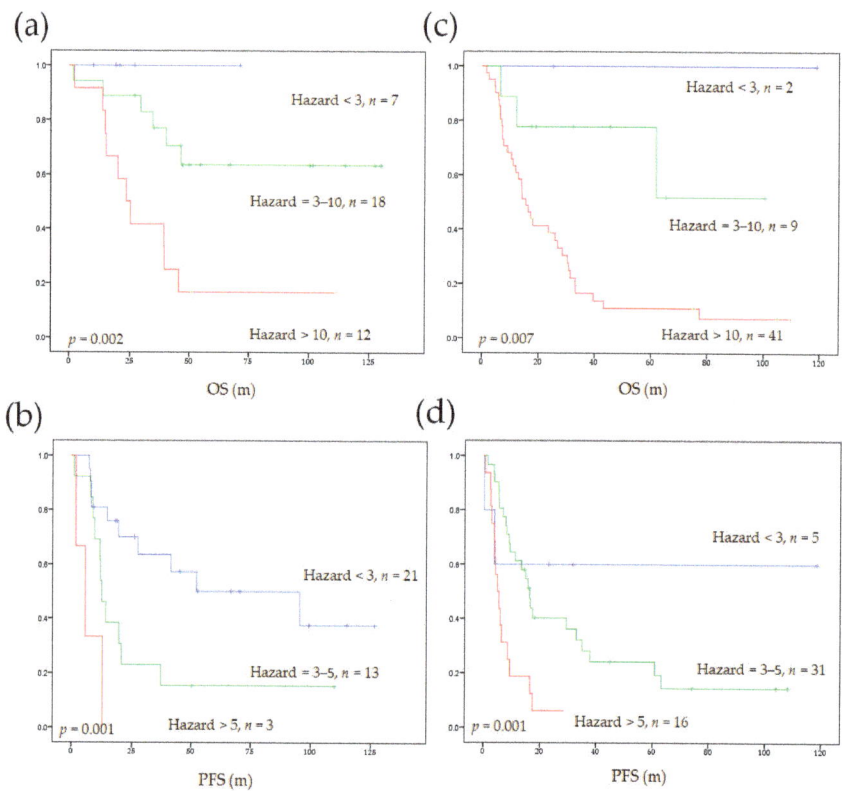

Figure 3. The Kaplan–Meier curves depicting OS and PFS stratified by our prediction model in subgroups of different initial treatments. The use of our model in subgroups that underwent curative surgery or neoadjuvant CCRT followed by surgery (**a,b**) and in initial non-surgical subgroup (**c,d**). OS, overall survival; PFS, progression-free survival; CCRT, concurrent chemoradiotherapy.

Table 4. A comparison of the c-indices of our model with the traditional cancer staging system in subgroups of different initial treatment strategies.

Model	c-Index for OS	p-Value	c-Index for PFS	p-value
Initial Surgery Group (n = 37) [a]				
Our Cox regression model	0.742	NA	0.657	NA
AJCC staging system [b]	0.513	<0.001	0.531	0.074
Initial non-surgery group (n = 52)				
Model	c-index for OS	p-value	c-index for PFS	p-Value
Our Cox regression model	0.667	NA	0.627	NA
AJCC staging system [b]	0.466	0.004	0.441	0.003

NA, not applicable; AJCC, American Joint Committee on Cancer. [a] Including initial curative surgery or neoadjuvant chemoradiation followed by curative surgery. [b] Staging according to 8th edition of AJCC manual.

4. Discussion

Regional lymph node metastasis is common in NSCLC patients without distant metastasis (M0 disease) and is associated with a worse survival prognosis [32]. Disease recurrence within 5 years after initial curative treatment occurs in over half of lung cancer patients with nodal metastasis, and these patients eventually die of recurrence [9,10,32]. The survival outcomes of M0 patients with regional nodal metastatic NSCLC vary widely, despite initial aggressive treatment [8,9,11]. Therefore, a more reliable prognostic stratification tool is an unmet need. The prognostic value of ^{18}F-FDG PET parameters derived from the primary tumor or the regional lymph node has been reported in patients with NSCLC [18–20,33,34]. However, the predictive power of combining the ^{18}F-FDG PET parameters from both primary tumor and metastatic nodes has not been well investigated. Although some studies have combined the ^{18}F-FDG PET volumetric parameters from the primary tumor and metastatic lesions, these study cohorts mixed locoregional disease cases with distant metastatic cases [35–38]. Thus, the results of these studies cannot be applied to patients with locoregional disease due to the diverse prognoses of patients with M0 or M1 diseases. In this study, we demonstrated that the total TLG derived from ^{18}F-FDG PET, a combination of TLGs from both the primary tumor and regional lymph nodes, is an independent risk factor for PFS and OS in patients of locoregional NSCLC. Incorporating the total TLG with traditional clinical risk factors improved survival stratification.

Although the AJCC staging system is currently the mainstay of decision making regarding treatment strategies in NSCLC, it does not simultaneously assess tumor biological activity and burden. In patients with regional nodal metastatic NSCLC without distant spreading, the ^{18}F-FDG PET metabolic parameters derived from primary tumor or metastatic nodes have been shown to be associated with survival outcomes in previous reports [18,33]. Because the primary tumor and metastatic nodes usually show different glucose metabolic profiles in ^{18}F-FDG PET images, a combination of the two may provide comprehensive biological information for predicting prognosis. In this study, we found that combining the TLG of the primary tumor and the metastatic nodes into a total TLG resulted in an independent risk factor with a higher prognostic significance. The TLG is calculated by multiplying the MTV by the mean SUV, which weights the volumetric burden and metabolic activity of tumors. Kim et al. and Park et al. showed that larger primary tumor MTV was associated with a higher likelihood of occult nodal metastases [39,40]. Accordingly, larger metabolic tumor burden in patients with nodal metastatic NSCLC may also be expected to bear a higher risk of occult metastases in the more remote lymph node stations or even in distant organs. These occult lesions may escape from the most intensive treatment in the locoregional area. In addition to describing the tumor burden per se, the TLG also depicts the viability and the glycolytic activity of the tumor. The glycolytic pathway elicits diverse non-glycolytic mechanisms related to the promotion of cancer survival, proliferation, invasiveness, and adaptation to therapeutic agents, which are associated with unfavorable prognoses in patients with cancer [41,42]. Therefore, being a surrogate marker for both disease burden and vicious tumor behavior, total TLG may facilitate the stratification of patients into different risk groups.

Older age (>75.5 years) was an independent prognosticator for poor OS and PFS in our study. ECOG was also a prognostic factor for OS. Age and performance status are associated with survival outcomes in lung cancer as well as other malignancies, such as aerodigestive tract and gynecologic cancers [10,43–46]. The aged population has more medical comorbidities. In addition, aged patients may experience more toxicities from anti-neoplastic agents and suffer more perioperative complications, which may increase treatment-related mortality [47]. Moreover, the function of the T-cell-mediated immune system declines with age and limits the cellular immune response against tumor cells in the elderly population, further explaining the unfavorable survival outcomes in patients with advanced age [48–51]. We also analyzed the effects of different histopathological types on survival. Similar to other reports, squamous cell pathology was associated with worse survival outcomes compared with outcomes in patients with other histopathological types in the univariate analysis, whereas no statistical significance was found in the multivariate Cox regression analysis [20]. The histopathological type of NSCLC may vary according to age [9,46], in line with the age distribution in our cohort (Supplementary Table S3). Thus, the survival differences according to histopathologic types in our study appear to depend on patient age. Nevertheless, whether histopathological types impact the outcome of nodal metastatic NSCLC requires a more uniform patient cohort for verification.

In our study, the total TLG is an independent risk factor depicting the disease, while the age and ECOG status characterize the host vitality. Survival outcomes in patients with cancer result from the complex interplay between the tumor and the host. Robust patient conditions with limited total TLG would have a higher chance of attaining disease-free status after curative treatment. On the other hand, vulnerable patient status and sizable total TLG are likely to experience treatment failure and eventually succumb to recurrence or disease progression (Figure 4). Therefore, incorporating both disease and host factors into one survival prediction model refines the prognostic stratification. Our survival stratification models also showed predictive value for survival outcomes in subgroups receiving different initial treatments. Because therapeutic decisions may vary from patient-to-patient based on clinical factors such as age, the baseline survival risk in subgroups receiving different initial treatment may vary as well [9,46]. For example, patients receiving curative surgery tend to be younger; thus, the surgical group has a lower baseline survival risk according to age. Nevertheless, the results of our study showed that our survival prediction model could be applied to different subgroups receiving different initial treatments, suggesting a wide utility of our survival stratification models in different treatment scenarios.

Despite the current therapeutic advances, treatment responses and survival times in nodal metastatic NSCLC patients are quite heterogeneous, and a reliable prognostic model for this patient group is still lacking [9–11]. For selected patients, salvage surgery for persistent or recurrent disease has been shown to improve disease control and may improve OS [52,53]. Furthermore, new therapeutic strategies have emerged that have improved disease control and prolonged survival in nodal metastatic NSCLC. For instance, adding adjuvant tyrosine kinase inhibitor in this patient group postpones recurrence in patients with an actionable epidermal growth factor receptor (EGFR) mutation [54]. Recently, preliminary data have suggested that neoadjuvant immunotherapy or chemoimmunotherapy may improve resectability and increase the pathological complete response rate [55–58]. However, sophisticated patient stratification before implementing these novel treatments is essential. Adding novel neoadjuvant or adjuvant therapy in patients with excellent survival outcomes after standard curative treatment may show little benefit and may result in undesirable adverse effects. Therefore, the survival prediction model in our study may aid in stratifying patients into different risk groups for tailored treatment decisions.

There were several limitations in our study. First, the patient cohort was not large and the study was conducted in a retrospective manner. In addition, heterogeneous patient characteristics such as the histopathological type of NSCLC and therapeutic strategies employed may introduce biases when analyzing survival data. Second, we did not include the EGFR mutation status in our survival analysis. Nonetheless, the meta-analysis by Zhang et al. showed that the EGFR mutation status was not predictive of the OS or disease-free survival in NSCLC with locoregional disease [59]. Furthermore, only 39 (43.8%) patients in our retrospective cohort were tested for EGFR mutation. Thus, we could not draw a clear conclusion on this issue. Finally, this study was performed in a single center and we only internally validated our results. Although external validation would be ideal before clinical implementation, external validation of a prognostic model requires a minimum of 100 events and ideally 200 events to produce reliable results [60]. Therefore, the generalizability of our survival prediction model warrants external validation in a larger prospective cohort.

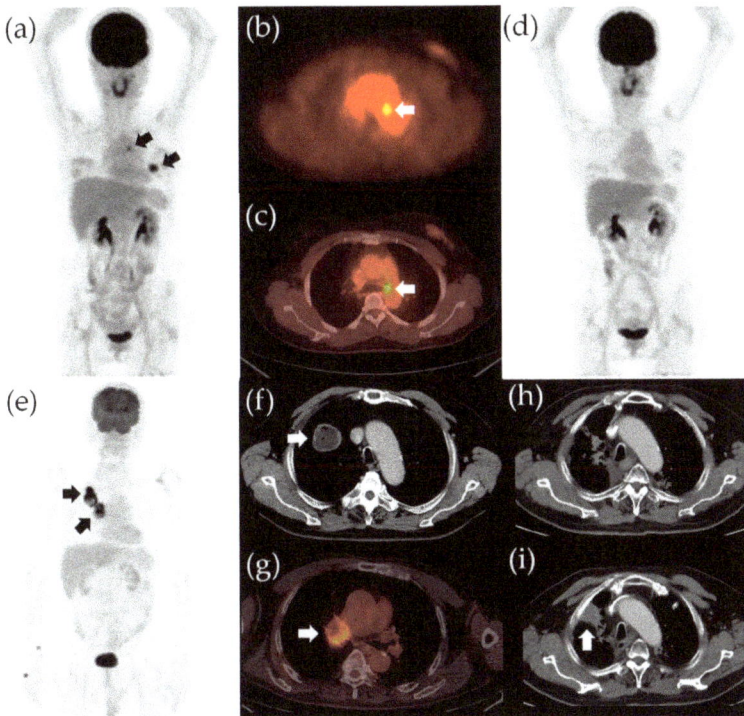

Figure 4. Survival stratification according to the independent risk factors in our study. The ^{18}F-FDG PET/CT images for a 50-year-old woman with adenocarcinoma in the left upper lobe and subaortic nodal metastasis, indicated by arrows in the panels (**a–c**). The clinical staging was cT2aN2M0, stage IIIA. The total TLG was 14.9 and the ECOG status was 0. The patient had no poor survival risk factor (hazards were both 1 for an unfavorable OS and poor PFS) and she underwent lobectomy of the left upper lobe and mediastinal lymph node dissection. The pathological staging was pT2aN2M0, stage IIIA. She underwent adjuvant chemotherapy and is now alive without recurrence (**d**). The OS and PFS were 116 and 115 months, respectively. A 75-year-old man with adenocarcinoma in the right lower lobe and ipsilateral hilar nodal metastasis, indicated by arrows in the panels (**e–g**). The clinical staging was cT2bN1M0, stage IIB. The total TLG was 246.6 (>81) and the ECOG status was 1 (the hazards for unfavorable OS and poor PFS were 16.8 and 3.3, respectively). The patient received definitive CCRT (2 Gy/fraction daily to a targeted dose of 66 Gy) and marked tumor shrinkage was observed (**h**). However, the patient experienced progression of the primary tumor 15.9 months after definitive CCRT, indicated by the arrow in the panel (**i**). The patient eventually died of lung cancer progression, with an OS of 24.0 months and PFS of 15.9 months. TLG, total lesion glycolysis; OS, overall survival; PFS, progression-free survival; CCRT, concurrent chemoradiotherapy.

5. Conclusions

Our preliminary results indicate that total TLG was a more significant independent prognostic factor than TLG when calculated from either primary tumor or metastatic nodes in predicting survival outcomes in patients with M0 NSCLC. Total TLG and age were predictive biomarkers for both OS and PFS, while ECOG status was an independent prognostic factor for OS. Combining total TLG with clinical factors yielded a survival stratification model that performed better than the traditional AJCC staging system. Our proposed survival stratification model may allow a more precise therapeutic approach in patients with nodal metastatic NSCLC without distant metastasis.

Supplementary Materials: The following are available online at https://www.mdpi.com/2075-4418/11/6/1065/s1: Table S1: Results of receiver operating characteristic curve analysis. Figure S1. In the OS model, the combination of three independent risk factors resulted in eight different patient hazards (from 1 to 43.8). The combination of two independent risk factors of the PFS model resulted in four different patient hazards (from 1 to 8.9). We further re-stratified patients with similar 5-year survival outcomes in the Kaplan–Meier curve analysis into one risk category. Finally, we obtained three separate risk categories in our survival models. OS, overall survival; PFS, progression-free survival. Table S2: The results of the bootstrapping validation of our survival analysis. Table S3: The mean age according to the histopathology and treatment strategy.

Author Contributions: Y.-H.C. and S.-C.C. (Sheng-Chieh Chan) have full access to all the study data; study design, Y.-H.C., S.-C.C. (Sung-Chao Chu), S.-C.C. (Sheng-Chieh Chan), and T.-F.W.; image analysis, Y.-H.C., S.-C.C. (Sheng-Chieh Chan), and S.-H.L.; image feature extraction, Y.-H.C. and K.-H.L.; statistical analysis and data curation, Y.-H.C. and L.-Y.W.; article drafting, Y.-H.C., L.-Y.W., and S.-C.C. (Sheng-Chieh Chan); critical revision of the article's important intellectual content, Y.-H.C., S.-C.C. (Sung-Chao Chu), T.-F.W., L.-Y.W., C.-B.L., B.-S.C., D.-W.L., K.-H.L., and S.-C.C. (Sheng-Chieh Chan). All authors have read and agreed to the published version of the manuscript.

Funding: This research was funded by The Ministry of Science and Technology in Taiwan, grant number 109-2314-B-303-015.

Institutional Review Board Statement: The study was conducted according to the guidelines of the Declaration of Helsinki and approved by the Institutional Review Board and Ethics Committee of Hualien Tzu Chi Hospital, Buddhist Tzu Chi Medical Foundation, Hualien, Taiwan (protocol code IRB109-235-B; date of approval: 22 September 2020).

Informed Consent Statement: Patient consent was waived due to the retrospective nature of this study.

Data Availability Statement: The data presented in this study are available on request from the corresponding author. The data are not publicly available due to privacy and ethical restrictions.

Acknowledgments: The authors wish to thank the staff from the Lung Cancer Research Team of Buddhist Tzu Chi General Hospital for their assistance in retrieving the data of patients with NSCLC.

Conflicts of Interest: The authors declare no conflict of interest.

References

1. Torre, L.A.; Bray, F.; Siegel, R.L.; Ferlay, J.; Lortet-Tieulent, J.; Jemal, A. Global cancer statistics, 2012. *CA Cancer J. Clin.* **2015**, *65*, 87–108. [CrossRef]
2. Ferlay, J.; Colombet, M.; Soerjomataram, I.; Mathers, C.; Parkin, D.M.; Pineros, M.; Znaor, A.; Bray, F. Estimating the global cancer incidence and mortality in 2018: GLOBOCAN sources and methods. *Int. J. Cancer* **2019**, *144*, 1941–1953. [CrossRef]
3. Siegel, R.L.; Miller, K.D.; Jemal, A. Cancer statistics, 2019. *CA Cancer J. Clin.* **2019**, *69*, 7–34. [CrossRef]
4. van Meerbeeck, J.P.; Fennell, D.A.; De Ruysscher, D.K.M. Small-cell lung cancer. *Lancet* **2011**, *378*, 1741–1755. [CrossRef]
5. Hirsch, F.R.; Suda, K.; Wiens, J.; Bunn, P.A. New and emerging targeted treatments in advanced non-small-cell lung cancer. *Lancet* **2016**, *388*, 1012–1024. [CrossRef]
6. Jin, F.; Qu, B.; Fu, Z.; Zhang, Y.; Han, A.; Kong, L.; Yu, J. Prognostic Value of Metabolic Parameters of Metastatic Lymph Nodes on (18)F-FDG PET/CT in Patients with Limited-stage Small-cell Lung Cancer with Lymph Node Involvement. *Clin. Lung Cancer* **2018**, *19*, e101–e108. [CrossRef]
7. Zhang, Y.K.; Chai, Z.D.; Tan, L.L.; Wang, Z.Y.; Chen, Z.J.; Le, H.B.; Zhu, W.Y. Association of lymph node involvement with the prognosis of pathological T1 invasive non-small cell lung cancer. *World J. Surg Oncol.* **2017**, *15*, 64. [CrossRef]
8. Katsumata, S.; Aokage, K.; Ishii, G.; Nakasone, S.; Sakai, T.; Okada, S.; Miyoshi, T.; Tane, K.; Tsuboi, M. Prognostic Impact of the Number of Metastatic Lymph Nodes on the Eighth Edition of the TNM Classification of NSCLC. *J. Thorac. Oncol.* **2019**, *14*, 1408–1418. [CrossRef]
9. Kim, H.C.; Ji, W.; Lee, J.C.; Kim, H.R.; Song, S.Y.; Choi, C.M.; Korean Association for Lung, C.; Korea Central Cancer, R. Prognostic Factor and Clinical Outcome in Stage III Non-Small Cell Lung Cancer: A Study Based on Real-World Clinical Data in the Korean Population. *Cancer Res. Treat.* **2021**. [CrossRef]
10. Aragaki, M.; Kato, T.; Fujiwara-Kuroda, A.; Hida, Y.; Kaga, K.; Wakasa, S. Preoperative identification of clinicopathological prognostic factors for relapse-free survival in clinical N1 non-small cell lung cancer: A retrospective single center-based study. *J. Cardiothorac. Surg.* **2020**, *15*, 229. [CrossRef]

11. Xu, L.; Su, H.; She, Y.; Dai, C.; Zhao, M.; Gao, J.; Xie, H.; Ren, Y.; Xie, D.; Chen, C. Which N Descriptor Is More Predictive of Prognosis in Resected Non-Small Cell Lung Cancer: The Number of Involved Nodal Stations or the Location-Based Pathological N Stage? *Chest* **2020**. [CrossRef]
12. Sakao, Y.; Okumura, S.; Mun, M.; Uehara, H.; Ishikawa, Y.; Nakagawa, K. Prognostic heterogeneity in multilevel N2 non-small cell lung cancer patients: Importance of lymphadenopathy and occult intrapulmonary metastases. *Ann. Thorac. Surg.* **2010**, *89*, 1060–1063. [CrossRef] [PubMed]
13. Detterbeck, F.C.; Chansky, K.; Groome, P.; Bolejack, V.; Crowley, J.; Shemanski, L.; Kennedy, C.; Krasnik, M.; Peake, M.; Rami-Porta, R.; et al. The IASLC Lung Cancer Staging Project: Methodology and Validation Used in the Development of Proposals for Revision of the Stage Classification of NSCLC in the Forthcoming (Eighth) Edition of the TNM Classification of Lung Cancer. *J. Thorac. Oncol.* **2016**, *11*, 1433–1446. [CrossRef] [PubMed]
14. Steinert, H.C. PET in lung cancer. *Chang. Gung Med. J.* **2005**, *28*, 296–305.
15. Cuaron, J.; Dunphy, M.; Rimner, A. Role of FDG-PET scans in staging, response assessment, and follow-up care for non-small cell lung cancer. *Front. Oncol.* **2012**, *2*, 208. [CrossRef]
16. Liu, F.; Ma, F.; Wang, Y.; Hao, L.; Zeng, H.; Jia, C.; Wang, Y.; Liu, P.; Ong, I.M.; Li, B.; et al. PKM2 methylation by CARM1 activates aerobic glycolysis to promote tumorigenesis. *Nat. Cell Biol.* **2017**, *19*, 1358–1370. [CrossRef]
17. Yu, M.; Chen, S.; Hong, W.; Gu, Y.; Huang, B.; Lin, Y.; Zhou, Y.; Jin, H.; Deng, Y.; Tu, L.; et al. Prognostic role of glycolysis for cancer outcome: Evidence from 86 studies. *J. Cancer Res. Clin. Oncol.* **2019**. [CrossRef]
18. Carvalho, S.; Leijenaar, R.T.H.; Troost, E.G.C.; van Timmeren, J.E.; Oberije, C.; van Elmpt, W.; de Geus-Oei, L.F.; Bussink, J.; Lambin, P. 18F-fluorodeoxyglucose positron-emission tomography (FDG-PET)-Radiomics of metastatic lymph nodes and primary tumor in non-small cell lung cancer (NSCLC)—A prospective externally validated study. *PLoS ONE* **2018**, *13*, e0192859. [CrossRef]
19. Chen, Y.H.; Wang, T.F.; Chu, S.C.; Lin, C.B.; Wang, L.Y.; Lue, K.H.; Liu, S.H.; Chan, S.C. Incorporating radiomic feature of pretreatment 18F-FDG PET improves survival stratification in patients with EGFR-mutated lung adenocarcinoma. *PLoS ONE* **2020**, *15*, e0244502. [CrossRef]
20. Roengvoraphoj, O.; Kasmann, L.; Eze, C.; Taugner, J.; Gjika, A.; Tufman, A.; Hadi, I.; Li, M.; Mille, E.; Gennen, K.; et al. Maximum standardized uptake value of primary tumor (SUVmax_PT) and horizontal range between two most distant PET-positive lymph nodes predict patient outcome in inoperable stage III NSCLC patients after chemoradiotherapy. *Transl. Lung Cancer Res.* **2020**, *9*, 541–548. [CrossRef]
21. Pellegrino, S.; Fonti, R.; Pulcrano, A.; Del Vecchio, S. PET-Based Volumetric Biomarkers for Risk Stratification of Non-Small Cell Lung Cancer Patients. *Diagnostics* **2021**, *11*, 210. [CrossRef] [PubMed]
22. Xu, C.W.; Wang, W.X.; Wu, M.J.; Zhu, Y.C.; Zhuang, W.; Lin, G.; Du, K.Q.; Huang, Y.J.; Chen, Y.P.; Chen, G.; et al. Comparison of the c-MET gene amplification between primary tumor and metastatic lymph nodes in non-small cell lung cancer. *Thorac. Cancer* **2017**, *8*, 417–422. [CrossRef]
23. Daniele, L.; Cassoni, P.; Bacillo, E.; Cappia, S.; Righi, L.; Volante, M.; Tondat, F.; Inghirami, G.; Sapino, A.; Scagliotti, G.V.; et al. Epidermal growth factor receptor gene in primary tumor and metastatic sites from non-small cell lung cancer. *J. Thorac. Oncol.* **2009**, *4*, 684–688. [CrossRef]
24. Hess, L.M.; Smith, D.; Cui, Z.L.; Montejano, L.; Liepa, A.M.; Schelman, W.; Bowman, L. The relationship between Eastern Cooperative Oncology Group performance status and healthcare resource utilization among patients with advanced or metastatic colorectal, lung or gastric cancer. *J. Drug Assess.* **2020**, *10*, 10–17. [CrossRef]
25. Albain, K.S.; Crowley, J.J.; Turrisi, A.T., 3rd; Gandara, D.R.; Farrar, W.B.; Clark, J.I.; Beasley, K.R.; Livingston, R.B. Concurrent cisplatin, etoposide, and chest radiotherapy in pathologic stage IIIB non-small-cell lung cancer: A Southwest Oncology Group phase II study, SWOG 9019. *J. Clin. Oncol.* **2002**, *20*, 3454–3460. [CrossRef]
26. Senan, S.; Brade, A.; Wang, L.H.; Vansteenkiste, J.; Dakhil, S.; Biesma, B.; Martinez Aguillo, M.; Aerts, J.; Govindan, R.; Rubio-Viqueira, B.; et al. PROCLAIM: Randomized Phase III Trial of Pemetrexed-Cisplatin or Etoposide-Cisplatin Plus Thoracic Radiation Therapy Followed by Consolidation Chemotherapy in Locally Advanced Nonsquamous Non-Small-Cell Lung Cancer. *J. Clin. Oncol.* **2016**, *34*, 953–962. [CrossRef]
27. Boellaard, R.; Delgado-Bolton, R.; Oyen, W.J.; Giammarile, F.; Tatsch, K.; Eschner, W.; Verzijlbergen, F.J.; Barrington, S.F.; Pike, L.C.; Weber, W.A.; et al. FDG PET/CT: EANM procedure guidelines for tumour imaging: Version 2.0. *Eur. J. Nucl. Med. Mol. Imaging* **2015**, *42*, 328–354. [CrossRef]
28. Okour, M.; Jacobson, P.A.; Israni, A.; Brundage, R.C. Comparative Evaluation of Median Versus Youden Index Dichotomization Methods: Exposure-Response Analysis of Mycophenolic Acid and Acyl-Glucuronide Metabolite. *Eur. J. Drug Metab. Pharm.* **2019**, *44*, 629–638. [CrossRef]
29. Chen, Y.H.; Lue, K.H.; Chu, S.C.; Chang, B.S.; Wang, L.Y.; Liu, D.W.; Liu, S.H.; Chao, Y.K.; Chan, S.C. Combining the radiomic features and traditional parameters of (18)F-FDG PET with clinical profiles to improve prognostic stratification in patients with esophageal squamous cell carcinoma treated with neoadjuvant chemoradiotherapy and surgery. *Ann. Nucl. Med.* **2019**, *33*, 657–670. [CrossRef]
30. Lue, K.H.; Wu, Y.F.; Lin, H.H.; Hsieh, T.C.; Liu, S.H.; Chan, S.C.; Chen, Y.H. Prognostic Value of Baseline Radiomic Features of (18)F-FDG PET in Patients with Diffuse Large B-Cell Lymphoma. *Diagnostics* **2020**, *11*, 36. [CrossRef]
31. Kang, L.; Chen, W.; Petrick, N.A.; Gallas, B.D. Comparing two correlated C indices with right-censored survival outcome: A one-shot nonparametric approach. *Stat. Med.* **2015**, *34*, 685–703. [CrossRef]

32. Dehing-Oberije, C.; De Ruysscher, D.; van der Weide, H.; Hochstenbag, M.; Bootsma, G.; Geraedts, W.; Pitz, C.; Simons, J.; Teule, J.; Rahmy, A.; et al. Tumor volume combined with number of positive lymph node stations is a more important prognostic factor than TNM stage for survival of non-small-cell lung cancer patients treated with (chemo)radiotherapy. *Int. J. Radiat. Oncol. Biol. Phys.* **2008**, *70*, 1039–1044. [CrossRef]
33. Roengvoraphoj, O.; Wijaya, C.; Eze, C.; Li, M.; Dantes, M.; Taugner, J.; Tufman, A.; Huber, R.M.; Belka, C.; Manapov, F. Analysis of primary tumor metabolic volume during chemoradiotherapy in locally advanced non-small cell lung cancer. *Strahlenther Onkol.* **2018**, *194*, 107–115. [CrossRef]
34. Kanyilmaz, G.; Benli Yavuz, B.; Aktan, M.; Sahin, O. Prognostic importance of (18)F-fluorodeoxyglucose uptake by positron emission tomography for stage III non-small cell lung cancer treated with definitive chemoradiotherapy. *Rev. Esp. Med. Nucl. Imagen Mol.* **2020**, *39*, 20–26.
35. Chen, H.H.; Chiu, N.T.; Su, W.C.; Guo, H.R.; Lee, B.F. Prognostic value of whole-body total lesion glycolysis at pretreatment FDG PET/CT in non-small cell lung cancer. *Radiology* **2012**, *264*, 559–566. [CrossRef]
36. Pellegrino, S.; Fonti, R.; Mazziotti, E.; Piccin, L.; Mozzillo, E.; Damiano, V.; Matano, E.; De Placido, S.; Del Vecchio, S. Total metabolic tumor volume by 18F-FDG PET/CT for the prediction of outcome in patients with non-small cell lung cancer. *Ann. Nucl. Med.* **2019**, *33*, 937–944. [CrossRef]
37. Lapa, P.; Oliveiros, B.; Marques, M.; Isidoro, J.; Alves, F.C.; Costa, J.M.N.; Costa, G.; de Lima, J.P. Metabolic tumor burden quantified on [(18)F]FDG PET/CT improves TNM staging of lung cancer patients. *Eur. J. Nucl. Med. Mol. Imaging* **2017**, *44*, 2169–2178. [CrossRef]
38. Pu, Y.; Zhang, J.X.; Liu, H.; Appelbaum, D.; Meng, J.; Penney, B.C. Developing and validating a novel metabolic tumor volume risk stratification system for supplementing non-small cell lung cancer staging. *Eur. J. Nucl. Med. Mol. Imaging* **2018**, *45*, 2079–2092. [CrossRef] [PubMed]
39. Park, S.Y.; Yoon, J.K.; Park, K.J.; Lee, S.J. Prediction of occult lymph node metastasis using volume-based PET parameters in small-sized peripheral non-small cell lung cancer. *Cancer Imaging* **2015**, *15*, 21. [CrossRef] [PubMed]
40. Kim, D.H.; Song, B.I.; Hong, C.M.; Jeong, S.Y.; Lee, S.W.; Lee, J.; Ahn, B.C. Metabolic parameters using (1)(8)F-FDG PET/CT correlate with occult lymph node metastasis in squamous cell lung carcinoma. *Eur. J. Nucl. Med. Mol. Imaging* **2014**, *41*, 2051–2057. [CrossRef] [PubMed]
41. Torresano, L.; Nuevo-Tapioles, C.; Santacatterina, F.; Cuezva, J.M. Metabolic reprogramming and disease progression in cancer patients. *Biochim. Biophys. Acta Mol. Basis Dis.* **2020**, *1866*, 165721. [CrossRef]
42. Gasmi, A.; Peana, M.; Arshad, M.; Butnariu, M.; Menzel, A.; Bjorklund, G. Krebs cycle: Activators, inhibitors and their roles in the modulation of carcinogenesis. *Arch. Toxicol.* **2021**, *95*, 1161–1178. [CrossRef] [PubMed]
43. Hosoya, K.; Fujimoto, D.; Morimoto, T.; Kumagai, T.; Tamiya, A.; Taniguchi, Y.; Yokoyama, T.; Ishida, T.; Matsumoto, H.; Hirano, K.; et al. Clinical factors associated with shorter durable response, and patterns of acquired resistance to first-line pembrolizumab monotherapy in PD-L1-positive non-small-cell lung cancer patients: A retrospective multicenter study. *BMC Cancer* **2021**, *21*, 346. [CrossRef]
44. Mallen, A.; Todd, S.; Robertson, S.E.; Kim, J.; Sehovic, M.; Wenham, R.M.; Extermann, M.; Chon, H.S. Impact of age, comorbidity, and treatment characteristics on survival in older women with advanced high grade epithelial ovarian cancer. *Gynecol. Oncol.* **2021**. [CrossRef] [PubMed]
45. Chen, Y.H.; Chang, K.P.; Chu, S.C.; Yen, T.C.; Wang, L.Y.; Chang, J.T.; Hsu, C.L.; Ng, S.H.; Liu, S.H.; Chan, S.C. Value of early evaluation of treatment response using (18)F-FDG PET/CT parameters and the Epstein-Barr virus DNA load for prediction of outcome in patients with primary nasopharyngeal carcinoma. *Eur. J. Nucl. Med. Mol. Imaging* **2019**, *46*, 650–660. [CrossRef] [PubMed]
46. Driessen, E.; Detillon, D.; Bootsma, G.; De Ruysscher, D.; Veen, E.; Aarts, M.; Janssen-Heijnen, M. Population-based patterns of treatment and survival for patients with stage I and II non-small cell lung cancer aged 65-74years and 75years or older. *J. Geriatr. Oncol.* **2019**, *10*, 547–554. [CrossRef]
47. Tew, W.P. Ovarian cancer in the older woman. *J. Geriatr. Oncol.* **2016**, *7*, 354–361. [CrossRef]
48. Dorshkind, K.; Montecino-Rodriguez, E.; Signer, R.A. The ageing immune system: Is it ever too old to become young again? *Nat. Rev. Immunol.* **2009**, *9*, 57–62. [CrossRef]
49. Nikolich-Zugich, J. Aging of the T cell compartment in mice and humans: From no naive expectations to foggy memories. *J. Immunol.* **2014**, *193*, 2622–2629. [CrossRef]
50. Briceno, O.; Lissina, A.; Wanke, K.; Afonso, G.; von Braun, A.; Ragon, K.; Miquel, T.; Gostick, E.; Papagno, L.; Stiasny, K.; et al. Reduced naive CD8(+) T-cell priming efficacy in elderly adults. *Aging Cell* **2016**, *15*, 14–21. [CrossRef]
51. Tubin, S.; Khan, M.K.; Gupta, S.; Jeremic, B. Biology of NSCLC: Interplay between Cancer Cells, Radiation and Tumor Immune Microenvironment. *Cancers* **2021**, *13*, 775. [CrossRef]
52. Dickhoff, C.; Dahele, M.; Paul, M.A.; van de Ven, P.M.; de Langen, A.J.; Senan, S.; Smit, E.F.; Hartemink, K.J. Salvage surgery for locoregional recurrence or persistent tumor after high dose chemoradiotherapy for locally advanced non-small cell lung cancer. *Lung Cancer* **2016**, *94*, 108–113. [CrossRef]
53. Hamada, A.; Soh, J.; Mitsudomi, T. Salvage surgery after definitive chemoradiotherapy for patients with non-small cell lung cancer. *Transl. Lung Cancer Res.* **2021**, *10*, 555–562. [CrossRef]

54. Zhong, W.Z.; Wang, Q.; Mao, W.M.; Xu, S.T.; Wu, L.; Wei, Y.C.; Liu, Y.Y.; Chen, C.; Cheng, Y.; Yin, R.; et al. Gefitinib Versus Vinorelbine Plus Cisplatin as Adjuvant Treatment for Stage II-IIIA (N1-N2) EGFR-Mutant NSCLC: Final Overall Survival Analysis of CTONG1104 Phase III Trial. *J. Clin. Oncol.* **2021**, *39*, 713–722. [CrossRef]
55. Liang, H.; Deng, H.; Liang, W.; Guo, K.; Gao, Z.; Wiesel, O.; Flores, R.M.; Song, K.; Redwan, B.; Migliore, M.; et al. Perioperative chemoimmunotherapy in a patient with stage IIIB non-small cell lung cancer. *Ann. Transl. Med.* **2020**, *8*, 245. [CrossRef]
56. Shu, C.A.; Gainor, J.F.; Awad, M.M.; Chiuzan, C.; Grigg, C.M.; Pabani, A.; Garofano, R.F.; Stoopler, M.B.; Cheng, S.K.; White, A.; et al. Neoadjuvant atezolizumab and chemotherapy in patients with resectable non-small-cell lung cancer: An open-label, multicentre, single-arm, phase 2 trial. *Lancet Oncol.* **2020**, *21*, 786–795. [CrossRef]
57. Provencio, M.; Nadal, E.; Insa, A.; Garcia-Campelo, M.R.; Casal-Rubio, J.; Domine, M.; Majem, M.; Rodriguez-Abreu, D.; Martinez-Marti, A.; De Castro Carpeno, J.; et al. Neoadjuvant chemotherapy and nivolumab in resectable non-small-cell lung cancer (NADIM): An open-label, multicentre, single-arm, phase 2 trial. *Lancet Oncol.* **2020**, *21*, 1413–1422. [CrossRef]
58. Uprety, D.; Mandrekar, S.J.; Wigle, D.; Roden, A.C.; Adjei, A.A. Neoadjuvant Immunotherapy for NSCLC: Current Concepts and Future Approaches. *J. Thorac. Oncol.* **2020**, *15*, 1281–1297. [CrossRef]
59. Zhang, Z.; Wang, T.; Zhang, J.; Cai, X.; Pan, C.; Long, Y.; Chen, J.; Zhou, C.; Yin, X. Prognostic value of epidermal growth factor receptor mutations in resected non-small cell lung cancer: A systematic review with meta-analysis. *PLoS ONE* **2014**, *9*, e106053. [CrossRef]
60. Collins, G.S.; Ogundimu, E.O.; Altman, D.G. Sample size considerations for the external validation of a multivariable prognostic model: A resampling study. *Stat. Med.* **2016**, *35*, 214–226. [CrossRef]

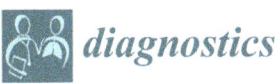

Article

Prognostic Value of Quantitative [^{18}F]FDG-PET Features in Patients with Metastases from Soft Tissue Sarcoma

Gijsbert M. Kalisvaart [1,*], Willem Grootjans [1], Judith V. M. G. Bovée [2], Hans Gelderblom [3], Jos A. van der Hage [4], Michiel A. J. van de Sande [5], Floris H. P. van Velden [1], Johan L. Bloem [1] and Lioe-Fee de Geus-Oei [1,6]

1. Department of Radiology, Leiden University Medical Centre, 2333 ZA Leiden, The Netherlands; W.Grootjans@lumc.nl (W.G.); F.H.P.van_Velden@lumc.nl (F.H.P.v.V.); J.L.Bloem@lumc.nl (J.L.B.); L.F.de_Geus-Oei@lumc.nl (L.-F.d.G.-O.)
2. Department of Pathology, Leiden University Medical Centre, 2333 ZA Leiden, The Netherlands; J.V.M.G.Bovee@lumc.nl
3. Department of Medical Oncology, Leiden University Medical Centre, 2333 ZA Leiden, The Netherlands; A.J.Gelderblom@lumc.nl
4. Department of Surgical Oncology, Leiden University Medical Centre, 2333 ZA Leiden, The Netherlands; J.A.van_der_Hage@lumc.nl
5. Department of Orthopaedic Surgery, Leiden University Medical Centre, 2333 ZA Leiden, The Netherlands; M.A.J.van_de_Sande@lumc.nl
6. Biomedical Photonic Imaging Group, University of Twente, 7522 NB Enschede, The Netherlands
* Correspondence: g.m.kalisvaart@lumc.nl

Abstract: Background: Prognostic biomarkers are pivotal for adequate treatment decision making. The objective of this study was to determine the added prognostic value of quantitative [^{18}F]FDG-PET features in patients with metastases from soft tissue sarcoma (STS). Methods: Patients with metastases from STS, detected by (re)staging [^{18}F]FDG-PET/CT at Leiden University Medical Centre, were retrospectively included. Clinical and histopathological patient characteristics and [^{18}F]FDG-PET features (SUVmax, SUVpeak, SUVmean, total lesion glycolysis, and metabolic tumor volume) were analyzed as prognostic factors for overall survival using a Cox proportional hazards model and Kaplan–Meier methods. Results: A total of 31 patients were included. SUVmax and SUVpeak were significantly predictive for overall survival (OS) in a univariate analysis ($p = 0.004$ and $p = 0.006$, respectively). Hazard ratios (HRs) were 1.16 per unit increase for SUVmax and 1.20 per unit for SUVpeak. SUVmax and SUVpeak remained significant predictors for overall survival after correction for the two strongest predictive clinical characteristics (number of lesions and performance status) in a multivariate analysis ($p = 0.02$ for both). Median SUVmax and SUVpeak were 5.7 and 4.9 g/mL, respectively. The estimated mean overall survival in patients with SUVmax > 5.7 g/mL was 14 months; otherwise, it was 39 months ($p < 0.001$). For patients with SUVpeak > 4.9 g/mL, the estimated mean overall survival was 18 months; otherwise, it was 33 months ($p = 0.04$). Conclusions: In this study, SUVmax and SUVpeak were independent prognostic factors for overall survival in patients with metastases from STS. These results warrant further investigation of metabolic imaging with [^{18}F]FDG-PET/CT in patients with metastatic STS.

Keywords: metastatic soft tissue sarcoma; [^{18}F]FDG-PET; prognosis

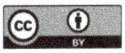

1. Introduction

Approximately 14% of patients with a soft tissue sarcoma (STS) present with metastatic disease [1]. Additionally, up to 34% of high-grade STS patients develop distant metastases within 5 years after resection of localized STS [2,3]. While several studies show an improvement in the survival of patients with metastatic STS over the last decades, the two-year survival rate remains less than 50% [4–6]. Indeed, treatment of these patients is complex due to the heterogeneous and aggressive nature of these tumors. Generally, therapies can consist of combinations of surgery, radiotherapy, and systemic treatment. Personalized decision making is important in designing treatment strategies, and a multitude of parameters is used for this purpose [7]. Prognostic factors play an important role among these parameters, and several studies have identified a group of characteristics that is associated with prognosis in these patients [4–6,8–10]. These studies strike the consensus that patient age, performance status, disease-free interval, and histological subtype are strong predictors for overall survival (OS). Nevertheless, stratification of patients on an individual level remains a difficult challenge and requires further insight in the link between tumor characteristics and prognosis.

The use of ^{18}F-fluorodeoxyglucose ([^{18}F]FDG) positron emission tomography (PET) for the characterization of malignant lesions is widely studied [11]. In STS patients, [^{18}F]FDG-PET imaging is regularly performed for (re)staging and follow-up [12]. Furthermore, in metastatic STS, specifically, a recent study has shown value of [^{18}F]FDG-PET in monitoring the response to systemic treatment [13]. The uptake of [^{18}F]FDG, as expressed by the standardized uptake value (SUV), reflects the degree of glucose metabolism of a lesion. High [^{18}F]FDG-uptake has shown to be connected to increased tumor aggressiveness in many STS subtypes. Especially in localized STS, several [^{18}F]FDG-PET features, such as maximum SUV (SUVmax), peak SUV (SUVpeak), metabolic tumor volume (MTV), and total lesion glycolysis (TLG), are found to have significant prognostic value [14,15]. Moreover, in other tumor types, these parameters have shown to be predictive for survival in metastatic disease and demonstrated to be valuable for the personalization of treatment decisions [16]. While the metabolic properties of lesions, as indicated by quantitative [^{18}F]FDG-PET features, might also provide valuable information for the prognosis of metastatic STS patients, no literature is readily available on the correlation between these features and survival. In the current study, we assessed the prognostic value of quantitative [^{18}F]FDG-PET features in patients diagnosed with metastases from STS.

2. Materials and Methods

2.1. Patients

Patients with biopsy-proven STS, who underwent a [^{18}F]FDG-PET/CT for (re)staging purposes on which metastatic disease was detected, were retrospectively included. Metastatic disease was defined as radiological evidence of systemic spread of tumor outside the primary tumor bed. Patients with GISTs (gastrointestinal stromal tumor) and primary uterine or retroperitoneal sarcomas were excluded to guarantee a relatively homogeneous population regarding tumor biology and treatment. Patients who received radiotherapy or systemic therapy for metastatic disease before [^{18}F]FDG-PET/CTs acquisition were also excluded. Furthermore, all [^{18}F]FDG-PET/CTs had to be performed between January 2017 and January 2021 at Leiden University Medical Center, which is a tertiary referral center for sarcoma care. Requirement to obtain patient consent was waived by the local ethical board, since clinical data were retrospectively collected and pseudo-anonymized.

2.2. Patient Characteristics

Clinical and histopathological characteristics, which were reported as independent prognostic factors of survival in previous studies, were collected for all included patients (Table 1). Primary tumor location was categorized based on the results of Lochner et al. to realize substantial group sizes for analysis [4]. Primary tumor localization in the deep trunk or upper extremity was categorized as high risk for impaired survival, while other locations were considered to be low risk. Since some patients were diagnosed with metastatic disease at first diagnosis of STS, the disease-free interval after resection of the primary tumor was not analyzed as a continuous variable but categorized in three groups based on the methods of Italiano et al. and Lochner et al. [4,5]. Patients who were diagnosed with metastatic disease at first diagnosis were categorized as 'synchronous'. Patients who developed metastases after resection of the primary tumor were dichotomized around the median number of months of the disease-free interval. Reported World Health Organization (WHO) scale and the Fédération Nationale des Centres de Lutte Contre le Cancer (FNCLCC) system scores were collected from patient files and used for analysis of performance status and tumor grade, respectively [17].

Table 1. Patient characteristics expressed as mean and standard deviation, median and quartile range, or as number and percentages of the whole population. * FNCLCC grade such as reported in pathologic reports. For round cell sarcoma, rhabdomyosarcoma, angiosarcoma, and intima sarcoma, grade was not reported in pathologic reports. These highly aggressive tumors were categorized as grade 3 in this study. In one patient with a morphologic myxoid liposarcoma, no FNCLCC classification was performed (not applicable), and this patient was excluded from the univariate analysis for FNCLCC grade. † Morphologically, this tumor resembled a myxoid liposarcoma, but a characteristic translocation could not be demonstrated.

	Characteristics, n = 31		
Age	59 ± 18	Histologic subtype	
Sex		Undifferentiated soft tissue sarcoma	8 (26%)
Male	20 (65%)	Myxofibrosarcoma	6 (19%)
Female	11 (35%)	MPNST	5 (16%)
WHO performance status		Leiomyosarcoma	3 (10%)
Unknown	8 (26%)	Dedifferentiated liposarcoma	2 (6%)
0	10 (32%)	Synovial sarcoma	2 (6%)
1	11 (35%)	Myxoid liposarcoma †	1 (3%)
2	2 (7%)	Round cell sarcoma	1 (3%)
Location of primary tumour		Rhabdomyosarcoma	1 (3%)
Lower extremity	18 (58%)	Angiosarcoma	1 (3%)
Upper extremity	3 (10%)	Intima sarcoma	1 (3%)
Trunk wall	3 (10%)	FNCLCC Grade *	
Deep trunk	6 (19%)	1	1 (3%)
Head/neck	1 (3%)	2	15 (48%)
Disease free interval		3	14 (45%)
Synchronous	7 (23%)	Not applicable	1 (3%)
<14 months	12 (39%)	Location of metastases	
>14 months	12 (39%)	Lung	7 (23%)
Number of lesions	3.3 ± 2.8	Lung and other	11 (35%)
Sum of lesion diameters per patient (cm)	7.5 (6.0–17.5)	Soft tissue only	9 (29%)
		Bone only	4 (13%)

2.3. [18F]FDG-PET/CT

All scans were acquired on a digital Vereos PET/CT scanner (Philips Healthcare, Best, The Netherlands) according to the most recent European Association for Nuclear Medicine (EANM) procedure guidelines for tumor imaging [18]. The PET/CT scanner was accredited by the Research4Life (EARL) initiative for quantitative PET/CT imaging. Patients fasted at least 6 h before imaging and were hydrated with 500 mL of water. [18F]FDG was administered 60 min before the acquisition of the PET scan. A low-dose CT scan (52 mAs, 120 kVp) was acquired prior to PET acquisition for the purpose of attenuation correction and anatomical reference. Standard [18F]FDG PET/CT scans were acquired from the skull base to mid-thigh or toes depending on the location of the primary tumor. Image acquisition time was 2 min per bed position. Image reconstruction was performed using a blob-based 3D iterative reconstruction algorithm (blobTOF; 3 iterations and 9 subsets) followed by a 5.5 mm full-width at half maximum (FWHM) post-reconstruction Gaussian filter. The image voxel size was $4 \times 4 \times 4$ mm^3. After reconstruction, all PET images were expressed in SUV by normalizing voxel radioactivity concentrations [kBq·mL^{-1}] to the injected dose of [18F]FDG [MBq] and the patient's body weight (kg).

2.4. [18F]]FDG-PET Features

Image analysis was performed using Philips Intellispace Portal software v10.1 (Philips Healthcare, Best, The Netherlands). Segmentation of all STS lesions was performed using an adaptive threshold algorithm. A segmentation threshold of 50% of the SUVpeak corrected for local background was used (Figure 1) [19]. After image segmentation, the resulting volumes of interest (VOIs) were used to calculate relevant uptake parameters in the PET images. For VOIs that covered normal tissue surrounding tumor lesions due to relatively high FDG uptake (e.g., heart tissue or urinary bladder), manual adjustment was performed to exclude normal tissue from the VOI. For every patient, the SUVmax and SUVpeak were calculated on the lesion with the highest SUVmax and with the highest SUVpeak, respectively. The SUVmax is defined as the voxel with the highest intensity within a tumor. The SUVpeak is defined as the largest mean value of a 1 cm^3 sphere positioned within a tumor. Furthermore, SUVmean, MTV, and TLG were calculated for all lesions combined per patient (whole body). The SUVmean is defined as the mean of all pixel values within all tumor lesions in a patient. The MTV is defined as the sum of the volume of all tumor lesions in a patient. The TLG is defined as the sum of the products of the SUVmean and its corresponding MTV of each lesion.

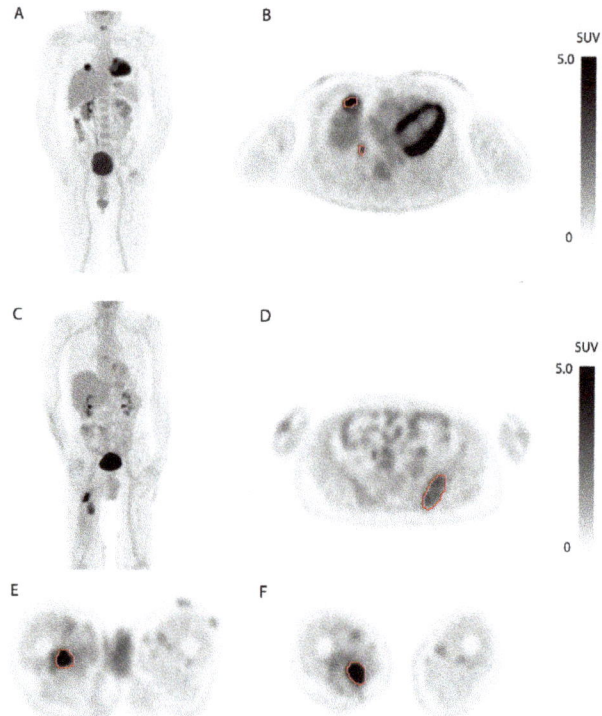

Figure 1. (**A**,**B**): [^{18}F]FDG-PET of a man 8 months after resection of a primary undifferentiated soft tissue sarcoma (grade 3). (**A**): Coronal view of a maximum-intensity projection (MIP) showing two metabolically active lesions in the right lung. (**B**): Axial plane showing two metastases in the right middle lobe and their VOIs outlined in red. (**C**–**F**): [^{18}F]FDG-PET of a man with three known tumor locations 6 months after resection of a primary myxofibrosarcoma (grade 2). (**C**): Coronal projection of a MIP showing two FDG-avid lesions in the right upper leg. (**D**): Axial plane showing a histologically proven metastasis in the left iliac bone and the corresponding VOI outlined in red. (**E**): Axial plane showing a tumor lesion and the corresponding VOI outlined in red in the adductor compartment of the right thigh just cranial of the primary tumor bed. (**F**): Axial plane showing local recurrence and corresponding VOI outlined in red in the adductor compartment of the right thigh.

2.5. Statistical Analyses

An univariate Cox proportional hazard model was used to determine the predictive value of clinical parameters and [^{18}F]FDG-PET features for OS. No analysis of histologic subtypes was performed in this heterogeneous population due to the small number of patients per subtype and previous studies reporting variable histologic subtypes to be correlated to survival. Due to the limited cohort size, not all variables were tested in the multivariate cox analysis. Therefore, multivariate Cox analysis was first performed using the 2 strongest prognostic clinical factors. Subsequently, the prognostic value of adding [^{18}F]FDG-PET features that were significant in univariate analysis was determined for each [^{18}F]FDG-PET feature separately. The [^{18}F]FDG-PET features that significantly added prognostic value to clinical parameters were stratified through the median and the Kaplan–Meier method, and log-rank test were used to estimate survival for the different groups. Statistical significance was defined as $p < 0.05$. The analysis was performed with IBM SPSS v.25 (IBM Corp., Armonk, NY, USA).

3. Results

3.1. Patients and Follow-Up

A total of 31 patients were included in this study, and segmentation of all STS lesions was performed (Figure 1). Patient characteristics are shown in Table 1. Median follow-up in survivors was 32 months. The two-year survival rate was 37%.

3.2. Univariate Analysis

The number of lesions was the only clinical parameter that was significantly predictive for survival in this population ($p = 0.006$) (Table 2). Furthermore, analysis of the [^{18}F]FDG-PET features showed SUVmax and SUVpeak to be significantly predictive for survival ($p = 0.004$ and 0.006, respectively) (Figure 2). Hazard ratios (HRs) were 1.16 per unit increase for SUVmax and 1.20 per unit increase for SUVpeak in univariate analysis.

3.3. Multivariate Analysis

The two strongest predictive clinical parameters were the number of lesions and the performance status. Adding SUVmax and SUVpeak separately to the multivariate model with these clinical parameters showed that both SUVmax and SUVpeak significantly improved the prediction ($p = 0.005$ and 0.004, respectively), independent of these clinical parameters. HRs were 1.29 per unit increase for SUVmax and 1.36 per unit increase for SUVpeak, independent of the number of lesions and the performance status.

Table 2. Clinical variables and PET features in univariate Cox proportional hazard analyses.

Variable	Overall Survival		p-value
Clinical variables	Hazard ratio	95% CI	
Age (years)	1.02	0.99–1.04	0.2
Grade (3 versus 2)	1.26	0.50–3.21	0.6
Location (Deep trunk or upper extr. versus other)	0.91	0.34–2.40	0.8
Number of lesions	1.28	1.07–1.52	0.006
WHO performance status (≥ 1 versus 0)	2.72	0.73–10.07	0.1
Disease free interval			0.2
Synchronous versus >14 months	3.36	0.94–12.0	
<14 months versus >14 months	1.44	0.47–4.47	
PET features			
SUVmax	1.16	1.05–1.29	0.004
SUVpeak	1.20	1.05–1.37	0.006
SUVmean	1.23	0.99–1.54	0.07
MTV	1.001	0.999–1.003	0.2
TLG	1.001	1.000–1.001	0.1

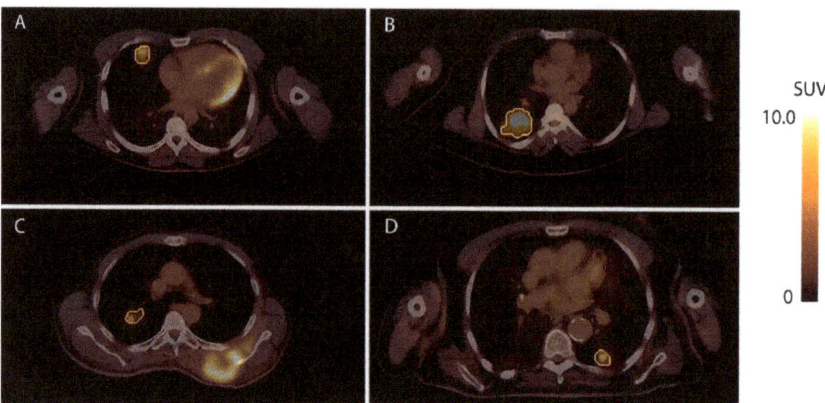

Figure 2. Examples of lung metastases with different metabolic characteristics. Axial planes of [18F]FDG-PET/CTs of four patients with lung metastases are shown with the corresponding VOIs outlined in orange. (**A**): A metastasis with a SUVmax of 6.1 detected 22 months after resection of an undifferentiated soft tissue sarcoma in the right deltoid muscle. (**B**): A metastasis with a SUVmax of 9.0 detected 34 months after resection of an undifferentiated soft tissue sarcoma in the right gluteus maximus. (**C**): A metastasis with a SUVmax of 5.2 detected synchronous with a myxofibrosarcoma originating from the left thoracic wall. (**D**): A metastasis with a SUVmax of 7.2 detected synchronous with local recurrence of a leiomyosarcoma in the right lower leg.

3.4. Survival Estimates

Median SUVmax and SUVpeak were 5.7 and 4.9 g/mL, respectively. The estimated mean overall survival in patients with SUVmax > 5.7 g/mL was 14 months, and that for patients with SUVmax < 5.7 g/mL was 39 months ($p < 0.001$). For patients with SUVpeak > 4.9 g/mL, the estimated mean overall survival was 18 months, while for those with SUVpeak < 4.9 g/mL, it was 33 months ($p = 0.04$) (Figure 3).

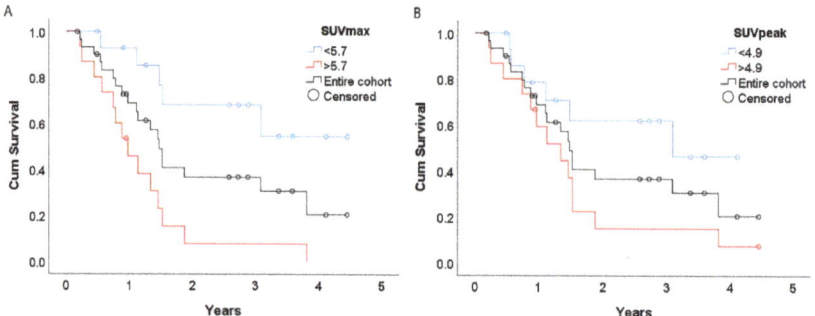

Figure 3. Survival curves with the cohort dichotomized at the median SUVmax (**A**) and median SUVpeak (**B**). The grey line represents the survival curve of the entire cohort. The estimated mean overall survival in patients with SUVmax > 5.7 g/mL was 14 months, and that for patients with SUVmax < 5.7 g/mL was 39 months ($p < 0.001$). For patients with SUVpeak > 4.9 g/mL, the estimated mean overall survival was 18 months, while for those with SUVpeak < 4.9 g/mL, it was 33 months ($p = 0.04$).

4. Discussion

In patients with STS, [18F]FDG-PET/CTs are often acquired for staging. Next to the identification of metastatic lesions, these scans provide quantitative information on the metabolic activity of the tumor tissue. The results in this study show that this biological characteristic has a prognostic value and turned out to be an independent predictor of overall survival in the soft tissue sarcoma patient group with metastatic disease. This information on tumor biology adds to the already known prognostic clinical parameters reported in the literature by Billingsley et al., Italiano et al., and Lochner et al., such as patient age, disease-free interval, number of lesions, FNCLCC grade, and histologic subtype [4–6].

In a systematic search that was conducted in preparation of this study, no report was found on the value of [^{18}F]FDG-PET features in metastatic STS patients (Appendix A), while prognosis is especially relevant in a cohort where cure might not be the primary goal of treatment. The prognostic value of [^{18}F]FDG-PET features in non-metastatic STS is studied more extensively. Original investigations focusing on this topic in patients with localized disease have found [^{18}F]FDG-PET features to be significantly predictive for progression-free and overall survival [20–23]. Nevertheless, in some of these studies, the added value of the features is not corrected for clinical parameters, such as resectability of the tumor, neoadjuvant treatment, etc., leaving the effect of [^{18}F]FDG-PET features difficult to interpret on an individual level. In studies performing multivariate analyses, results are variable and partly clouded due to the limited statistical power caused by small cohort sizes [24–26].

In the current study, the overall survival of the whole cohort was comparable with survival in recent larger studies, suggesting the current study population is representative, and our findings might add to the ability to accurately predict survival in patient with metastases from STS [4,5]. Our results show both SUVmax and SUVpeak to have prognostic value, and therefore, are in line with the results in patients with localized disease. For SUVmean, TLG, and MTV, however, studies in localized STS patients typically find significant correlations with overall survival, while no predictive value was found in the metastatic cohort in our study [22,23,25]. Partially, this could be caused by the limited cohort size. Another plausible reason for this discrepancy is found in the composition of these features and the biological background they resemble. All [^{18}F]FDG-PET features investigated in this study, i.e., SUVmax, SUVpeak, SUVmean, TLG, and MTV, quantify the metabolism in selected tumor tissue, but SUVmean and inherently TLG and MTV are strongly dependent on tumor size next to metabolism and thus altered after resection of the primary tumor. In contrast, SUVmax and SUVpeak are not dependent on lesion size and thus resemble the metabolic potential of tumor cells accurately, even after surgical volume reduction. Thus, the results suggest that the prognosis of a metastatic STS patient is determined by the most aggressive tumor clone in the body.

Research in other tumor types, such as breast, colorectal, and lung carcinoma, also shows added prognostic value of [^{18}F]FDG-PET features next to clinical parameters in cohorts of patients with metastasized disease [16,27,28]. In contrast with the current results, TLG and MTV generally also show a correlation to survival in these cohorts. An explanation for this discrepancy is the relative heterogeneous population in our study, including both patients with synchronous diagnosis of the primary tumor and metastasis and patients with diagnosis of metastasis after resection of the primary tumor. In addition, differences in tumor biology, such as pattern and interval of spread, might cause deviation between results in different tumor types.

A strength of this study is the use of a multivariate analysis to determine the added value of the PET features in addition to prognostic clinical parameters that are readily available. This multiparametric analysis showed that both SUVmax and SUVpeak provide prognostic value, next to the two strongest predictive clinical characteristics. Furthermore, the [^{18}F]FDG-PET scans are often performed in standard clinical practice for staging of disease, and therefore, the features can be determined without extra costs and distress for the patients [7]. There are some limitations to this study. Due to the retrospective nature, the performance status of some patients could not be determined accurately. Moreover, the limited cohort size and the heterogeneity in tumor subtypes prohibited definitive conclusions about [^{18}F]FDG-PET features when correcting for all known clinical parameters.

In this regard, especially the link with the wide variety of histological subtype remains unexplored to some extent.

In larger studies investigating prognosis in metastatic STS patients, correlations with subtype are typically found [4–6]. These results are, however, partly contradicting regarding which subtypes are causing poor survival rates. With metastatic leiomyosarcoma as a reference, both Italiano et al. and Lochner et al. concluded that patients with metastatic undifferentiated soft tissue sarcoma or malignant peripheral nerve sheath tumors have an impaired survival but reported conflicting results regarding liposarcoma and synovial sarcoma patients [4,5]. This leads to the conclusion that a correlation between histologic subtype and survival in metastatic patients exists but is difficult to define. Several reasons for this complexity are rarity of subtypes, heterogeneity within sarcoma subtypes, and shifts in histologic definitions of subtypes over the years. In the current study, the biological differences between histologic subtypes might have amplified the predictive value of quantitative [^{18}F]FDG-PET features on survival. In literature, relatively aggressive subtypes, such as undifferentiated soft tissue sarcoma, are found to show high FDG avidity. Other specific subtypes, such as (myxoid) liposarcomas, tend to show relatively low avidity [29,30]. Nevertheless, these studies report varying and non-specific SUVmax values within subtypes, suggesting [^{18}F]FDG-PET features could provide additional prognostic information. Figure 2 presents examples of differences in SUVmax between and within STS subtypes. Future studies validating the prognostic value of quantitative [^{18}F]FDG-PET features in metastatic STS patients should aim to address the link with histologic subtypes.

Furthermore, the use of multimodality imaging should be considered in research aiming to identify more prognostic biomarkers in patients with metastatic STS. Magnetic resonance (MR) imaging is widely used for the characterization of localized soft tissue tumors. Quantitative diffusion-weighted imaging (DWI) and dynamic contrast-enhanced (DCE) MR features are linked to tumor grade, response to treatment, and survival [31,32]. Multimodality imaging with [^{18}F]FDG-PET/MR showed increased usefulness over [^{18}F]FDG-PET alone in several studies on localized STS [33,34]. This raises the hypothesis that the addition of quantitative MR parameters to clinical and [^{18}F]FDG-PET parameters could improve the characterization of tumor biology in patients with metastases from STS even further.

Personalized treatment in patients with metastases from STS is complex, and prognostic factors are important for multiple considerations during the development of treatment strategies. For example, factors linked to an impaired prognosis support the addition of chemotherapy to surgery in patients with resectable metastases. A high number of tumor lesions and a short recurrence-free interval are factors that are typically used for this purpose, as stated in the recent ESMO-EURACAN-GENTURIS guidelines [7]. The current study shows added value of [^{18}F]FDG-PET features to these clinical factors. Moreover, in treatment strategies with a palliative intent specifically, periods without active treatment can be desirable to warrant the quality of life of patients. Prognostic factors are decisive in the timing of these treatment-free periods, as they are partly guided by the expected time to progression of disease [35].

5. Conclusions

In conclusion, personalized medicine is especially challenging and important in this patient group with strongly impaired survival rates. Therefore, accurate information about individual patient prognosis should be pursued before individual patient management decision making. Next to clinical and pathological characteristics, biological tumor characteristics such as metabolic parameters on [^{18}F]FDG-PET scans can be considered for this purpose. In this regard, the current study finds SUVmax and SUVpeak to be significantly predictive for overall survival in patients with metastases from STS. Furthermore, both features add prognostic value to the best performing clinical parameters.

Author Contributions: Conceptualization, G.M.K., W.G. and L.-F.d.G.-O.; methodology, G.M.K., W.G., J.L.B. and L.-F.d.G.-O.; software, G.M.K. and F.H.P.v.V.; validation, G.M.K., W.G. and F.H.P.v.V.; formal analysis, G.M.K., W.G. and L.-F.d.G.-O.; investigation, G.M.K., J.V.M.G.B., H.G., J.A.v.d.H., M.A.J.v.d.S., J.L.B. and L.-F.d.G.-O.; resources, G.M.K., J.V.M.G.B., H.G., J.A.v.d.H., M.A.J.v.d.S., F.H.P.v.V., J.L.B. and L.-F.d.G.-O.; data curation, G.M.K., W.G., J.V.M.G.B. and L.-F.d.G.-O.; writing—original draft preparation, G.M.K. and L.-F.d.G.-O.; writing—review and editing, G.M.K., W.G., J.V.M.G.B., H.G., J.A.v.d.H., M.A.J.v.d.S., F.H.P.v.V., J.L.B. and L.-F.d.G.-O.; visualization, G.M.K., F.H.P.v.V. and L.-F.d.G.-O.; supervision, W.G., J.L.B. and L.-F.d.G.-O.; project administration, G.M.K.; funding acquisition, W.G., J.L.B. and L.-F.d.G.-O. All authors have read and agreed to the published version of the manuscript.

Funding: We declare the following financial interests/personal relationships which may be considered as potential competing interests: G.M. Kalisvaart was the recipient of an educational grant from Philips Electronics Nederland B.V, Eindhoven, The Netherlands, during writing of this manuscript. Furthermore, the research presented in the manuscript was supported by a public grant from Health~Holland TKI Life Sciences & Health.

Institutional Review Board Statement: The study was conducted according to the guidelines of the Declaration of Helsinki and approved by the Ethics Committee Leiden Den Haag Delft (METC LDD) (protocol code: B19.050, date of approval 14 January 2020).

Informed Consent Statement: Patient consent was waived due to due to the retrospective nature of the study. Patients who objected to the use of their data were excluded.

Data Availability Statement: The datasets generated during and/or analyzed during the current study are available from the corresponding author upon reasonable request.

Acknowledgments: The authors would like to thank Jan W. Schoones for his contribution to the search strategy.

Conflicts of Interest: The authors have declared that no competing interest exist.

Appendix A. Literature Search

A systematic literature search was performed to identify available articles describing original research attending to our hypothesis. A search strategy based on our hypothesis was designed with the assistance of a medical librarian and conducted in PubMed on 1 September 2021. A total of 182 records were identified. After screening the titles, 32 records were excluded. In addition, after reading the abstracts and/or full articles, another 150 records were excluded. No articles that investigated our hypothesis were found (Figure A1).

Search strategy: ((("advanced soft tissue sarcoma"[tw] OR "advanced soft tissue sarcomas"[tw] OR "advanced sarcoma"[tw] OR "advanced sarcomas"[tw] OR "metastatic soft tissue sarcoma"[tw] OR "metastatic soft tissue sarcomas"[tw] OR "metastatic sarcoma"[tw] OR "metastatic sarcomas"[tw] OR "metastasized sarcoma"[tw] OR (("soft tissue sarcomas"[tw] OR "soft tissue sarcoma"[tw] OR (("Sarcoma"[Mesh:NoExp] OR "sarcoma"[tw] OR "sarcomas"[tw]) AND ("soft tissue"[tw] OR "soft tissues"[tw])) OR "Adenosarcoma"[mesh] OR "Carcinosarcoma"[mesh] OR "Fibrosarcoma"[mesh] OR "Hemangiosarcoma"[mesh] OR "Histiocytoma, Malignant Fibrous"[mesh] OR "Leiomyosarcoma"[mesh] OR "Liposarcoma"[mesh] OR "Lymphangiosarcoma"[mesh] OR "Mixed Tumor, Mesodermal"[mesh] OR "Myosarcoma"[mesh] OR "Myxosarcoma"[mesh] OR "Sarcoma, Alveolar Soft Part"[mesh] OR "Sarcoma, Clear Cell"[mesh] OR "Sarcoma, Myeloid"[mesh] OR "Sarcoma, Small Cell"[mesh] OR "Sarcoma, Synovial"[mesh] OR "Adenosarcoma"[tw] OR "Adenosarcomas"[tw] OR "Alveolar Soft Part Sarcoma"[tw] OR "Alveolar Soft Part Sarcomas"[tw] OR "Carcinosarcoma"[tw] OR "Carcinosarcomas"[tw] OR "Clear Cell Sarcoma"[tw] OR "Clear Cell Sarcomas"[tw] OR "Dermatofibrosarcoma"[tw] OR "Dermatofibrosarcomas"[tw] OR "Fibrosarcoma"[tw] OR "Fibrosarcomas"[tw] OR "Hemangiosarcoma"[tw] OR "Hemangiosarcomas"[tw] OR "Leiomyosarcoma"[tw] OR "Leiomyosarcomas"[tw] OR "Liposarcoma"[tw] OR "Liposarcomas"[tw] OR "Lymphangiosarcoma"[tw] OR "Lymphangiosarcomas"[tw] OR "Malignant Fibrous

Histiocytoma"[tw] OR "Malignant Fibrous Histiocytomas"[tw] OR "Mesodermal Mixed Tumor"[tw] OR "Mesodermal Mixed Tumors"[tw] OR "Mesodermal Mixed Tumour"[tw] OR "Mesodermal Mixed Tumours"[tw] OR "Myeloid Sarcoma"[tw] OR "Myeloid Sarcomas"[tw] OR "Myosarcoma"[tw] OR "Myosarcomas"[tw] OR "Myxosarcoma"[tw] OR "Myxosarcomas"[tw] OR "Neurofibrosarcoma"[tw] OR "Neurofibrosarcomas"[tw] OR "Rhabdomyosarcoma"[tw] OR "Rhabdomyosarcomas"[tw] OR "Small Cell Sarcoma"[tw] OR "Small Cell Sarcomas"[tw] OR "Synovial Sarcoma "[tw] OR "Synovial Sarcomas"[tw] OR "Walker Carcinoma 256"[tw]) AND ("Neoplasm Metastasis"[Mesh] OR "Metastasis"[tw] OR "metasta*"[tw] OR "advanced"[tw])) AND ("FDG-PET"[tw] OR "FDG-PET"[tw] OR "18FDG-PET"[tw] OR "18FDGPET"[tw] OR "Positron-Emission Tomography"[Mesh] OR "Positron-Emission Tomography"[tw] OR "Positron-Emission"[tw] OR "PET"[tw] OR "PETCT"[tw] OR "Fluorodeoxyglucose F18"[Mesh] OR "Fluorodeoxyglucose F18"[tw] OR "FDG"[tw] OR "18F-FDG"[tw] OR "Fluorodeoxyglucose F 18"[tw] OR "Fludeoxyglucose F 18"[tw] OR "Fluorine 18 fluorodeoxyglucose"[tw] OR "18F Fluorodeoxyglucose"[tw] OR "18FDG"[tw] OR "2 Fluoro 2 deoxy D glucose"[tw] OR "2 Fluoro 2 deoxyglucose"[tw] OR "4-fluoro-4-deoxyglucose"[Supplementary Concept]) AND ("Mortality"[Mesh] OR "mortality"[Subheading] OR "Disease-Free Survival"[Mesh] OR "Survival Analysis"[Mesh] OR "Survival Rate"[Mesh] OR "Progression-Free Survival"[Mesh] OR "mortality"[tw] OR "survival"[tw] OR "death"[tw] OR "deaths"[tw] OR "Prognosis"[Mesh] OR "Prognosis"[tw] OR "prognos*"[tw] OR "outcome"[tw] OR "outcomes"[tw]) NOT ((("Case Reports"[ptyp] OR "case report"[ti]) NOT ("Clinical Study"[ptyp] OR "trial"[ti] OR "RCT"[ti]))).

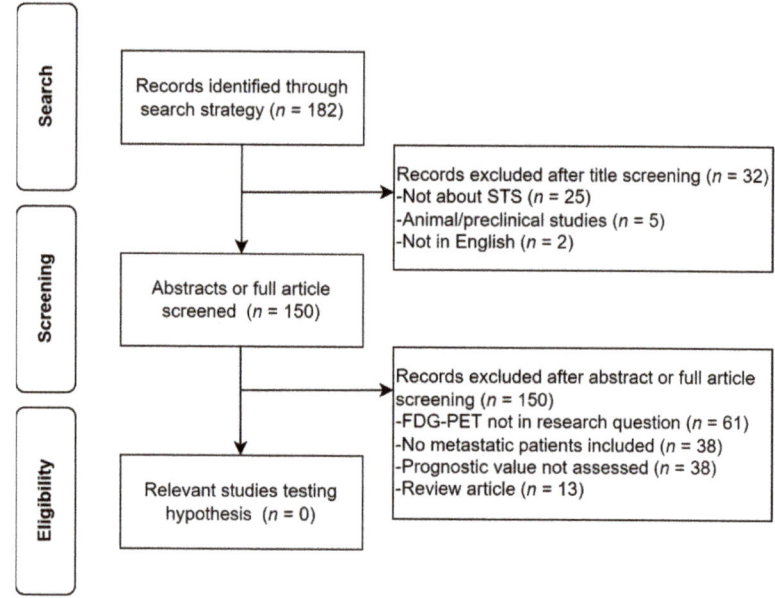

Figure A1. Flowchart of the performed literature search.

References

1. Society, A.C. *Cancer Facts & Figures 2017*; American Cancer Society: Atlanta, GA, USA, 2017.
2. Callegaro, D.; Miceli, R.; Bonvalot, S.; Ferguson, P.; Strauss, D.C.; Levy, A.; Griffin, A.; Hayes, A.J.; Stacchiotti, S.; Pechoux, C.L.; et al. Development and external validation of two nomograms to predict overall survival and occurrence of distant metastases in adults after surgical resection of localised soft-tissue sarcomas of the extremities: A retrospective analysis. *Lancet Oncol.* **2016**, *17*, 671–680. [CrossRef]

3. Acem, I.; Verhoef, C.; Rueten-Budde, A.J.; Grunhagen, D.J.; van Houdt, W.J.; van de Sande, M.A.; Aston, W.; Bonenkamp, H.; Desar, I.M.; Ferguson, P.C.; et al. Age-related differences of oncological outcomes in primary extremity soft tissue sarcoma: A multistate model including 6260 patients. *Eur. J. Cancer* **2020**, *141*, 128–136. [CrossRef]
4. Lochner, J.; Menge, F.; Vassos, N.; Hohenberger, P.; Kasper, B. Prognosis of Patients with Metastatic Soft Tissue Sarcoma: Advances in Recent Years. *Oncol. Res. Treat.* **2020**, *43*, 613–619. [CrossRef] [PubMed]
5. Italiano, A.; Mathoulin-Pelissier, S.; Cesne, A.L.; Terrier, P.; Bonvalot, S.; Collin, F.; Michels, J.J.; Blay, J.Y.; Coindre, J.M.; Bui, B. Trends in survival for patients with metastatic soft-tissue sarcoma. *Cancer* **2011**, *117*, 1049–1054. [CrossRef] [PubMed]
6. Billingsley, K.G.; Lewis, J.J.; Leung, D.H.; Casper, E.S.; Woodruff, J.M.; Brennan, M.F. Multifactorial analysis of the survival of patients with distant metastasis arising from primary extremity sarcoma. *Cancer* **1999**, *85*, 389–395. [CrossRef]
7. Gronchi, A.; Miah, A.B.; Dei Tos, A.P.; Abecassis, N.; Bajpai, J.; Bauer, S.; Biagini, R.; Bielack, S.; Blay, J.Y.; Bolle, S.; et al. Soft tissue and visceral sarcomas: ESMO-EURACAN-GENTURIS Clinical Practice Guidelines for diagnosis, treatment and follow-up ☆. *Ann. Oncol.* **2021**, *32*, 1348–1365. [CrossRef]
8. Van Glabbeke, M.; van Oosterom, A.T.; Oosterhuis, J.W.; Mouridsen, H.; Crowther, D.; Somers, R.; Verweij, J.; Santoro, A.; Buesa, J.; Tursz, T. Prognostic factors for the outcome of chemotherapy in advanced soft tissue sarcoma: An analysis of 2,185 patients treated with anthracycline-containing first-line regimens—A European Organization for Research and Treatment of Cancer Soft Tissue and Bone Sarcoma Group Study. *J. Clin. Oncol.* **1999**, *17*, 150–157. [CrossRef] [PubMed]
9. Rueten-Budde, A.J.; van Praag, V.M.; van de Sande, M.A.; Fiocco, M.; Group, P.S. External validation and adaptation of a dynamic prediction model for patients with high-grade extremity soft tissue sarcoma. *J. Surg. Oncol.* **2021**, *123*, 1050–1056. [CrossRef] [PubMed]
10. Rueten-Budde, A.J.; Van Praag, V.M.; Jeys, L.M.; Laitinen, M.K.; Pollock, R.; Aston, W.; van der Hage, J.A.; Dijkstra, P.S.; Ferguson, P.C.; Griffin, A.M.; et al. Dynamic prediction of overall survival for patients with high-grade extremity soft tissue sarcoma. *Surg. Oncol.* **2018**, *27*, 695–701. [CrossRef]
11. Kalisvaart, G.M.; Bloem, J.L.; Bovee, J.; van de Sande, M.A.; Gelderblom, H.; van der Hage, J.A.; Hartgrink, H.H.; Krol, A.D.; de Geus-Oei, L.F.; Grootjans, W. Personalising sarcoma care using quantitative multimodality imaging for response assessment. *Clin. Radiol.* **2021**, *76*, 313.e1–313.e13. [CrossRef]
12. Annovazzi, A.; Rea, S.; Zoccali, C.; Sciuto, R.; Baldi, J.; Anelli, V.; Petrongari, M.G.; Pescarmona, E.; Biagini, R.; Ferraresi, V. Diagnostic and Clinical Impact of 18F-FDG PET/CT in Staging and Restaging Soft-Tissue Sarcomas of the Extremities and Trunk: Mono-Institutional Retrospective Study of a Sarcoma Referral Center. *J. Clin. Med.* **2020**, *9*, 2549. [CrossRef] [PubMed]
13. Vlenterie, M.; Oyen, W.J.; Steeghs, N.; Desar, I.M.; Verheijen, R.B.; Koenen, A.M.; Grootjans, W.; De Geus-Oei, L.F.; Van Erp, N.P.; Van Der Graaf, W.T. Early Metabolic Response as a Predictor of Treatment Outcome in Patients with Metastatic Soft Tissue Sarcomas. *Anticancer Res.* **2019**, *39*, 1309–1316. [CrossRef]
14. Reyes Marles, R.H.; Navarro Fernandez, J.L.; Puertas Garcia-Sandoval, J.P.; Santonja Medina, F.; Mohamed Salem, L.; Frutos Esteban, L.; Contreras Gutierrez, J.F.; Castellon Sanchez, M.I.; Ruiz Merino, G.; Claver Valderas, M.A. Clinical value of baseline ^{18}F-FDG PET/CT in soft tissue sarcomas. *Eur. J. Hybrid Imaging* **2021**, *5*, 16. [CrossRef]
15. Chen, J.; Wu, X.; Ma, X.; Guo, L.; Zhu, C.; Li, Q. Prognostic value of 18F-FDG PET-CT-based functional parameters in patients with soft tissue sarcoma: A meta-analysis. *Medicine* **2017**, *96*, e5913. [CrossRef]
16. De Geus-Oei, L.F.; Wiering, B.; Krabbe, P.F.; Ruers, T.J.; Punt, C.J.; Oyen, W.J. FDG-PET for prediction of survival of patients with metastatic colorectal carcinoma. *Ann. Oncol.* **2006**, *17*, 1650–1655. [CrossRef] [PubMed]
17. Trojani, M.; Contesso, G.; Coindre, J.M.; Rouesse, J.; Bui, N.B.; de Mascarel, A.; Goussot, J.F.; David, M.; Bonichon, F.; Lagarde, C. Soft-tissue sarcomas of adults; study of pathological prognostic variables and definition of a histopathological grading system. *Int. J. Cancer* **1984**, *33*, 37–42. [CrossRef] [PubMed]
18. Boellaard, R.; Delgado-Bolton, R.; Oyen, W.J.; Giammarile, F.; Tatsch, K.; Eschner, W.; Verzijlbergen, F.J.; Barrington, S.F.; Pike, L.C.; Weber, W.A.; et al. FDG PET/CT: EANM procedure guidelines for tumour imaging: Version 2.0. *Eur. J. Nucl. Med. Mol. Imaging* **2015**, *42*, 328–354. [CrossRef] [PubMed]
19. Frings, V.; van Velden, F.H.; Velasquez, L.M.; Hayes, W.; van de Ven, P.M.; Hoekstra, O.S.; Boellaard, R. Repeatability of metabolically active tumor volume measurements with FDG PET/CT in advanced gastrointestinal malignancies: A multicenter study. *Radiology* **2014**, *273*, 539–548. [CrossRef]
20. Singh, T.P.; Sharma, A.; Sharma, A.; Bakhshi, S.; Patel, C.; Pandey, A.K.; Dhamija, E.; Batra, A.; Kumar, R. Utility of 18F-FDG-PET/CT in management and prognostication of treatment naive late-stage soft tissue sarcomas. *Nucl. Med. Commun.* **2021**, *42*, 818–825. [CrossRef]
21. Fuglø, H.M.; Jørgensen, S.M.; Loft, A.; Hovgaard, D.; Petersen, M.M. The diagnostic and prognostic value of ^{18}F-FDG PET/CT in the initial assessment of high-grade bone and soft tissue sarcoma. A retrospective study of 89 patients. *Eur. J. Nucl. Med. Mol. Imaging* **2012**, *39*, 1416–1424. [CrossRef] [PubMed]
22. Lee, J.W.; Heo, E.J.; Moon, S.H.; Lee, H.; Cheon, G.J.; Lee, M.; Kim, H.S.; Chung, H.H. Prognostic value of total lesion glycolysis on preoperative ^{18}F-FDG PET/CT in patients with uterine carcinosarcoma. *Eur. Radiol.* **2016**, *26*, 4148–4154. [CrossRef] [PubMed]
23. Chang, K.J.; Lim, I.; Park, J.Y.; Jo, A.R.; Kong, C.B.; Song, W.S.; Jo, W.H.; Lee, S.Y.; Koh, J.S.; Kim, B.I.; et al. The Role of ^{18}F-FDG PET/CT as a Prognostic Factor in Patients with Synovial Sarcoma. *Nucl. Med. Mol. Imaging* **2015**, *49*, 33–41. [CrossRef]
24. Lisle, J.W.; Eary, J.F.; O'Sullivan, J.; Conrad, E.U. Risk assessment based on FDG-PET imaging in patients with synovial sarcoma. *Clin. Orthop. Relat. Res.* **2009**, *467*, 1605–1611. [CrossRef] [PubMed]

25. Choi, E.S.; Ha, S.G.; Kim, H.S.; Ha, J.H.; Paeng, J.C.; Han, I. Total lesion glycolysis by 18F-FDG PET/CT is a reliable predictor of prognosis in soft-tissue sarcoma. *Eur. J. Nucl. Med. Mol. Imaging* **2013**, *40*, 1836–1842. [CrossRef] [PubMed]
26. Baum, S.H.; Frühwald, M.; Rahbar, K.; Wessling, J.; Schober, O.; Weckesser, M. Contribution of PET/CT to prediction of outcome in children and young adults with rhabdomyosarcoma. *J. Nucl. Med.* **2011**, *52*, 1535–1540. [CrossRef]
27. Satoh, Y.; Nambu, A.; Ichikawa, T.; Onishi, H. Whole-body total lesion glycolysis measured on fluorodeoxyglucose positron emission tomography/computed tomography as a prognostic variable in metastatic breast cancer. *BMC Cancer* **2014**, *14*, 525. [CrossRef]
28. Lim, Y.; Bang, J.I.; Han, S.W.; Paeng, J.C.; Lee, K.H.; Kim, J.H.; Kang, G.H.; Jeong, S.Y.; Park, K.J.; Kim, T.Y. Total lesion glycolysis (TLG) as an imaging biomarker in metastatic colorectal cancer patients treated with regorafenib. *Eur. J. Nucl. Med. Mol. Imaging* **2017**, *44*, 757–764. [CrossRef]
29. Macpherson, R.E.; Pratap, S.; Tyrrell, H.; Khonsari, M.; Wilson, S.; Gibbons, M.; Whitwell, D.; Giele, H.; Critchley, P.; Cogswell, L.; et al. Retrospective audit of 957 consecutive ^{18}F-FDG PET-CT scans compared to CT and MRI in 493 patients with different histological subtypes of bone and soft tissue sarcoma. *Clin. Sarcoma Res.* **2018**, *8*, 9. [CrossRef]
30. Charest, M.; Hickeson, M.; Lisbona, R.; Novales-Diaz, J.A.; Derbekyan, V.; Turcotte, R.E. FDG PET/CT imaging in primary osseous and soft tissue sarcomas: A retrospective review of 212 cases. *Eur. J. Nucl. Med. Mol. Imaging* **2009**, *36*, 1944–1951. [CrossRef]
31. Spinnato, P.; Kind, M.; Le Loarer, F.; Bianchi, G.; Colangeli, M.; Sambri, A.; Ponti, F.; van Langevelde, K.; Crombe, A. Soft Tissue Sarcomas: The Role of Quantitative MRI in Treatment Response Evaluation. *Acad. Radiol.* **2021**. [CrossRef]
32. Casali, P.G.; Abecassis, N.; Aro, H.T.; Bauer, S.; Biagini, R.; Bielack, S.; Bonvalot, S.; Boukovinas, I.; Bovee, J.; Brodowicz, T.; et al. Soft tissue and visceral sarcomas: ESMO-EURACAN Clinical Practice Guidelines for diagnosis, treatment and follow-up. *Ann. Oncol.* **2018**, *29*, iv268–iv269. [CrossRef] [PubMed]
33. Chodyla, M.; Demircioglu, A.; Schaarschmidt, B.M.; Bertram, S.; Morawitz, J.; Bauer, S.; Podleska, L.; Rischpler, C.; Forsting, M.; Herrmann, K.; et al. Evaluation of the Predictive Potential of 18F-FDG PET and DWI Data Sets for Relevant Prognostic Parameters of Primary Soft-Tissue Sarcomas. *Cancers* **2021**, *13*, 2753. [CrossRef]
34. Chodyla, M.; Demircioglu, A.; Schaarschmidt, B.M.; Bertram, S.; Bruckmann, N.M.; Haferkamp, J.; Li, Y.; Bauer, S.; Podleska, L.; Rischpler, C.; et al. Evaluation of ^{18}F-FDG PET and DWI Datasets for Predicting Therapy Response of Soft-Tissue Sarcomas Under Neoadjuvant Isolated Limb Perfusion. *J. Nucl. Med.* **2021**, *62*, 348–353. [CrossRef] [PubMed]
35. Dangoor, A.; Seddon, B.; Gerrand, C.; Grimer, R.; Whelan, J.; Judson, I. UK guidelines for the management of soft tissue sarcomas. *Clin. Sarcoma Res.* **2016**, *6*, 20. [CrossRef] [PubMed]

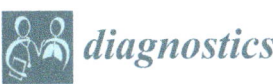

Article

The Use of ^{18}F-FDG PET/CT Metabolic Parameters in Predicting Overall Survival in Patients Undergoing Restaging for Malignant Melanoma

Khanyisile N. Hlongwa [1], Kgomotso M. G. Mokoala [1], Zvifadzo Matsena-Zingoni [2], Mariza Vorster [1,3] and Mike M. Sathekge [1,3,*]

1. Department of Nuclear Medicine, University of Pretoria and Steve Biko Academic Hospital, Pretoria 0001, South Africa; khanyi29@gmail.com (K.N.H.); kgomotso.mokoala@up.ac.za (K.M.G.M.); marizavorster@gmail.com (M.V.)
2. Division of Epidemiology and Biostatistics, School of Public Health, University of Witwatersrand, Johannesburg 2193, South Africa; zvifadzo.matsenazingoni@wits.ac.za
3. Nuclear Medicine Research Infrastructure (NuMeRI), Steve Biko Academic Hospital, Pretoria 0001, South Africa
* Correspondence: mike.sathekge@up.ac.za or sathekgemike@gmail.com; Tel.: +27-12-354-1794

Abstract: Malignant melanoma is one of the more aggressive cancers in the skin, with an increasing incidence every year. Melanoma has a better prognosis if diagnosed early and survival tends to decrease once the disease has metastasized. Positron emission tomography (PET) with 2-[^{18}F]fluoro-2-deoxy-D-glucose (^{18}F-FDG) has been used extensively over the past two decades in staging and assessing responses to therapy in patients with melanoma. Metabolic PET parameters have been demonstrated to be independent prognostic factors for progression-free survival (PFS) and overall survival (OS) in different malignancies, melanoma included. In our study, we evaluated the metabolic parameters of ^{18}F-FDG PET/CT (flourodeoxyglucose positron emission tomography/computed tomography) in predicting the overall survival in patients with malignant melanoma who presented for restaging. Metabolic PET parameters (maximum standardized uptake value (SUVmax), metabolic tumor volume (MTV) and total lesion glycolysis (TLG)) of the primary tumor, as well as whole-body MTV and TLG of the metastatic disease, were measured. Survival curves for OS were constructed and mortality rates were determined using the different PET variables. Forty-nine patients who presented for a PET/CT restaging in melanoma were included in this study. We found that non-survivors had significantly higher median MTV (11.86 cm^3 vs. 5.68 cm^3; p-value = 0.022), TLG (3125 vs. 14; p-value = 0.0357), whole-body MTV (53.9 cm^3 vs. 14.4 cm^3; p-value = 0.0076) and whole-body TLG (963.4 vs. 114.6; p-value = 0.0056). This demonstrated that high MTV and TLG values of the primary tumor and whole-body TLG as quantified by ^{18}F-FDG PET/CT were prognostic factors for overall survival. The findings may potentially guide clinicians in decision making and identifying patients with a poorer prognosis.

Keywords: ^{18}F-FDG PET/CT (fluorodeoxyglucose positron emission tomography/computed tomography); metabolic parameters; metabolic tumor volume (MTV); total lesion glycolysis (TLG); maximum standard uptake value (SUVmax); oncology; malignant melanoma (MM); overall survival (OS); restaging

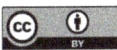

1. Introduction

Melanoma is a malignant tumor that arises from the uncontrolled and rapid growth of the melanocytes, which are the pigment-producing cells of the body [1]. The most common form is cutaneous melanoma; however, the tumor can occur in mucosal surfaces, the eye or the brain [1]. Malignant melanoma is one of the aggressive cancers in the skin, with an increasing incidence every year. It is known to represent a small proportion of all cutaneous malignancies but causes a higher rate of fatalities in comparison to other deaths related to skin cancer [1]. Melanoma has a better prognosis if diagnosed early and survival tends to decrease once the disease has metastasized. The cost of management of melanoma contributes significantly to public health and several strategies are being implemented worldwide to improve outcomes via prevention, assessing the at-risk population and improving management strategies [1].

In the South African setting, a country with a diverse population, melanoma is commonly seen in fair-skinned people rather than darker individuals. A retrospective observational study done between 2005 and 2013 from the national cancer registry found that the incidence of melanoma was 2.7 per 100,000 [2]. The different population groups are affected by varying histological subtypes of melanoma, with the superficial spreading subtype being more common in fair individuals and the acral lentiginous subtype seen more in pigmented individuals [2].

Positron emission tomography (PET) with 2-[^{18}F]fluoro-2-deoxy-D-glucose (^{18}F-FDG) has been used extensively over the past two decades in staging and assessing responses to therapy in patients with melanoma; this has been due to a significant relationship between ^{18}F-FDG uptake and glucose metabolism [3]. Flourodeoxyglucose positron emission tomography/computed tomography (^{18}F-FDG PET/CT) has been demonstrated to be more reliable in the assessment of survival prognosis in comparison to morphological staging. This is because ^{18}F-FDG uptake demonstrates malignant potential, which has been associated with reduced survival [4].

^{18}F-FDG uptake has been demonstrated as an excellent substrate in measuring the malignant potential for melanoma; when compared to immunohistochemistry, it demonstrated a positive correlation between glucose transporters (GLUT)-1 and GLUT-3, which is the mechanism that ^{18}F-FDG uses to demonstrate malignant tissues in patients with melanoma [5].

The sensitivity, specificity and accuracy of ^{18}F-FDG PET to detect metastatic and distant melanoma range from 70 to 100% [6]. The findings in ^{18}F-FDG PET studies have been shown to better stage patients, guide further management and provide a better prognosis of patients. This was demonstrated in a study by Reinhardt et al. whereby 250 patients imaged with ^{18}F-FDG PET/CT demonstrated more nodal and visceral metastases in comparison to CT alone [6]. A smaller study in South Africa also demonstrated how ^{18}F-FDG PET/CT altered staging in patients with malignant melanoma, which further changed the management by treating physicians [7].

Recently, the use of metabolic parameters of ^{18}F-FDG PET/CT has been investigated as a tool to risk-stratify patients and to determine prognostic value in patients prior to management, either by surgery or immune therapy, or to detect recurrence [8–11].

In this study, we investigated the association of metabolic parameters of ^{18}F-FDG PET/CT in patients with melanoma undergoing restaging with overall survival.

2. Materials and Methods

2.1. Patients

^{18}F-FDG PET/CT scans of patients presenting for restaging of melanoma were retrospectively reviewed.

Patients were included in the study if they had a suspicion of recurrent or progressive disease as deemed by the referring clinician. The decision to refer a patient for an ^{18}F-FDG PET/CT scan and the frequency of imaging were at the discretion of the managing physician. Patients were excluded if they had no disease demonstrable on ^{18}F-FDG PET/CT, had advanced primary cancers other than melanoma, were below 18 years of age and had incomplete records.

This retrospective study was approved by the Research Ethics Committee, University of Pretoria (Reference no. 875/2020) and was carried out in accordance with the Declaration of Helsinki.

2.2. ^{18}F-FDG PET/CT Imaging

Imaging was acquired on a dedicated PET/CT scanner (Biograph 40, Siemens). Standard patient preparation was observed. All patients had a minimum of 4 h of fasting, blood sugar was ≤11.0 mmol/L and activity of ^{18}F-FDG injected was calculated based on weight using the formula: [(body weight ÷ 10) + 1] × 37 MBq. Vertex-to-mid-thigh imaging was commenced after 60 min of uptake time. A separate lower limb imaging was done if the initial primary lesion was from the lower limb. PET acquisition was in 3D mode at 3 min per bed position. Except where a contraindication existed, CT was done with intravenous contrast using non-ionic contrast material (Omnipaque) injected at a rate of 2 mL/second. Images were reconstructed using OSEM (ordered subsets expectation maximization) to yield axial, sagittal and coronal slices of PET, CT and fused PET/CT images. Both attenuation-corrected and non-corrected images were reviewed for interpretation. CT data was used for the attenuation correction of PET data according to camera manufacturer specifications. A diagnostic CT with intravenous and/or oral contrast agents was done according to our departmental protocols and guidelines and was in line with EANM procedure guidelines, which were followed by our department [12].

2.3. Image Interpretation and PET/CT Data Analysis

Image interpretation was performed by two experienced nuclear medicine physicians. The reconstructed images were displayed on a dedicated workstation equipped with syngo software (Siemens Medical Solutions, Buffalo Grove, IL, USA).

A positive finding was defined as a focus of increased ^{18}F-FDG uptake as compared with surrounding normal tissue corresponding to the primary tumor site and metastatic disease. Increased ^{18}F-FDG uptake due to normal physiology or benign uptake was excluded from the analysis. Benign disease was characterized as a disease that did not anatomically represent metastatic disease, e.g., inflammatory lung changes.

Metabolic PET parameters (maximum standardized uptake value (SUVmax), metabolic tumor volume (MTV) and total lesion glycolysis (TLG)) of the primary tumor, as well as whole-body MTV and TLG of the metastatic disease, were measured. To obtain SUVmax, we drew a semi-automatic spherical volume of interest (VOI) around the primary tumor on PET images. We used an SUV threshold of 2.5 and a 3D isocontour of 41%. MTV and SUVmean were automatically computed by the software from the VOI. The TLG was calculated as the MTV multiplied by the SUVmean of the lesion (TLG = MTV × SUVmean). Whole-body MTV was calculated by adding the sum of all the VOI of the metastatic lesions (whole-body MTV = Σ (VOI of all metastatic lesions)), which were obtained on PET images. Whole-body TLG was calculated by adding the sum of all whole-body MTVs and SUVmeans of all the metastatic lesions (whole-body TLG = Σ (all whole-body MTVs and SUVmeans of all metastatic lesions)). ^{18}F-FDG PET metabolic parameters were measured as previously described in our facility [13–15]. Findings on the images were verified using a combination of histological confirmation and medical records.

2.4. Clinical Endpoints and Follow-Ups

Overall survival was the time from PET/CT date to the date of death due to any cause or the last time the patient was known to be alive. Patient files were reviewed from the referral clinics that sent them for PET/CT. Overall survival was measured in months, as the patient follow-up in our institution is every 3 months, depending on the condition of the patient. Should patients need an additional follow-up, they may present earlier, and should their conditions remain stable, follow-up is increased to 6 monthly and yearly intervals.

2.5. Statistical Analysis

Time-dependent receiver operating characteristic (ROC) curve analysis was performed to determine the optimal cut-off values for the prediction of death. However, the optimal values selected by this method did not give a clear cut-off as the cut-off of choice gave unbalanced data. As a result, a median point was used to create bivariate data for the PET parameters. Numerical data are expressed as median (interquartile range (IQR)). Since the data was non-normal, the Mann–Whitney test was used to compare the median values of the SUVmax, MTV, TLG, whole-body MTV and whole-body TLG between the survivors and the non-survivors. Categorical data were summarized using frequencies and percentages. Survival curves for OS were constructed using the Kaplan–Meier method and the log-rank test was used to determine as mortality rates significant differences between groups of the PET bivariate variables. Univariate and multivariate Cox proportional hazards models were fitted for OS to determine independent demographic and clinicopathologic prognostic factors for OS. Cox models results are expressed as a hazard ratio (HR) with corresponding 95% confidence intervals (CI). Statistical significance was set at 5%. Statistical analyses were performed using the STATA package (version 16).

3. Results

3.1. Patient Characteristics

This study focused on patients who had restaging PET/CT scans and met the inclusion criteria. Their demographic and clinicopathologic characteristics are shown in Table 1.

Table 1. Patient demographic and clinicopathologic characteristics.

Variables	Restaging		Total n (%)
	Survivors n (%)	Non-Survivors n (%)	
Age (years)			
<65	13 (76.47)	17 (53.13)	30 (61.22)
≥65	4 (23.53)	15 (46.88)	19 (38.78)
Sex			
Female	11 (64.71)	12 (37.5)	23 (46.94)
Male	6 (35.29)	20 (62.5)	26 (53.06)
Site of the primary tumor			
Upper limb	2 (11.76)	2 (6.25)	4 (8.16)
Lower limb	7 (41.18)	14 (43.75)	21 (42.86)
Head and neck	4 (23.53)	12 (37.5)	16 (32.65)
Chest and back	4 (23.53)	4 (12.5)	8 (16.33)
Histology			
Acral lentiginous	0	1 (3.13)	1 (2.04)
Amelanotic	2 (11.76)	0	2 (4.08)
Choroidal melanoma	0	1 (3.13)	1 (2.04)
Malignant melanoma	9 (52.94)	26 (81.25)	35 (71.43)
Nodular	5 (29.41)	4 (12.5)	9 (18.37)
Superficial spreading	1 (5.88)	0	1 (2.04)
Clinical staging			
II	3 (17.65)	2 (6.25)	5 (10.2)
III	8 (47.06)	6 (18.75)	14 (28.57)
IV	6 (35.29)	24 (75.0)	30 (61.22)

A total of 167 patients presented for restaging; after excluding those that did not meet the inclusion criteria, 49 patients remained. This study consisted of 23 (46.9%) females and 26 (53.1%) males. Most of the patients (61.22%, n = 30) were less than 65 years old. The lower limb primary tumors were the most common, observed in 42.86% (n = 21) of the patients; the remainder were distributed in the upper limbs, head and neck, chest and back. The histological types reported among these patients included unspecified malignant melanoma present in 71.43% (n = 35) patients and nodular type (18.37%, n = 9). The majority of the patients had stage IV disease (61.22%, n = 30).

The AJCC clinical stage at the time of referral was documented. Treatment received by the patients prior to the restaging PET was surgery (n = 36) and chemotherapy (n = 13). Patients were then restaged based on clinical and imaging findings. Patients in stages II and III were upstaged and those in stage IV either progressed or had stable disease. Based on the new stages, nine patients proceeded to receive immunotherapy, three received chemotherapy and the rest were followed up by observation and/or referral to palliative care.

The median follow-up time for survival was 12 months (interquartile range (IQR) of 3–32 months). High mortality rates were observed among males, those aged <65 years and those in clinical stage IV.

3.2. Metabolic PET Parameters

The median (IQR) SUVmax, MTV, TLG, whole-body MTV and whole-body TLG for the patients were 6.62 (3.1–12.6), 8.06 cm^3 (2.9–21.0), 19.49 (6.8–118.3), 33.36 (10.2–100.2) and 462.89 (59.3–1553.3), respectively. Compared to the survivors, non-survivors had a significantly higher median MTV (11.86 cm^3 vs. 5.68 cm^3; p-value = 0.022), TLG (31.25 vs. 14; p-value = 0.0357), whole-body MTV (53.9 cm^3 vs. 14.4 cm^3; p-value = 0.0076) and whole-body TLG (963.4 vs. 114.6; p-value = 0.0056) (Table 2).

Table 2. Metabolic PET parameters of survivors and non-survivors.

PET Parameter	Total Median (IQR)	Restaging Group		p-Value
		Survivors Median (IQR)	Non-Survivors Median (IQR)	
SUVmax	6.62 (3.1–12.6)	3.66 (2.9–8.7)	8.65 (3.27–13.6)	0.0661
MTV (cm^3)	8.06 (2.9–21.0)	5.68 (2.5–12.2)	11.86 (4.1–191.6)	0.022
TLG	19.49 (6.8–118.3)	14.3 (5.0–23.9)	31.25 (9.9–191.6)	0.0357
Whole-body MTV (cm^3)	33.36 (10.2–100.2)	14.4 (8.3–34.7)	53.91 (21.4–547.7)	0.0076
Whole-body TLG	462.89 (59.3–1553.3)	114.6 (23.9–479.5)	963.44 (167.9–11523.2)	0.0056

IQR: Interquartile range; SUVmax: maxiumum standard uptake value; MTV: metabolic tumor volume; TLG: total lesion glycolysis.

3.3. Survival Analysis

The Kaplan–Meier plots showed that there was no significant difference between patients with SUVmax $\leq$ median (6.62) compared to those with SUVmax > median (6.62), p-value = 0.0905 (Figure 1).

The bivariate log-rank test showed significant difference in predicting survival using the log-rank test: MTV $\leq$ median (8.06 cm^3) vs. MTV > median (8.06 cm^3) (p-value = 0.0506); TLG $\leq$ median (19.49) vs. TLG > median (19.49) (p-value < 0.0291); whole-body MTV $\leq$ median (33.36 cm^3) vs. whole-body MTV > median (33.36 cm^3) (p-value = 0.0001) and whole-body TLG $\leq$ median (462.89) vs. whole-body TLG > median (462.89) (p-value < 0.001). Higher MTV, TLG, whole-body MTV and whole-body TLG were associated with lower survival (see Figures 2–4).

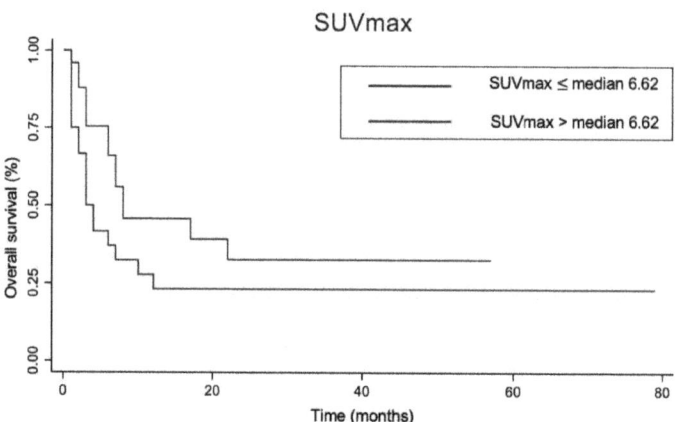

Figure 1. Kaplan–Meier curves for overall survival in restaging melanoma with respect to maximum standard uptake value (SUVmax).

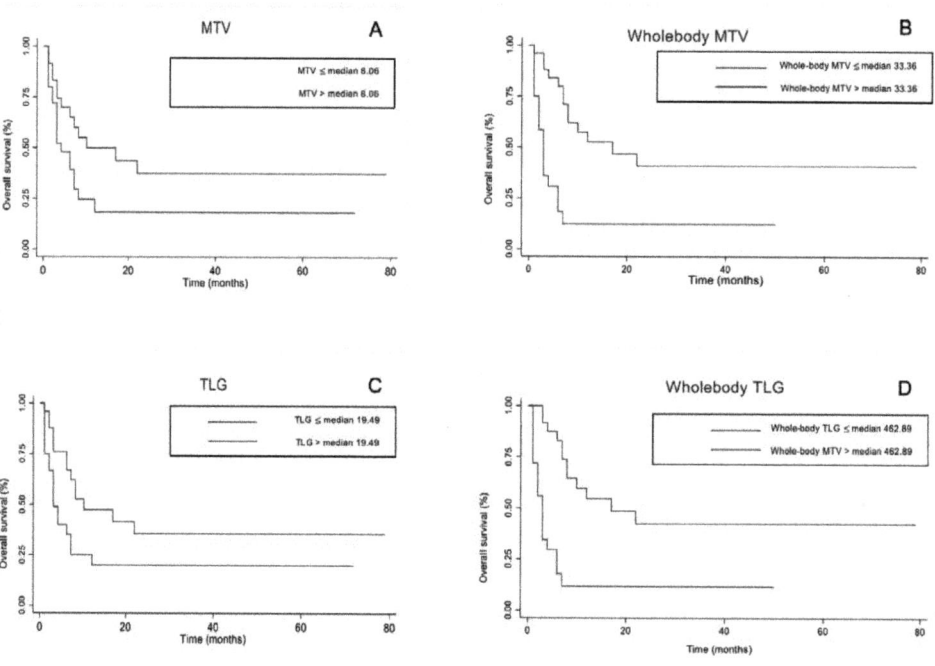

Figure 2. Kaplan–Meier curves for overall survival in restaging melanoma with respect to metabolic tumor volume (MTV) (**A**), whole-body MTV (**B**), total lesion glycolysis (TLG) (**C**), and whole-body TLG (**D**).

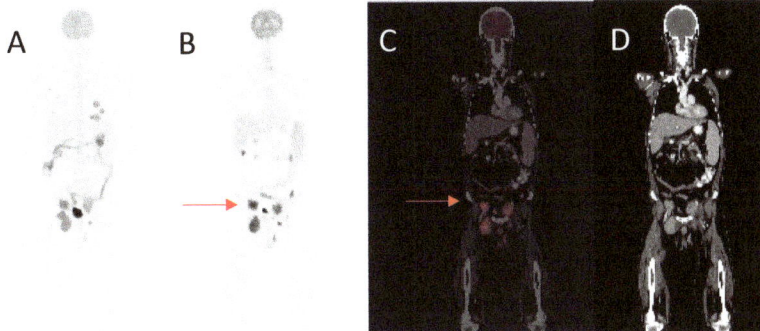

Figure 3. A 50-year-old male, diagnosed with malignant melanoma of the right groin with inguinal lymph node metastases, excision and resection of metastatic inguinal nodes, presented with right groin recurrence. Maximal intensity projection image (**A**), coronal ^{18}F-FDG- PET (**B**), fused (**C**) and CT (**D**) images demonstrating right inguinal recurrence (arrow). He also had abdominal and retroperitoneal lesions. MTV 174.59 cm^3, TLG 1611.46, SUVmax 22.12, whole-body MTV 780.55 cm^3 and whole-body TLG 28,279.33. Overall survival was 5 months.

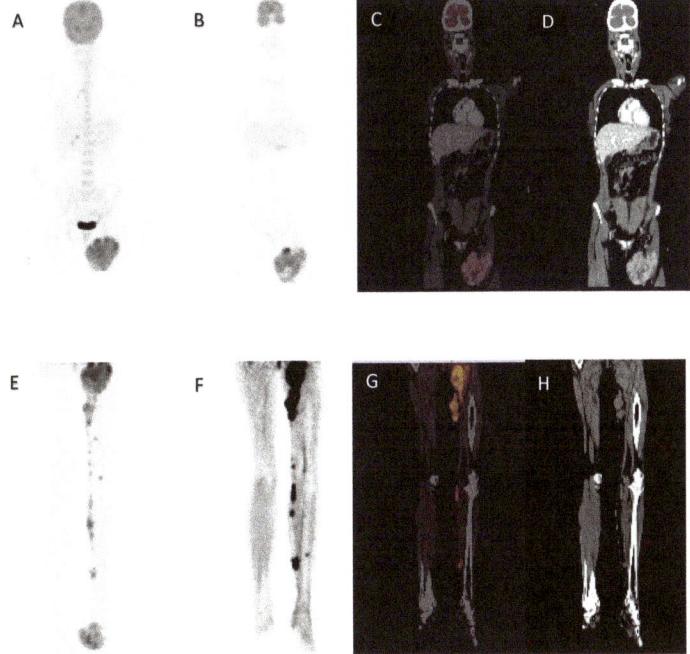

Figure 4. A 32-year-old female, acral lentiginous melanoma resected from the left foot, presented with a recurrence and nodal metastases. Maximal intensity projection image (**A**), coronal ^{18}F-FDG PET (**B**), fused (**C**) and CT (**D**) images demonstrating large inguinal node metastases. Maximal intensity projection image (**E**), Coronal ^{18}F-FDG PET of lower limbs (**F**), fused (**G**) and CT (**H**) images demonstrating left foot primary with subcutaneous and nodal metastases in the left leg. MTV 126.73 cm^3, TLG 567.75, SUVmax 10.78, whole-body MTV 635.48 cm^3 and whole-body TLG 9964.33. Overall survival was 8 months.

3.4. Univariate Analysis of Demographic and Clinicopathology in Relation to Overall Survival

In relation to overall survival, patients aged >65 years had a 1.88-fold statistically significant increased risk of death compared to those who were aged <65 years (p-value = 0.08). Male patients had a 2.26-fold increased risk of death compared to females (p-value = 0.027). Patients with MTV > 12.39 cm^3 were 2.53 times more likely to die compared to those with MTV $\leq$ 12.39 cm^3 (p-value = 0.01), while patients with TLG > 36.84 had an increased risk factor of 2.43 compared to TLG $\leq$ 36.84 (p-value < 0.014). The risk of mortality was 4.09 times higher amongst patients with a whole-body MTV > 51.15 cm^3 compared to those with a whole-body MTV $\leq$ 51.15 cm^3 (p-value < 0.001), while patients with a whole-body TLG > 564.47 were 4.33 times more likely to die compared to those with a whole-body TLG $\leq$ 564.47 (p-value < 0.001). This is shown in Table 3.

Table 3. Univariate analysis of demographic and clinicopathology in relation to overall survival.

Variables	Overall Survival	
	HR (95%CI)	p-Value
Age (years)		
<65	1 (base)	
$\geq$65	1.88 (0.93.82)	0.08
Sex		
Female	1 (base)	
Male	2.26 (1.09–4.67)	0.027
Clinical staging		
2	1 (base)	
3	1.21 (0.24–5.99)	0.818
4	3.41 (0.800–14.57)	0.097
SUVmax		
$\leq$8.61	1 (base)	
>8.61	1.78 (0.88–3.58)	0.108
MTV (cm^3)		
$\leq$12.39	1 (base)	
>12.39	2.53 (1.25–5.15)	0.01
TLG		
$\leq$36.84	1 (base)	
>36.84	2.43 (1.19–4.91)	0.014
Whole-body MTV (cm^3)		
$\leq$51.15	1 (base)	
>51.15	4.09 (1.97–8.48)	<0.001
Whole-body TLG		
$\leq$564.47	1 (base)	
>564.47	4.33 (2.05–913)	<0.001

HR: Hazards ratio; CI: Confidence interval.

4. Discussion

In this study, we evaluated the significance of metabolic ^{18}F-FDG PET/CT volumetric parameters in predicting the overall survival of patients presenting for restaging. Our patient cohort had a recurrence in the primary site of disease, as well as distant disease. Regarding the multivariate and univariate parameters, patients that demonstrated higher MTV and TLG were at a higher risk of death. In relation to survival, only whole-body TLG was significantly associated. Our data did not demonstrate a positive correlation with other variables, such as age or the site of the primary tumor, and survival.

Metabolic PET parameters have been discussed as a potential benefit in the prognosis of solid tumors. This has been seen in head and neck cancers, lung cancer and gynecological malignancies [16]. There are several metabolic parameters measured in ^{18}F-FDG PET/CT. A high metabolic volume in ^{18}F-FDG PET scans is associated with poor prognosis and changes in metabolic activity can be used to monitor response to therapy [17]. Metabolic PET parameters have been demonstrated to be independent prognostic factors for progression-free survival (PFS) and overall survival (OS) [18]. Metabolic PET parameters that are tumor-based, namely, MTV and TLG, have been shown to better represent the entire tumor and are closely associated with prognosis in various malignancies [18]. MTV and TLG have also been demonstrated to have a greater association with PFS and OS when compared to SUVmax. Metabolic parameters of tumor volumes have been demonstrated to be associated with prognostic values of overall survival and progression-free survival in esophageal cancer [19], head and neck cancer [20] and small cell lung cancer [21].

A study by Son et al. looked at the prognostic relevance of MTV and TLG in patients with malignant melanoma and found that pre-treatment MTV and TLG may be useful in risk-stratifying patients for likelihood of death and recurrence, with TLG being the best predictor [9]. Our findings were similar, where those patients with higher MTV, TLG and whole-body TLG were associated with overall survival. The difference between our study and theirs is that they looked at patients who presented for initial staging and our cohort of patients presented for restaging. Our study did not focus on progression-free survival, as a large proportion of our patients already had stage IV disease. The findings did however agree that metabolic parameters played a role in prognosis.

Another study by Ito et al., which looked at tumor volumes, demonstrated that whole-body MTV is a strong independent prognostic factor in determining which melanoma patients will respond to immunotherapy [8]. Our study did not look at the response to therapy but demonstrated that a higher whole-body MTV was associated with poorer survival. This agrees with another study that looked at treatment response and reported that those with more tumor involvement faired more poorly than those with less tumor involvement. This demonstrates that tumor volumes can be used to see which patients are more likely to benefit from intervention.

More recently, a study by Reinert et al. demonstrated the prognostic value of metabolic parameters in patients with melanoma regarding progression-free and overall survival [22]. This study demonstrated a positive correlation between MTV and TLG with overall and progression-free survival [22]. These findings were almost similar to our findings; however, this was done on a European population that presumably has better access to healthcare. In our population, patients typically present late and with more advanced disease [2]; therefore, in our population, having an additional risk stratification tool may guide clinicians regarding which therapies to use, more frequent follow-ups or earlier palliative treatment if necessary. The study also looked at other parameters, such as serological markers, lactate dehydrogenase and C-reactive protein. These specific parameters were not commonly reviewed in our patient cohort. Prognostication using ^{18}F-FDG PET/CT was also reviewed by Schweigoffer-Zwink et al., who demonstrated that metabolic parameters in patients with advanced cutaneous melanoma were predictive for survival in melanoma patients undergoing immunotherapy [23]. This study also found that tumor-to-background values had a stronger predictive value than MTV and TLG. Our study did not look at tumor-to-background ratios but similarly demonstrated that metabolic PET parameters can be predictive in a resource-constrained setting such as ours.

As our study specifically looked at restaging, our findings were somewhat similar to the Albano et al. group in Italy, which reviewed patients with ^{18}F-FDG PET/CT after surgery with suspicion for recurrence or metastatic disease post-surgical intervention; they found that imaging a positive scan was associated with an increased risk of disease progression and a negative study demonstrated longer survival than a positive one [24]. Metabolic parameters were not reviewed in this study; however, findings agree that a positive PET has prognostic outcomes in survival [24]. ^{18}F-FDG PET/CT also has the added advantage that it can detect melanoma recurrence in asymptomatic patients prior to clinical detection and this was demonstrated in a study done at our center [25].

Survival in melanoma is dependent on the stage at diagnosis. The different factors that encompass staging, namely, tumor size, nodal involvement and metastases, have been evaluated for melanoma-specific survival. Overall survival tends to be poorer depending on the stage at diagnosis [26]. This correlates with our data, as most of our patients presented for restaging at a later stage and had poorer outcomes. Due to mostly delayed presentation in our patient population, our study evaluated patients that demonstrated disease in the primary tumor at restaging with distant metastases. Our patients had significantly higher tumor volumes compared to what has been described by other authors [11,22].

The strength of this study was in demonstrating the value of metabolic parameters ^{18}F-FDG PET/CT in restaging patients with malignant melanoma for prognostic purposes. The role in recurrent melanoma is yet to be defined in a prospective study and would be beneficial to guide clinicians on potential clinical outcomes of patients, especially in recurrent disease.

The limitations of this study are that it is retrospective with a limited sample size of patients that presented to our hospital for restaging. Our study sample was based on the hospital records, which were not intended for research; therefore, challenges with incomplete records were encountered. A large proportion of our patients were also lost to follow-up, which also influenced our results. Difficulties in record keeping have been described in a resource-constrained setting similar to ours by Pirkle et al., who found that researchers in diverse settings struggle with record keeping. The authors mentioned that illegible notes or missing records can affect hospital care and research and mentioned the need for electronic records, which may assist with improving this [27]. Unfortunately, in our setting, medical records are still done on paper and only imaging is available electronically. A study done in a first-world setting, namely, in Taiwan, by Li et al. found that, although electronic medical records were available, most retrospective studies had a case number of fewer than 100 patients, with the average being 41 [28]. The lower case numbers were speculated to be due to the authors' preference of accessing paper records despite the availability of electronic records [28]. These studies demonstrate that lower case numbers in retrospective data are not unique to our population alone, but are seen in low-income and first-world countries with access to better record keeping [27,28]. Another limitation is the inability to correlate the histology of all the metastatic lesions to truly confirm melanoma metastases despite anatomical features of metastases. Our data demonstrated a positive correlation with tumor volumes and overall survival in this retrospective analysis of patients presenting for restaging. Prospective studies in patients with melanoma preventing for staging would be beneficial, as the bulk of known literature is retrospective.

5. Conclusions

In this patient cohort that presented for restaging, we found that a high MTV and TLG of the primary tumor and whole-body TLG were prognostic for overall survival. These findings may assist clinicians in evaluating and recognizing patients with a poorer prognosis in a similar population group.

Author Contributions: Conceptualization: K.N.H., K.M.G.M., M.V. and M.M.S.; data curation: K.N.H., K.M.G.M., Z.M.-Z., M.V. and M.M.S.; methodology, K.N.H., K.M.G.M., M.V., Z.M.-Z. and M.M.S.; software: K.N.H., K.M.G.M. and M.M.S.; formal analysis: K.N.H., K.M.G.M., Z.M.-Z., M.V. and M.M.S.; validation: K.N.H., K.M.G.M., Z.M.-Z. and M.M.S.; investigation: K.N.H., K.M.G.M., Z.M.-Z., M.V. and M.M.S.; writing—original draft preparation: K.N.H., K.M.G.M., Z.M.-Z., M.V. and M.M.S.; writing—review and editing: K.N.H., K.M.G.M., Z.M.-Z. and M.M.S.; supervision: K.M.G.M., M.V. and M.M.S. All authors have read and agreed to the published version of the manuscript.

Funding: This research received no external funding.

Institutional Review Board Statement: The study was conducted in accordance with the Declaration of Helsinki, and approved by the Research Ethics Committee, University of Pretoria (protocol code 875/2020 on 21 January 2021).

Informed Consent Statement: Patient consent was waived due to the retrospective nature of the study, as granted by the Research Ethics Committee.

Data Availability Statement: The data presented in this study are available on request from the corresponding author. The data is not publicly available due to patient confidentiality.

Acknowledgments: The authors wish to acknowledge Susan Botha (Medical Oncology) and Frans Mothapo (Nuclear Medicine) for the many hours spent accessing clinical records for data collection.

Conflicts of Interest: The authors declare no conflict of interest.

References

1. Matthews, N.H.; Li, W.Q.; Qureshi, A.A.; Weinstock, M.A.; Cho, E. Epidemiology of melanoma. In *Cutaneous Melanoma: Etiology and Therapy*; Ward, W.H., Farma, J.M., Eds.; Codon Publications: Brisbane, Australia, 2017.
2. Tod, B.M.; Kellett, P.E.; Singh, E.; Visser, W.I.; Lombard, C.J.; Wright, C.Y. The incidence of melanoma in South Africa: An exploratory analysis of National Cancer Registry data from 2005 to 2013 with a specific focus on melanoma in black Africans. *S. Afr. Med. J.* **2019**, *109*, 246–253. [CrossRef] [PubMed]
3. Aktolun, C.; Goldsmith, S.J. *Nuclear Oncology*; Wolters Kluwer: Philadelphia, PA, USA, 2015.
4. Pleiss, C.; Risse, J.H.; Biersack, H.-J.; Bender, H. Role of FDG-PET in the assessment of survival prognosis in melanoma. *Cancer Biother. Radiopharm.* **2007**, *22*, 740–747. [CrossRef] [PubMed]
5. Park, S.G.; Lee, J.H.; Lee, W.A.; Han, K.M. Biologic correlation between glucose transporters, hexokinase-ii, ki-67 and FDG uptake in malignant melanoma. *Nucl. Med. Biol.* **2012**, *39*, 1167–1172. [CrossRef] [PubMed]
6. Reinhardt, M.J.; Joe, A.Y.; Jaeger, U.; Huber, A.; Matthies, A.; Bucerius, J.; Roedel, R.; Strunk, H.; Bieber, T.; Biersack, H.J.; et al. Diagnostic performance of whole body dual modality 18F-FDG PET/CT imaging for N- and M-staging of malignant melanoma: Experience with 250 consecutive patients. *J. Clin. Oncol.* **2006**, *24*, 1178–1187. [CrossRef]
7. Twycross, S.H.; Burger, H.; Holness, J. The utility of PET-CT in the staging and management of advanced and recurrent malignant melanoma. *S. Afr. J. Surg. Suid-Afrik. Tydskr. Chir.* **2019**, *57*, 44–49. [CrossRef]
8. Ito, K.; Schöder, H.; Teng, R.; Humm, J.L.; Ni, A.; Wolchok, J.D.; Weber, W.A. Prognostic value of baseline metabolic tumor volume measured on ^{18}F-fluorodeoxyglucose positron emission tomography/computed tomography in melanoma patients treated with ipilimumab therapy. *Eur. J. Nucl. Med. Mol. Imaging* **2019**, *46*, 930–939. [CrossRef]
9. Joyce, K.M. Surgical management of melanoma. In *Cutaneous Melanoma: Etiology and Therapy*; Ward, W.H., Farma, J.M., Eds.; Codon Publications: Brisbane, Australia, 2017.
10. Kang, S.; Ahn, B.-C.; Hong, C.; Song, B.; Lee, H.; Jeong, S.; Lee, S.; Lee, J.; Lee, S. Can (18)F-FDG PET/CT predict recurrence in patients with cutaneous malignant melanoma? *Nuclearmedizin* **2011**, *50*, 116–121. [CrossRef]
11. Son, S.H.; Kang, S.M.; Jeong, S.Y.; Lee, S.W.; Lee, S.J.; Lee, J.; Ahn, B.C. Prognostic Value of Volumetric Parameters Measured by Pretreatment 18F FDG PET/CT in Patients with Cutaneous Malignant Melanoma. *Clin. Nucl. Med.* **2016**, *41*, e266–e273. [CrossRef]
12. Boellaard, R.; Delgado-Bolton, R.; Oyen, W.J.; Giammarile, F.; Tatsch, K.; Eschner, W.; Verzijlbergen, F.J.; Barrington, S.F.; Pike, L.C.; Weber, W.A.; et al. FDG PET/CT: EANM procedure guidelines for tumour imaging: Version 2.0. *Eur. J. Nucl. Med. Mol. Imaging* **2015**, *42*, 328–354. [CrossRef]
13. Mokoala, K.M.G.; Lawal, I.O.; Lengana, T.; Popoola, G.O.; Boshomane, T.M.G.; Mokgoro, N.P.; Vorster, M.; Sathekge, M.M. The association of tumor burden by ^{18}F-FDG PET/CT and survival in vulvar carcinoma. *Clin. Nucl. Med.* **2021**, *46*, 375–381. [CrossRef]
14. Lawal, I.O.; Ankrah, A.O.; Popoola, G.O.; Nyakale, N.E.; Boshomane, T.G.; Reyneke, F.; Lengana, T.; Vorster, M.; Sathekge, M.M. ^{18}F-FDG-PET metabolic metrics and international prognostic score for risk assessment in HIV-infected patients with Hodgkin Lymphoma. *Nucl. Med. Commun.* **2018**, *39*, 1005–1012. [CrossRef] [PubMed]
15. Lawal, I.O.; Nyakale, N.E.; Harry, L.M.; Modiselle, M.R.; Ankrah, A.O.; Msomi, A.P.; Mokgoro, N.P.; Boshomane, T.G.; de Wiele, C.V.; Sathekge, M.M. The role of F-18 FDG PET/CT in evaluating the impact of HIV infection on tumor burden and therapy outcome in patients with Hodgkin Lymphoma. *Eur. J. Nucl. Med. Mol. Imaging* **2017**, *44*, 2025–2033. [CrossRef]
16. Van de Wiele, C.; Kruse, V.; Smeets, P.; Sathekge, M.; Maes, A. Predictive and prognostic value of metabolic tumour volume and total lesion glycolysis in solid tumours. *Eur. J. Nucl. Med. Mol. Imaging* **2013**, *40*, 290–301. [CrossRef]
17. Im, H.; Bradshaw, T.; Solaiyappan, M.; Cho, S. Current Methods to Define Metabolic Tumor Volume in Positron Emission Tomography: Which one is better? *Nucl. Med. Mol. Imaging* **2018**, *52*, 5–15. [CrossRef] [PubMed]
18. Steiger, S.; Arvanitakis, M.; Sick, B.; Weder, W.; Hillinger, S.; Burger, I.A. Analysis of Prognostic Values of Various PET Metrics in Preoperative ^{18}F-FDG PET for Early-Stage Bronchial Carcinoma for Progression-Free and Overall Survival: Significantly Increased Glycolysis Is a Predictive Factor. *J. Nucl. Med.* **2017**, *58*, 1925–1930. [CrossRef] [PubMed]
19. Han, S.; Kim, Y.; Woo, S.; Suh, C.; Lee, J. Prognostic Value of Volumetric Parameters of Pretreatment 18F-FDG PET/CT in Esophageal Cancer: A Systematic Review and Meta-analysis. *Clin. Nucl. Med.* **2018**, *43*, 887–894. [CrossRef] [PubMed]
20. Wang, L.; Bai, J.; Duan, P. Prognostic value of 18F-FDG PET/CT functional parameters in patients with head and neck cancer: A meta-analysis. *Nucl. Med. Commun.* **2019**, *40*, 361–369. [CrossRef]
21. Kim, H.; Yoo, I.R.; Boo, S.H.; Park, H.L.; O, J.H.; Kim, S.H. Prognostic Value of Pre- and Post-Treatment FDG PET/CT Parameters in Small Cell Lung Cancer Patients. *Nucl. Med. Mol. Imaging* **2018**, *52*, 31–38. [CrossRef]

22. Reinert, C.; Gatidis, S.; Sekler, J.; Dittmann, H.; Pfannenberg, C.; la Fougère, C.; Nikolaou, K.; Forschner, A. Clinical and prognostic value of tumor volumetric parameters in melanoma patients undergoing ^{18}F-FDG-PET/CT: A comparison with serologic markers of tumor burden and inflammation. *Cancer Imaging* **2020**, *20*, 44. [CrossRef]
23. Schweighofer-Zwink, G.; Manafi-Farid, R.; Kölblinger, P.; Hehenwarter, L.; Harsini, S.; Pirich, C.; Beheshti, M. Prognostic value of 2-[18f]FDG PET-CT in metastatic melanoma patients receiving immunotherapy. *Eur. J. Radiol.* **2022**, *146*, 110107. [CrossRef]
24. Albano, D.; Familiari, D.; Fornito, C.M.; Scalisi, S.; Laudicella, R.; Galia, M.; Grassedonio, E.; Ruggeri, A.; Ganduscio, G.; Messina, M.; et al. Clinical and Prognostic Value of ^{18}F-FDG-PET/CT in the Restaging Process of Recurrent Cutaneous Melanoma. *Curr. Radiopharm.* **2020**, *13*, 42–47. [CrossRef] [PubMed]
25. Lawal, I.; Lengana, T.; Ololade, K.; Boshomane, T.; Reyneke, F.; Modiselle, M.; Vorster, M.; Sathekge, M. ^{18}F-FDG PET/CT in the detection of asymptomatic malignant melanoma recurrence. *Nuklearmedizin* **2017**, *56*, 83–89. [CrossRef] [PubMed]
26. Gershenwald, J.E.; Scolyer, R.A. Melanoma Staging: American Joint Committee on Cancer (AJCC) 8th Edition and Beyond. *Ann. Surg. Oncol.* **2018**, *25*, 2105–2110. [CrossRef]
27. Pirkle, C.M.; Dumont, A.; Zunzunegui, M.-V. Medical recordkeeping, essential but overlooked aspect of quality of care in resource-limited settings. *Int. J. Qual. Health Care* **2012**, *24*, 564–567. [CrossRef] [PubMed]
28. Li, H.-C.; Chen, Y.-W.; Chen, T.-J.; Chiou, S.-H.; Hwang, S.-J. The role of patient records in research: A bibliometric analysis of publications from an academic medical center in Taiwan. *J. Chin. Med. Assoc.* **2021**, *84*, 718–721. [CrossRef]

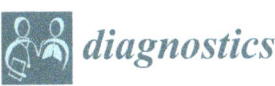

Article

The Influence of the Exclusion of Central Necrosis on [18F]FDG PET Radiomic Analysis

Wyanne A. Noortman [1,2,*], Dennis Vriens [1], Charlotte D. Y. Mooij [1,3], Cornelis H. Slump [2], Erik H. Aarntzen [4], Anouk van Berkel [5], Henri J. L. M. Timmers [5], Johan Bussink [6], Tineke W. H. Meijer [7], Lioe-Fee de Geus-Oei [1,2] and Floris H. P. van Velden [1]

1. Section of Nuclear Medicine, Department of Radiology, Leiden University Medical Center, 2333 ZA Leiden, The Netherlands; d.vriens@lumc.nl (D.V.); c.d.y.mooij@lumc.nl (C.D.Y.M.); l.f.de_geus-oei@lumc.nl (L.-F.d.G.-O.); f.h.p.van_velden@lumc.nl (F.H.P.v.V.)
2. TechMed Centre, University of Twente, 7522 NB Enschede, The Netherlands; c.h.slump@utwente.nl
3. Technical Medicine, Delft University of Technology, 2628 CD Delft, The Netherlands
4. Department of Radiology and Nuclear Medicine, Radboud University Medical Center, 6525 GA Nijmegen, The Netherlands; erik.aarntzen@radboudumc.nl
5. Division of Endocrinology, Department of Internal Medicine, Radboud University Medical Center, 6525 GA Nijmegen, The Netherlands; anouk.vanberkel@radboudumc.nl (A.v.B.); henri.timmers@radboudumc.nl (H.J.L.M.T.)
6. Radiotherapy and OncoImmunology Laboratory, Department of Radiation Oncology, Radboud University Medical Center, 6525 GA Nijmegen, The Netherlands; jan.bussink@radboudumc.nl
7. Department of Radiation Oncology, University Medical Center Groningen, 9713 GZ Groningen, The Netherlands; t.van.zon@umcg.nl
* Correspondence: w.a.noortman@lumc.nl

Citation: Noortman, W.A.; Vriens, D.; Mooij, C.D.Y.; Slump, C.H.; Aarntzen, E.H.; van Berkel, A.; Timmers, H.J.L.M.; Bussink, J.; Meijer, T.W.H.; de Geus-Oei, L.-F.; et al. The Influence of the Exclusion of Central Necrosis on [18F]FDG PET Radiomic Analysis. *Diagnostics* **2021**, *11*, 1296. https://doi.org/10.3390/diagnostics11071296

Academic Editor: Giorgio Treglia

Received: 1 June 2021
Accepted: 15 July 2021
Published: 19 July 2021

Publisher's Note: MDPI stays neutral with regard to jurisdictional claims in published maps and institutional affiliations.

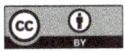

Copyright: © 2021 by the authors. Licensee MDPI, Basel, Switzerland. This article is an open access article distributed under the terms and conditions of the Creative Commons Attribution (CC BY) license (https://creativecommons.org/licenses/by/4.0/).

Abstract: Background: Central necrosis can be detected on [18F]FDG PET/CT as a region with little to no tracer uptake. Currently, there is no consensus regarding the inclusion of regions of central necrosis during volume of interest (VOI) delineation for radiomic analysis. The aim of this study was to assess how central necrosis affects radiomic analysis in PET. Methods: Forty-three patients, either with non-small cell lung carcinomas (NSCLC, $n = 12$) or with pheochromocytomas or paragangliomas (PPGL, $n = 31$), were included retrospectively. VOIs were delineated with and without central necrosis. From all VOIs, 105 radiomic features were extracted. Differences in radiomic features between delineation methods were assessed using a paired *t*-test with Benjamini–Hochberg multiple testing correction. In the PPGL cohort, performances of the radiomic models to predict the noradrenergic biochemical profile were assessed by comparing the areas under the receiver operating characteristic curve (AUC) for both delineation methods. Results: At least 65% of the features showed significant differences between $VOI_{vital-tumour}$ and $VOI_{gross-tumour}$ (65%, 79% and 82% for the NSCLC, PPGL and combined cohort, respectively). The AUCs of the radiomic models were not significantly different between delineation methods. Conclusion: In both tumour types, almost two-third of the features were affected, demonstrating that the impact of whether or not to include central necrosis in the VOI on the radiomic feature values is significant. Nevertheless, predictive performances of both delineation methods were comparable. We recommend that radiomic studies should report whether or not central necrosis was included during delineation.

Keywords: radiomics; [18F]FDG PET/CT; tumour delineation; central necrosis

1. Introduction

Tumour morphology might be heterogeneous with alternating regions of relatively vital tumour tissue, mild hypoxia, severe hypoxia and necrosis [1]. Tumour hypoxia manifests itself predominantly in solid tumours [2]. Central necrosis of tumours occurs as a result of hypoxia and is caused by uncontrolled oncogene-driven proliferation without efficient vasculature, inducing a nutrient and oxygen shortage [1]. As a morphological marker, central necrosis is associated with poor prognosis in a variety of cancers [3–5], including non-small cell lung carcinomas (NSCLC) [6,7]. Larger regions of necrosis can be detected on 2-[^{18}F]fluoro-2-deoxy-D-glucose positron emission tomography ([^{18}F]FDG PET/CT) as an often centrally located region with little to no tracer uptake.

Radiomics aims to quantify the geometry and tracer uptake, including uptake heterogeneity, of tumours by using first order, shape and texture features and hypothesizing that these features can be used for tumour characterisation, prognostic stratification and response prediction in precision medicine [8]. It is uncertain whether regions of central necrosis should be added to the delineation of the tumour, since the effect of delineation methods on the predictive value of the radiomic signature remains unknown [9]. Semi-automatic tumour delineation methods used in radiomic analysis apply isocontours by using fixed or adaptive thresholds [10,11] or more advanced algorithms, such as the fuzzy locally adaptive Bayesian (FLAB) algorithm [12]. Although these methods have shown to be highly reproducible [10,13], they often underestimate the true (anatomical) tumour volume by excluding (up to a certain degree) regions of low tracer uptake. Some studies manually add the excluded regions of low tracer uptake to the volume of interest (VOI), but this is not always clearly reported. It is hypothesised that the addition of a region of central necrosis to the VOI may influence all three radiomic feature classes numerically. First order features might be affected by the addition of voxels with low grey levels and this skews the intensity histogram. Shape features might be influenced by the different 3D morphology of the VOI when central necrosis is included. Texture features, representing spatial relationships between voxels in terms of run lengths or size zones of the same voxel values or combinations of neighbouring voxel values, might change as well. The introduction of an area of central necrosis might, for instance, result in long runs with low values that will change the run length matrix and, as a result, the feature values. The Image Biomarker Standardisation Initiative (IBSI), which is an independent international collaboration working towards standardising the extraction of image biomarkers, provides reporting guidelines for radiomic studies but, up to this point, does not specify the need to report on the inclusion/exclusion of necrosis while describing the used segmentation method [14]. Moreover, the effect of the delineation method, including whether or not to include central necrosis, on the performance of the radiomic signature for predicting underlying tumour biology remains unknown [9].

This study explores how central necrosis influences PET radiomic analysis by assessing the differences in radiomic features and the predictive performance of features extracted from VOIs delineated using an isocontour method with and without the manual addition of the region of central necrosis for two datasets of NSCLC and pheochromocytomas or paragangliomas (PPGL), catecholamine-producing neuroendocrine tumours that arise from the chromaffin cells of the adrenal medulla and extra-adrenal sympathetic paraganglia [15].

2. Materials and Methods

2.1. Patient Population, Data Acquisition and Image Reconstruction

Subjects from two cohorts of patients who underwent an [^{18}F]FDG PET/CT in a single academic centre were retrospectively included to study the effect of different aspects of central necrosis on the radiomic analysis. A cohort of patients with non-small cell lung-carcinomas (NSCLC, $n = 35$), generally presenting a high tumour-to-background ratio, and a cohort of patients with pheochromocytomas or paragangliomas (PPGL, $n = 77$), generally presenting a low tumour-to-background ratio, were included.

The NSCLC cohort is a previously published prospective cohort [16]. Patients underwent a dynamic [^{18}F]FDG PET/CT scan with the primary tumour located centrally in the field of view using the Biograph Duo or Biograph 40 mCT (Siemens Healthineers, Erlangen, Germany) at the Radboud University Medical Center between 2009 and 2014. Only tumours with a diameter larger than 30 mm were included to minimise the influence of partial volume effects and to be able to reliably quantify uptake heterogeneity [17]. Imaging was in accordance with European Association of Nuclear Medicine (EANM) guidelines for tumour PET imaging [18]. Patients fasted for at least 6 h before imaging and serum glucose levels were below 8 mmol/L. Directly after the start of the acquisition, a standardised infusion of 3.45 MBq of [^{18}F]FDG per kilogram of body weight started. The final time frame (50–60 min p.i.) of the dynamic series was used in the current study. Voxel sizes were 2.56 × 2.56 × 3.38 and 1.59 × 1.59 × 2.03 mm^3 for the Biograph Duo PET/CT and Biograph 40 mCT PET/CT, respectively. This study has been reviewed and approved by the Commission on Medical Research Involving Human Subjects Region Arnhem-Nijmegen, the Netherlands. All patients signed an informed consent form.

The PPGL patients who underwent a [^{18}F]FDG PET/CT scan in the Radboud University Medical Center between 2011 and 2018 were retrospectively included. A selection of these patients has previously been described [15,19]. Static PET/CT images were acquired using the Biograph 40 mCT (Siemens Healthineers, Erlangen, Germany), in accordance with aforementioned EANM guidelines [18]. Patients fasted for at least 6 h and serum glucose levels were below 8 mmol/L. Image acquisition (3 or 4 min per bed position) started 60 (55–75) minutes after intravenous administration of [^{18}F]FDG (dosage according to a non-linear dosage regimen based on body weight; details can be found in Supplementary File S1). The reconstructed voxel size was 3.18 × 3.18 × 3.00 mm^3. This retrospective database study has been reviewed and approved by the Commission on Medical Research Involving Human Subjects Region Arnhem-Nijmegen, the Netherlands. Informed consent was waived due to the retrospective nature of the study. Patients that objected to the use of their anonymised data were excluded.

Additional details on patient preparation, data acquisition, image reconstruction, image processing and radiomic analysis can be found in Supplementary File S1: the IBSI reporting guidelines [14].

2.2. Image Analysis
2.2.1. Image Processing

For NSCLC, images were interpolated to isotropic voxels of 3.38 × 3.38 × 3.38 mm^3 using trilinear interpolation with the grids aligned by the centre using MATLAB version 2017b (Mathworks, Natick, MA, USA) [14]. PPGL images were not interpolated since the voxels were almost isotropic (3.18 × 3.18 × 3.00 mm^3).

2.2.2. Volumes of Interest Delineation

VOIs were delineated semi-automatically using 3DSlicer version 4.11 (www.slicer.org, accessed on 1 March 2021) [20] and in-house built software implemented in Python version 3.7 (Python Software Foundation, Wilmington, Delaware). The often peripheral region of the tumour showing increased [^{18}F]FDG uptake (VOI$_{vital-tumour}$) was delineated using a semi-automatic threshold-based method and corrected for local background [10]. A threshold of 41% of the peak standardised uptake value (SUV$_{peak}$) that was obtained using a sphere of 12 mm diameter [21] was selected, since the delineated tumour sizes of this method agreed best with pathological tumour sizes [22]. As tumours in the PPGL cohort showed low contrast between the tumour and surrounding tissue, boxing was applied to exclude the surrounding [^{18}F]FDG-avid tissues. VOI$_{gross-tumour}$ was generated by manually adding the volumes of central necrosis to VOI$_{vital-tumour}$, using the low-dose CT as a visual reference. The necrotic tumour fraction (NTF) was determined using Equation (1):

$$\text{NTF} = 1 - \text{VOI}_{vital-tumour} / \text{VOI}_{gross-tumour} \quad (1)$$

where a NTF of 0 indicates no central necrosis and a higher NTF indicates larger volumes of necrosis. Patients were selected when NTF > 0.

2.2.3. Radiomic Feature Extraction

For each selected patient, 105 radiomic features were extracted from VOI$_{vital-tumour}$ and VOI$_{gross-tumour}$ using PyRadiomics version 3.0 in Python version 3.7 (Python Software Foundation, Wilmington, DE, USA) [23]: 18 first order features, 14 shape features, 22 grey level cooccurrence matrix (GLCM) features, 16 grey level run length matrix (GLRLM) features, 16 grey level size zone matrix (GLSZM) features, 14 grey level dependence matrix (GLDM) features and 5 neighbouring grey tone difference matrix (NGTDM) features. A fixed bin size of 0.5 g/mL was applied.

2.3. Statistical Analysis

Statistical analyses were performed in SPSS version 25 (IBM Statistics, Chicago, IL, USA). Per cohort and for both cohorts together, differences in radiomic features extracted from $VOI_{vital-tumour}$ and $VOI_{gross-tumour}$ were assessed using a Wilcoxon signed-rank test or a paired t-test after testing for (log-)normality. Since over one hundred features are tested simultaneously, some features may show a significant difference between both delineation methods by chance, which increases the false discovery rate [24]. Therefore, the Benjamini–Hochberg multiple testing correction was performed [25]. The Benjamini–Hochberg correction determines the significance level for specific feature (p_i) using Equation (2):

$$p_i < \left(\frac{i}{n}\right)a \qquad (2)$$

where i is the ranking of a feature when ranking all features based on the significance level of the paired *t*-test from smallest to largest, n is the total number of features and a is the original significance level ($a = 0.05$). Additional subset analyses of all patients based on the NTF and SUV_{max} were performed by creating three equally-sized groups for low, medium and high values: NTF: ≤ 0.12, $0.12 < NTF \leq 0.36$, >0.36; SUV_{max}: ≤ 4.61, $4.61 < SUV_{max} \leq 12.09$, >12.09 g/mL. Differences in numbers of affected features per cohort and subgroup were assessed using the Fisher's exact test. Overlaps in the affected features per cohort and subgroup were visualised using Venn diagrams.

For the PPGL cohort, the predictive performance for the underlying tumour biology of the radiomic models based on features derived from the different delineation methods was assessed by binary logistic regression in R version 3.6.0 (R Foundation for Statistical Computing, Vienna, Austria). Moreover, a radiomic model was created out of features from both delineation methods, assuming that both features contain different information. The response variable in regression was the noradrenergic biochemical profile of the PPGLs. Unsupervised feature selection or dimension reduction was performed to deal with multicollinearity and high dimensionality, which occurs when the number of features largely exceeds the number of patients. As a rule of thumb, 1 feature was selected for every 10 subjects [26] and 3 features were selected to be tested (PPGL dataset: $n = 31$ patients). The predictive performance of the radiomic models was not assessed for the NSCLC cohort since this cohort consisted of only 12 patients, which corresponds to only 1 feature to be tested and is inadequate to explain sufficient variance of the dataset. Dimension reduction in the PPGL dataset using redundancy filtering and factor analysis was performed using the FMradio (Factor Modeling for Radiomics Data) R-package version 1.1.1 [27]. Features were scaled (centred around 0, variance of 1), avoiding that features with the largest scale dominated the analysis. Redundancy filtering of the Pearson correlation matrix of features is performed with a threshold of $\tau = 0.95$ and, from each group, one feature is retained. Factor analysis of the redundancy filtered correlation matrix with an orthogonal rotation was executed so that the first factor explained the largest possible variance in the dataset; the succeeding factors explained the largest variance in orthogonal directions. The sampling adequacy of the model, which is quantified by the Kaiser-Meier-Olkin (KMO) statistic, was predefined to be ≥ 0.9. The feature with the highest loading on a single factor was selected for regression analysis. The three selected features are associated with the noradrenergic biochemical profile using multiple binary logistic regression. Areas under the curve (AUC) of the receiver operating characteristic (ROC) of the radiomic models based on the three selected features for $VOI_{vital-tumour}$, $VOI_{gross-tumour}$ and combined were computed and compared using DeLong's test for paired ROC curves. A sham experiment was conducted to validate the findings by randomisation of the outcome labels (noradrenergic biochemical profile) [28]. This takes into account the prevalence of the outcome and the distributions and multicollinearity of the radiomic features but uncouples their hypothesised relation. Binary logistic regression was performed and the sham experiment was repeated 100 times to calculate the mean AUCs.

3. Results

Patient characteristics of included patients with central necrosis (n = 43) are presented in Table 1. In the NSCLC cohort, central necrosis was observed in 12 out of 35 patients (34%). In the PPGL cohort, central necrosis was observed in 31 of 77 patients (40%; Figure 1).

Table 1. Clinical characteristics of 31 PPGL and 12 NSCLC patients with central necrosis. SUV: standardised uptake value, MTV: metabolic tumour volume, NTF: necrotic tumour fraction, NSCLC: non-small cell lung carcinomas, PPGL: pheochromocytomas and paragangliomas.

	NSCLC (n = 12)	PPGL (n = 31)
Age (years), median (range)	65 (44–80)	62 (23–80)
Sex (M/F)	11/1	10/21
Histology	Adenocarcinoma: 4 Squamous cell carcinoma: 7 Other: 1	Pheochromocytoma: 26 Paraganglioma: 5
Noradrenergic biochemical profile (yes/no)	-	13/18
SUV_{max} (g/mL), median (range)	16.00 (9.05–29.77)	5.00 (2.54–36.01)
$MTV_{vital\text{-}tumour}$ (cm^3), median (range)	36.3 (15.2–173.4)	58.3 (16.6–388.8)
$MTV_{gross\text{-}tumour}$ (cm^3), median (range)	45.1 (18.7–327.3)	103.8 (28.7–611.2)
NTF, median (range)	0.19 (0.03–0.77)	0.23 (0.01–0.97)

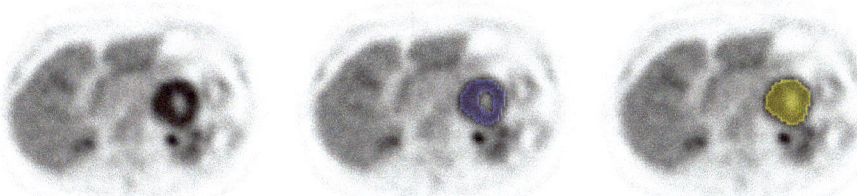

Figure 1. Example of a [^{18}F]FDG PET/CT scan of a patient with a pheochromocytoma with central necrosis in the left adrenal gland, with $VOI_{vital\text{-}tumour}$ in blue and $VOI_{gross\text{-}tumour}$ in yellow. The NTF is 0.05.

At least 65% of the features were affected by the choice of delineation (Table 2). The PPGL population was influenced the most with 79% of affected features, compared to 65% in the NSCLC population, which is a significant difference between the populations (p = 0.031). Out of the 105 features, 61% were affected in the NSCLC cohort as well as the PPGL cohort. For all patients taken together, even 82% of the features were affected.

First order features were affected substantially, with at least 72% of features, followed by texture features with at least 66% of features. Shape features were affected the least, with 50% of affected features in both datasets. Of all texture feature classes, GLCM features were affected the least, with a maximum of 68% of features. For all other classes, the maximum number of affected features was at least 80%.

Table 2. Numbers and percentages of features affected by the delineation method ($VOI_{vital-tumour}$ vs. $VOI_{gross-tumour}$) per feature class for the different cohorts and both cohorts together. Differences in the number of affected features between cohorts were assessed using the Fisher's exact test. NSCLC: non-small cell lung carcinoma, PPGL: pheochromocytoma and paraganglioma, GLCM: grey level cooccurrence matrix, GLRLM: grey level run length matrix, GLSZM: grey level size zone matrix, GLDM: grey level dependence matrix, NGTDM: neighbouring grey tone difference matrix.

Feature Class	All (n = 43)	NSCLC (n = 12)	PPGL (n = 31)	p-Value
First order (18)	17 (94%)	13 (72%)	16 (89%)	0.402
Shape (14)	11 (79%)	7 (50%)	7 (50%)	1.000
Texture (73)	58 (79%)	48 (66%)	60 (82%)	0.024
GLCM (22)	15 (68%)	12 (55%)	15 (68%)	0.537
GLRLM (16)	15 (94%)	12 (75%)	15 (94%)	0.333
GLSZM (16)	12 (75%)	11 (69%)	13 (81%)	0.685
GLDM (14)	12 (86%)	9 (64%)	13 (93%)	0.165
NGTDM (5)	4 (80%)	4 (80%)	4 (80%)	1.000
Total (105)	86 (82%)	68 (65%)	83 (79%)	0.031

The size of the NTF appeared to influence the number of affected shape features (nonsignificant; Table 3). For a small NTF, 36% of the features were affected, increasing to 57% and 71% for medium and large NTFs, respectively. Moreover, for small and medium NTFs 100% of the NGTDM features were affected compared to only 40% for a large NTF.

Table 3. Numbers and percentages of features affected by the delineation method ($VOI_{vital-tumour}$ vs. $VOI_{gross-tumour}$) per feature class for the subgroups based on NTF. Differences in the number of affected features between subgroups were assessed using the Fisher's exact test. NTF: necrotic tumour fraction, GLCM: grey level cooccurrence matrix, GLRLM: grey level run length matrix, GLSZM: grey level size zone matrix, GLDM: grey level dependence matrix, NGTDM: neighbouring grey tone difference matrix.

Feature Class	All (n = 43)	Small NTF (NTF $\leq$ 0.12, n = 14)	Medium NTF (0.12 < NTF $\leq$ 0.36, n = 15)	Large NTF (NTF > 0.36, n = 14)	p-Value
First order (18)	17 (94%)	14 (78%)	16 (89%)	14 (78%)	0.745
Shape (14)	11 (79%)	5 (36%)	8 (57%)	10 (71%)	0.199
Texture (73)	58 (79%)	52 (71%)	60 (82%)	51 (70%)	0.170
GLCM (22)	15 (68%)	13 (59%)	15 (68%)	15 (68%)	0.850
GLRLM (16)	15 (94%)	12 (75%)	14 (88%)	14 (88%)	0.701
GLSZM (16)	12 (75%)	12 (75%)	15 (94%)	9 (94%)	0.058
GLDM (14)	12 (86%)	10 (71%)	11 (79%)	11 (79%)	1.000
NGTDM (5)	4 (80%)	5 (100%)	5 (100%)	2 (40%)	0.066
Total (105)	86 (82%)	71 (68%)	84 (80%)	75 (71%)	0.116

Although nonsignificant, the value of the SUV_{max} appeared to influence the number of affected features (Table 4) and a higher value resulted in more affected features (56%, 66% and 70% for low, medium and high values, respectively). This increasing trend could also be observed for all texture feature classes except for GLCM features, where the number of affected features decreased with an increasing SUV_{max}.

Overlap in affected features between cohorts and subgroups is generally high (Figure 2), yet the affected shape features varied largely between cohorts and for different-sized NTFs. It can be observed that many features that were affected in one subset or cohort, were also affected in most of the other subsets or cohorts (Supplementary Table S1).

Table 4. Numbers and percentages of features affected by the delineation method (VOI$_{vital\text{-}tumour}$ vs. VOI$_{gross\text{-}tumour}$) per feature class for the different subgroups based on SUV$_{max}$. Differences in the number of affected features between subgroups were assessed using the Fisher's exact test. SUV$_{max}$: maximum standardised uptake value, GLCM: grey level co-occurrence matrix, GLRLM: grey level run length matrix, GLSZM: grey level size zone matrix, GLDM: grey level dependence matrix, NGTDM: neighbouring grey tone difference matrix.

Feature Class	All (n = 43)	Low SUV$_{max}$ (SUV$_{max} \leq 4.61$, n = 14)	Medium SUV$_{max}$ (4.61 < SUV$_{max} \leq 12.09$, n = 15)	High SUV$_{max}$ (SUV$_{max}$ > 12.09, n = 14)	p-Value
First order (18)	17 (94%)	14 (78%)	15 (83%)	16 (89%)	0.898
Shape (14)	11 (79%)	4 (29%)	5 (36%)	4 (29%)	1.000
Texture (73)	58 (79%)	41 (56%)	49 (67%)	53 (73%)	0.106
GLCM (22)	15 (68%)	15 (68%)	12 (55%)	12 (55%)	0.610
GLRLM (16)	15 (94%)	9 (56%)	13 (81%)	15 (94%)	0.051
GLSZM (16)	12 (75%)	7 (44%)	11 (69%)	12 (75%)	0.249
GLDM (14)	12 (86%)	8 (57%)	9 (64%)	10 (71%)	0.919
NGTDM (5)	4 (80%)	2 (40%)	4 (80%)	4 (80%)	0.500
Total (105)	86 (82%)	59 (56%)	69 (66%)	73 (70%)	0.120

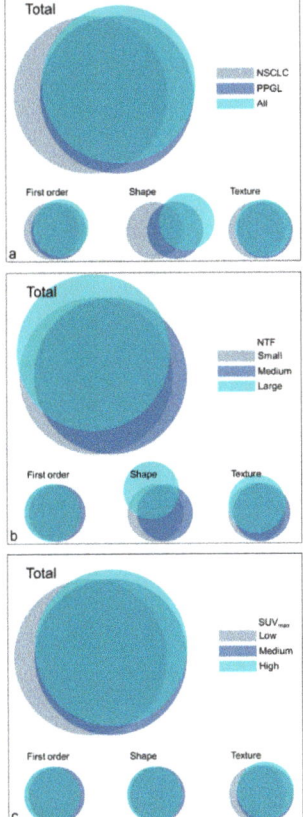

Figure 2. Venn diagrams representing the overlap in affected features per feature class for the cohorts (**a**) and subgroups ((**b**): NTF, (**c**): SUV$_{max}$). NSCLC: non-small cell lung carcinoma, PPGL: pheochromocytoma and paraganglioma, NTF: necrotic tumour fraction, SUV$_{max}$: maximum standardised uptake value.

For each of the three radiomic models evaluating predictive performance ($VOI_{vital-tumour}$, $VOI_{gross-tumour}$ and combined) for the PPGL dataset, three factors were retained and the three best corresponding features were selected (Table 5). The KMOs of the models were excellent (>0.96). AUCs varied 0.791–0.829, but were not significantly different between the radiomic models ($VOI_{vital-tumour}$ vs. $VOI_{gross-tumour}$: $p = 0.775$; $VOI_{vital-tumour}$ vs. combined: $p = 0.625$; $VOI_{gross-tumour}$ vs. combined: $p = 0.874$; Figure 3). The mean AUCs of the sham experiments were lower (0.645–0.655) than the AUCs of the radiomic models, indicating the validity of the findings.

Table 5. Results of dimension reduction and predictive performance of the $VOI_{vital-tumour}$, $VOI_{gross-tumour}$ and combined model for the noradrenergic biochemical profile in the PPGL cohort. For each model, 3 features were selected corresponding to the factors with the highest loadings. AUCs of the radiomic models and the mean AUC of the sham experiment are reported. Features marked with * are not significantly different between delineation methods in the PPGL dataset. KMO: Kaiser–Meier–Olkin (KMO) measure, AUC: area under the receiver operating characteristic curve.

	$VOI_{vital-tumour}$	$VOI_{gross-tumour}$	Combined
Features retained after filtering ($\tau = 0.95$)	53/105	57/105	103/210
KMO	0.970	0.969	0.986
Cumulative variance	0.63	0.58	0.53
Selected features	- First order Minimum - Shape Surface Area * - GLCM Informational Measure of Correlation 2	- Shape Surface Area * - NGTDM Complexity - GLDM Dependence Entropy	- $VOI_{gross-tumour}$ GLCM Sum entropy - $VOI_{vital-tumour}$ Shape maximum 3D diameter * - $VOI_{vital-tumour}$ Shape Surface Volume ratio
AUC (95% CI)	0.829 (0.677–0.981)	0.803 (0.640–0.967)	0.791 (0.618–0.963)
Mean AUC sham experiment (100 iterations)	0.643	0.660	0.666

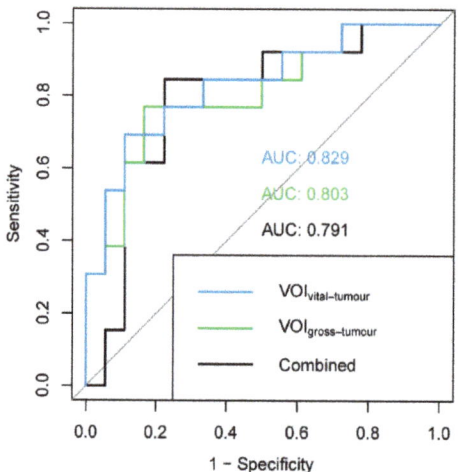

Figure 3. ROC curves and AUCs for the different radiomic models: blue: $VOI_{vital-tumour}$ (features: first order minimum, shape surface area and GLCM informational measure of correlation 2); green: $VOI_{gross-tumour}$ (features: shape surface area, NGTDM complexity and GLDM dependence entropy); black: combined (features: $VOI_{gross-tumour}$ GLCM sum entropy, $VOI_{vital-tumour}$ shape maximum 3D diameter and $VOI_{vital-tumour}$ shape surface volume ratio). ROC: receiver operating characteristic, AUC: area under the ROC curve.

4. Discussion

In this study, we assessed the effect of the inclusion of central necrosis during tumour delineation on radiomic analysis in two cohorts of patients with NSCLC and PPGL. Around two-third of radiomic features showed significant differences between adaptive threshold delineation with and without manual addition of the region of central necrosis. Nevertheless, the predictive performance of radiomic models with and without central necrosis for the noradrenergic biochemical profile of PPGLs was not significantly different. Due to the low number of subjects, the predictive performance was not assessed for the NSCLC cohort.

At least 65% of all features were significantly affected after adjustment for multiple-testing by the difference in delineation method. Less features were affected in the NSCLC cohort compared to the PPGL cohort (65% versus 82%, respectively), which is likely a result of lower power of the test due to a smaller cohort (12 versus 31, respectively).

More than 72% of the first order features, describing the distribution of voxel intensities in a histogram, significantly changed when central necrosis, i.e., lower intensity values, was added to the VOI. The number of affected first order features increases with a higher SUV_{max}, which can be explained by the larger range of voxel values in the intensity histogram in the case of a high SUV_{max} after the addition of a region with central necrosis.

At least 66% of the texture features, describing the spatial relationships between individual voxels in terms of run lengths, size zones of the same voxel values or combinations of neighbouring voxel values, were affected by central necrosis, which resulted in a change of the spatial relationships between the voxels. It is beyond the scope of this study to dive into the mathematical definition of all texture features, but we will highlight some of our findings and possible explanations.

Similarly to first order features, the number of affected texture features also increased with increasing SUV_{max}. The introduction of a region with low grey levels might result in longer run lengths and size zones with low values. In a tumour with relatively high grey levels, this might result in a larger run length or size zone matrix, with high incidences for the low grey values (central necrosis) and for the high grey levels (edge of the tumour) and low incidences in the middle range. For a tumour with a lower SUV_{max}, the matrices remain smaller, with incidences in the low and middle ranges and this results in different feature values.

Furthermore, it is remarkable that almost all normalised texture features were significantly different for both delineation methods for the NSCLC cohort, the PPGL cohort and all patients combined: The *normalised* GLCM inverse difference and inverse difference moment, the GLRLM grey level non-uniformity and run length non-uniformity and the GLSZM grey level non-uniformity and size zone non-uniformity were significantly different between both delineation methods. The normalised GLDM dependence non-uniformity was only different in the PPGL cohort and the combined cohort. Normalisation of GLCM features is performed to improve classification accuracy [29]. Normalised features are standardised for the number of elements in their respective matrix, i.e., the GLCM consists of the square of the number of discretised grey levels and the GLRLM consist of the product of the number of discretised grey levels and the maximal run length [14]. Since the number of discretised grey levels and the maximal run length increase by the addition of the region of central necrosis, it could result in a decrease in feature values, resulting in differences in feature values between delineation methods.

Compared to other features classes, shape features were affected least frequently by the choice of the delineation method, but 50% of shape features were still affected. Some shape features consider the outer diameter or morphology of the VOI, which, in most cases, did not expressively change when adding the region of central necrosis. Nevertheless, in some cases the region of central necrosis touched the outer surface of the volume of interest (3D U-shape) and caused some features to change. The number of affected shape features increased with the NTF as a result of a larger additional region of necrosis.

Several studies on repeatability and reproducibility showed that radiomic feature values are affected by delineation methods [30]. Unfortunately, overviews of repeatability and reproducibility on a feature level are scarce and are often limited to feature classes. Traverso et al. wrote a systematic review on repeatability and reproducibility of radiomic features and assessed to what extent (highly likely/probable/less likely) the different feature classes were affected by different processing steps of the radiomic pipeline [31]. They found that it is probable that semi-automatic VOI delineation exerts an adverse effect on repeatability and reproducibility of texture features. Moreover, in the case of shape features, this adverse effect is probable but when compared to shape features derived from CT, PET shape features are more reproducible. According to Traverso et al., first order features are less likely to be affected by the delineation method, which is in sharp contrast with our study that shows that first order features are affected in particular by the delineation method. They also present that entropy was consistent among the most repeatable and reproducible first order features [31]. However, in our study it can be observed that entropy is one of the features that is significantly affected by the delineation method in all cohorts and subgroups. Coarseness and contrast (GLCM as well as NGTDM), on the other hand, are considered among the least reproducible features [31,32], whereas our results show that coarseness and GLCM contrast are affected in only two and zero out of nine subgroups (Supplementary Table S1), respectively. This shows that non-repeatable or non-reproducible features are not the only features affected by central necrosis and therefore the choice of the delineation method concerning central necrosis should be considered in the design of radiomic studies.

Our study analysed the differences in radiomic features in two cohorts with different tumour types, showing a different tumour-to-background ratio. While the same image analysis (VOI delineation and radiomic feature extraction) was performed, acquisition and reconstruction settings were different between cohorts even though both protocols were in accordance with the EANM guidelines. The features affected by the delineation method, however, were highly similar between both cohorts, indicating that the effect of the delineation method concerning central necrosis is independent of the tumour type. Therefore, whether or not to include central necrosis in the tumour delineation is an important factor to consider when performing clinical radiomic studies. We hypothesise that this might also apply to other tumour types, but the number of affected features might vary as a result of tumour characteristics such as the tracer uptake and distribution, tumour geometry and NTF.

While almost two-third of radiomic feature values were significantly affected by the choice of delineation method, the predictive performances of the radiomic models, as assessed in the PPGL cohort, were not affected accordingly. The predictive performances, as assessed by the AUCs for the noradrenergic biochemical profile of PPGLs and found valid in a sham experiment, were not significantly different between radiomic features derived from VOIs with and without central necrosis. An explanation for this could be that the radiomic feature set describes many different types of heterogeneity and, as a result, feature sets from both delineation methods contain useful features in terms of predictive performance. Multicollinearity within one feature set is high, but might also be high between feature sets of different delineation methods. Additionally, the combination of radiomic features from both delineation methods resulted in an AUC similar to the ones of the different delineation methods seperately. This indicates that, in this small dataset, the combination of features from the two delineation methods does not result in additional information that is favorable for the predictive performance. It should be taken into account that, in order to prevent overfitting of the model, only three features could be retained in factor analysis. In other tumour types, multicollinearity in and between feature sets of different delineation methods is expected to be high as well, but further research is needed to confirm this effect in a larger population as well as for different tumour types.

This study showed that the effect of inclusion or exclusion of the region of central necrosis in the delineation significantly impacts radiomic feature values in PPGL and

NSCLC, but does not impact the predictive performance of the PPGL radiomic model. A guideline on the choice to add or leave out central necrosis in delineation could not be provided. From a biological perspective, regions of central necrosis are part of the tumour and should therefore be included in the VOI, especially considering that central necrosis is associated with poor prognosis [6]. On the other hand, from a data-driven perspective, some features might already capture the presence of central necrosis without our awareness, since the features are investigated exploratively and without biological rationale. Both delineation methods can be used in radiomic studies, but feature values vary largely between both methods. For reproducibility purposes, especially in the setting of external validation [33], future studies should report whether regions of central necrosis were included in the delineation.

5. Conclusions

Central necrosis of tumours on [^{18}F]FDG PET significantly impacts radiomic feature values. Almost two-third of the features were affected, demonstrating that the influence of whether or not to include regions of central necrosis in the delineation of the tumour on the radiomic feature values is significant. However, no significant difference in the predictive performance of both delineation methods was observed. In order to advance reproducibility of radiomic research, radiomic studies should report on whether or not central necrosis was (manually) included during delineation.

Supplementary Materials: The following are available online at https://www.mdpi.com/2075-4418/11/7/1296/s1, Supplementary File S1: Image Biomarker Standardisation Initiative Reporting Guidelines, Supplementary Table S1: Features affected by the choice of delineation method (VOI$_{vital-tumour}$ vs. VOI$_{gross-tumour}$) for the different cohorts and subgroups based on NTF and SUV$_{max}$.

Author Contributions: Conceptualisation, W.A.N., D.V., C.H.S., L.-F.d.G.-O. and F.H.P.v.V.; methodology, W.A.N., D.V., L.-F.d.G.-O. and F.H.P.v.V.; software, W.A.N. and F.H.P.v.V.; validation, W.A.N., D.V., L.-F.d.G.-O. and F.H.P.v.V.; formal analysis, W.A.N. and C.D.Y.M.; investigation, W.A.N. and C.D.Y.M.; resources, D.V., E.H.A., A.v.B., H.J.L.M.T., J.B., T.W.H.M. and L.-F.d.G.-O.; data curation, W.A.N., D.V., L.-F.d.G.-O. and F.H.P.v.V.; writing—original draft preparation, W.A.N.; writing—Review and Editing, D.V., C.D.Y.M., C.H.S., E.H.A., A.v.B., H.J.L.M.T., J.B., T.W.H.M., L.-F.d.G.-O. and F.H.P.v.V.; visualisation, W.A.N.; supervision, D.V., L.-F.d.G.-O. and F.H.P.v.V.; project administration, D.V., L.-F.d.G.-O. and F.H.P.v.V.; funding acquisition, L.-F.d.G.-O. and F.H.P.v.V. All authors have read and agreed to the published version of the manuscript.

Funding: Dennis Vriens was supported in part by the Netherlands Organisation for Health Research and Development (ZonMw) stipends for a Clinical Research Fellowship (AGIKO) (project no. 92003552) for design and data collection of the original clinical NSCLC study. The costs of the additional dynamic PET scans were covered by the Department of Radiology and Nuclear Medicine, Radboud University Medical Center, Nijmegen. The PPGL study [19] was supported by the European Union Seventh Framework Programme (FP7/2007–2013) under grant agreement 259735 (ENSAT CANCER). No additional funding was received for this study.

Institutional Review Board Statement: The studies were conducted according to the guidelines of the Declaration of Helsinki. The NSCLC study has been reviewed and approved by the Commission on Medical Research Involving Human Subjects Region Arnhem-Nijmegen, the Netherlands (protocol code: NL24886.091.08, date of approval: 8 December 2008). The PPGL retrospective database study has been reviewed and approved by the Commission on Medical Research Involving Human Subjects Region Arnhem-Nijmegen, the Netherlands (protocol code: 2018-4655, date of approval: 10 December 2018).

Informed Consent Statement: All NSCLC patients signed an informed consent form. For the PPGL study, informed consent was waived due to the retrospective nature of the study. Patients that objected to the use of their anonymised data were excluded.

Data Availability Statement: The datasets generated during and/or analysed during the current study are available from the corresponding author upon reasonable request.

Acknowledgments: The authors want to thank the PET/CT technologists from the Radboud University Medical Center for their assistance with the PET/CT scans.

Conflicts of Interest: The authors have declared that no competing interests exist.

References

1. Eales, K.L.; Hollinshead, K.E.R.; Tennant, D.A. Hypoxia and metabolic adaptation of cancer cells. *Oncogenesis* **2016**, *5*, e190. [CrossRef]
2. Hanahan, D.; Weinberg, R.A. Hallmarks of Cancer: The Next Generation. *Cell* **2011**, *144*, 646–674. [CrossRef]
3. Bredholt, G.; Mannelqvist, M.; Stefansson, I.M.; Birkeland, E.; Bø, T.H.; Oyan, A.M.; Trovik, J.; Kalland, K.-H.; Jonassen, I.; Salvesen, H.B.; et al. Tumor necrosis is an important hallmark of aggressive endometrial cancer and associates with hypoxia, angiogenesis and inflammation responses. *Oncotarget* **2015**, *6*, 39676–39691. [CrossRef]
4. Lam, J.S.; Shvarts, O.; Said, J.W.; Pantuck, A.J.; Seligson, D.B.; Aldridge, M.E.; Bui, M.H.T.; Liu, X.; Horvath, S.; Figlin, R.A.; et al. Clinicopathologic and molecular correlations of necrosis in the primary tumor of patients with renal cell carcinoma. *Cancer* **2005**, *103*, 2517–2525. [CrossRef]
5. Maiorano, E.; Regan, M.M.; Viale, G.; Mastropasqua, M.G.; Colleoni, M.; Castiglione-Gertsch, M.; Price, K.N.; Gelber, R.D.; Goldhirsch, A.; Coates, A.S. Prognostic and predictive impact of central necrosis and fibrosis in early breast cancer: Results from two International Breast Cancer Study Group randomized trials of chemoendocrine adjuvant therapy. *Breast Cancer Res. Treat.* **2010**, *121*, 211–218. [CrossRef]
6. Swinson, D.E.; Jones, J.; Richardson, D.; Cox, G.; Edwards, J.G.; O'Byrne, K.J. Tumour necrosis is an independent prognostic marker in non-small cell lung cancer: Correlation with biological variables. *Lung Cancer* **2002**, *37*, 235–240. [CrossRef]
7. Sahni, V.; Guvenc-Tuncturk, S.; Paintal, H.S.; Kuschner, W.G. Bronchogenic Squamous Cell Carcinoma Mass with Central Photopenia on FDG-PET Scan. *Clin. Med. Res.* **2012**, *10*, 36–37. [CrossRef] [PubMed]
8. Noortman, W.A.; Vriens, D.; Grootjans, W.; Tao, Q.; de Geus-Oei, L.F.; Van Velden, F.H. Nuclear medicine radiomics in precision medicine: Why we can't do without artificial intelligence. *Q. J. Nucl. Med. Mol. Imaging* **2020**, *64*, 278–290. [CrossRef]
9. Cook, G.J.; Azad, G.; Owczarczyk, K.; Siddique, M.; Goh, V. Challenges and Promises of PET Radiomics. *Int. J. Radiat. Oncol. Biol. Phys.* **2018**, *102*, 1083–1089. [CrossRef] [PubMed]
10. Frings, V.; Van Velden, F.H.P.; Velasquez, L.M.; Hayes, W.; Van De Ven, P.M.; Hoekstra, O.S.; Boellaard, R. Repeatability of Metabolically Active Tumor Volume Measurements with FDG PET/CT in Advanced Gastrointestinal Malignancies: A Multicenter Study. *Radiology* **2014**, *273*, 539–548. [CrossRef] [PubMed]
11. Bashir, U.; Azad, G.; Siddique, M.M.; Dhillon, S.; Patel, N.; Bassett, P.; Landau, D.; Goh, V.; Cook, G. The effects of segmentation algorithms on the measurement of 18F-FDG PET texture parameters in non-small cell lung cancer. *EJNMMI Res.* **2017**, *7*, 60. [CrossRef]
12. Hatt, M.; Visvikis, D.; Albarghach, N.M.; Tixier, F.; Pradier, O.; Rest, C.C.-L. Prognostic value of 18F-FDG PET image-based parameters in oesophageal cancer and impact of tumour delineation methodology. *Eur. J. Nucl. Med. Mol. Imaging* **2011**, *38*, 1191–1202. [CrossRef]
13. Cheebsumon, P.; Van Velden, F.H.; Yaqub, M.; Frings, V.; De Langen, A.J.; Hoekstra, O.S.; Lammertsma, A.A.; Boellaard, R. Effects of Image Characteristics on Performance of Tumor Delineation Methods: A Test-Retest Assessment. *J. Nucl. Med.* **2011**, *52*, 1550–1558. [CrossRef] [PubMed]
14. Zwanenburg, A.; Leger, S.; Vallieres, M.; Lock, S. Image biomarker standardisation initiative—Feature definitions v11. *arXiv* **2016**, arXiv:1612.07003.
15. Van Berkel, A.; Rao, J.U.; Kusters, B.; Demir, T.; Visser, E.; Mensenkamp, A.; van der Laak, J.A.; Oosterwijk, E.; Lenders, J.W.; Sweep, F.C.; et al. Correlation Between In Vivo 18F-FDG PET and Immunohistochemical Markers of Glucose Uptake and Metabolism in Pheochromocytoma and Paraganglioma. *J. Nucl. Med.* **2014**, *55*, 1253–1259. [CrossRef] [PubMed]
16. Meijer, T.W.H.; de Geus-Oei, L.-F.; Visser, E.P.; Oyen, W.J.; Looijen-Salamon, M.G.; Visvikis, D.; Verhagen, A.F.T.M.; Bussink, J.; Vriens, D. Tumor Delineation and Quantitative Assessment of Glucose Metabolic Rate within Histologic Subtypes of Non–Small Cell Lung Cancer by Using Dynamic 18F Fluorodeoxyglucose PET. *Radiology* **2017**, *283*, 547–559. [CrossRef]
17. Hatt, M.; Majdoub, M.; Vallières, M.; Tixier, F.; Le Rest, C.C.; Groheux, D.; Hindié, E.; Martineau, A.; Pradier, O.; Hustinx, R.; et al. 18F-FDG PET Uptake Characterization Through Texture Analysis: Investigating the Complementary Nature of Heterogeneity and Functional Tumor Volume in a Multi–Cancer Site Patient Cohort. *J. Nucl. Med.* **2015**, *56*, 38–44. [CrossRef]
18. Boellaard, R.; O'Doherty, M.J.; Weber, W.A.; Mottaghy, F.M.; Lonsdale, M.N.; Stroobants, S.; Oyen, W.J.; Kotzerke, J.; Hoekstra, O.S.; Pruim, J.; et al. FDG PET and PET/CT: EANM procedure guidelines for tumour PET imaging: Version 1.0. *Eur. J. Nucl. Med. Mol. Imaging* **2009**, *37*, 181–200. [CrossRef]
19. Van Berkel, A.; Vriens, D.; Visser, E.P.; Janssen, M.J.; Gotthardt, M.; Hermus, A.R.; de Geus-Oei, L.-F.; Timmers, H.J. Metabolic Subtyping of Pheochromocytoma and Paraganglioma by 18F-FDG Pharmacokinetics Using Dynamic PET/CT Scanning. *J. Nucl. Med.* **2019**, *60*, 745–751. [CrossRef]
20. Kikinis, R.; Pieper, S.D.; Vosburgh, K.G. 3D Slicer: A Platform for Subject-Specific Image Analysis, Visualization, and Clinical Support. In *Intraoperative Imaging and Image-Guided Therapy*; Jolesz, F., Ed.; Springer: New York, NY, USA, 2014; pp. 277–289. [CrossRef]

21. Wahl, R.L.; Jacene, H.; Kasamon, Y.; Lodge, M.A. From RECIST to PERCIST: Evolving Considerations for PET Response Criteria in Solid Tumors. *J. Nucl. Med. Off. Publ. Soc. Nucl. Med.* **2009**, *50*, 122S–150S. [CrossRef]
22. Cheebsumon, P.; Boellaard, R.; De Ruysscher, D.; Van Elmpt, W.; Van Baardwijk, A.; Yaqub, M.; Hoekstra, O.S.; Comans, E.F.; Lammertsma, A.A.; Van Velden, F.H. Assessment of tumour size in PET/CT lung cancer studies: PET- and CT-based methods compared to pathology. *EJNMMI Res.* **2012**, *2*, 56. [CrossRef]
23. Van Griethuysen, J.J.M.; Fedorov, A.; Parmar, C.; Hosny, A.; Aucoin, N.; Narayan, V.; Beets-Tan, R.G.H.; Fillion-Robin, J.-C.; Pieper, S.; Aerts, H.J.W.L. Computational Radiomics System to Decode the Radiographic Phenotype. *Cancer Res.* **2017**, *77*, e104–e107. [CrossRef]
24. Chalkidou, A.; O'Doherty, M.J.; Marsden, P.K. False Discovery Rates in PET and CT Studies with Texture Features: A Systematic Review. *PLoS ONE* **2015**, *10*, e0124165. [CrossRef]
25. Benjamini, Y.; Hochberg, Y. Controlling the False Discovery Rate: A Practical and Powerful Approach to Multiple Testing. *J. R. Stat. Soc.* **1995**, *57*, 289–300. [CrossRef]
26. Gillies, R.J.; Kinahan, P.E.; Hricak, H. Radiomics: Images Are More than Pictures, They Are Data. *Radiology* **2016**, *278*, 563–577. [CrossRef] [PubMed]
27. Peeters, C.F.; Übelhör, C.; Mes, S.W.; Martens, R.; Koopman, T.; de Graaf, P.; van Velden, F.H.; Boellaard, R.; Castelijns, J.A.; Beest, D.E.t.; et al. Stable prediction with radiomics data. *arXiv* **2019**, arXiv:1903.11696.
28. Buvat, I.; Orlhac, F. The Dark Side of Radiomics: On the Paramount Importance of Publishing Negative Results. *J. Nucl. Med.* **2019**, *60*, 1543–1544. [CrossRef] [PubMed]
29. Clausi, D.A. An analysis of co-occurrence texture statistics as a function of grey level quantization. *Can. J. Remote. Sens.* **2002**, *28*, 45–62. [CrossRef]
30. Van Velden, F.H.; Kramer, G.M.; Frings, V.; Nissen, I.A.; Mulder, E.R.; de Langen, A.J.; Hoekstra, O.S.; Smit, E.F.; Boellaard, R. Repeatability of Radiomic Features in Non-Small-Cell Lung Cancer [(18)F]FDG-PET/CT Studies: Impact of Reconstruction and Delineation. *Mol. Imaging Biol.* **2016**, *18*, 788–795. [CrossRef]
31. Traverso, A.; Wee, L.; Dekker, A.; Gillies, R. Repeatability and Reproducibility of Radiomic Features: A Systematic Review. *Int. J. Radiat. Oncol.* **2018**, *102*, 1143–1158. [CrossRef]
32. Desseroit, M.-C.; Tixier, F.; Weber, W.A.; Siegel, B.A.; Le Rest, C.C.; Visvikis, D.; Hatt, M. Reliability of PET/CT Shape and Heterogeneity Features in Functional and Morphologic Components of Non–Small Cell Lung Cancer Tumors: A Repeatability Analysis in a Prospective Multicenter Cohort. *J. Nucl. Med.* **2016**, *58*, 406–411. [CrossRef] [PubMed]
33. Lambin, P.; Leijenaar, R.T.H.; Deist, T.M.; Peerlings, J.; de Jong, E.E.C.; van Timmeren, J.; Sanduleanu, S.; Larue, R.T.H.M.; Even, A.J.G.; Jochems, A.; et al. Radiomics: The bridge between medical imaging and personalized medicine. *Nat. Rev. Clin. Oncol.* **2017**, *14*, 749–762. [CrossRef] [PubMed]

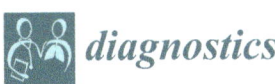

Article

Image Quantification for TSPO PET with a Novel Image-Derived Input Function Method

Yu-Hua Dean Fang [1,2,*], Jonathan E. McConathy [1], Talene A. Yacoubian [2], Yue Zhang [3], Richard E. Kennedy [3] and David G. Standaert [2]

[1] Department of Radiology, Heersink School of Medicine, University of Alabama at Birmingham, Birmingham, AL 35294, USA; jmcconathy@uabmc.edu
[2] Center for Neurodegeneration and Experimental Therapeutics, Department of Neurology, Heersink School of Medicine, University of Alabama at Birmingham, Birmingham, AL 35294, USA; tyacoubian@uabmc.edu (T.A.Y.); dstandaert@uabmc.edu (D.G.S.)
[3] Department of Medicine, Heersink School of Medicine, University of Alabama at Birmingham, Birmingham, AL 35294, USA; yuezhang@uabmc.edu (Y.Z.); richardkennedy@uabmc.edu (R.E.K.)
* Correspondence: yfang@uab.edu; Tel.: +1-205-934-5377; Fax: +1-205-996-2031

Abstract: There is a growing interest in using ^{18}F-DPA-714 PET to study neuroinflammation and microglial activation through imaging the 18-kDa translocator protein (TSPO). Although quantification of ^{18}F-DPA-714 binding can be achieved through kinetic modeling analysis with an arterial input function (AIF) measured with blood sampling procedures, the invasiveness of such procedures has been an obstacle for wide application. To address these challenges, we developed an image-derived input function (IDIF) that noninvasively estimates the arterial input function from the images acquired for ^{18}F-DPA-714 quantification. Methods: The method entails three fully automatic steps to extract the IDIF, including a segmentation of voxels with highest likelihood of being the arterial blood over the carotid artery, a model-based matrix factorization to extract the arterial blood signal, and a scaling optimization procedure to scale the extracted arterial blood signal into the activity concentration unit. Two cohorts of human subjects were used to evaluate the extracted IDIF. In the first cohort of five subjects, arterial blood sampling was performed, and the calculated IDIF was validated against the measured AIF through the comparison of distribution volumes from AIF ($V_{T,AIF}$) and IDIF ($V_{T,IDIF}$). In the second cohort, PET studies from twenty-eight healthy controls without arterial blood sampling were used to compare $V_{T,IDIF}$ with $V_{T,REF}$ measured using a reference region-based analysis to evaluate whether it can distinguish high-affinity (HAB) and mixed-affinity (MAB) binders. Results: In the arterial blood-sampling cohort, V_T derived from IDIF was found to be an accurate surrogate of the V_T from AIF. The bias of $V_{T,IDIF}$ was $-5.8 \pm 7.8\%$ when compared to $V_{T,AIF}$, and the linear mixed effect model showed a high correlation between $V_{T,AIF}$ and $V_{T,IDIF}$ ($p < 0.001$). In the nonblood-sampling cohort, $V_{T,IDIF}$ showed a significance difference between the HAB and MAB healthy controls. $V_{T,IDIF}$ and standard uptake values (SUV) showed superior results in distinguishing HAB from MAB subjects than $V_{T,REF}$. Conclusions: A novel IDIF method for ^{18}F-DPA-714 PET quantification was developed and evaluated in this study. This IDIF provides a noninvasive alternative measurement of V_T to quantify the TSPO binding of ^{18}F-DPA-714 in the human brain through dynamic PET scans.

Keywords: TSPO PET; neuroinflammation; image-derived input function; kinetic modeling analysis

Citation: Fang, Y.-H.D.; McConathy, J.E.; Yacoubian, T.A.; Zhang, Y.; Kennedy, R.E.; Standaert, D.G. Image Quantification for TSPO PET with a Novel Image-Derived Input Function Method. *Diagnostics* **2022**, *12*, 1161. https://doi.org/10.3390/diagnostics12051161

Academic Editors: Lioe-Fee de Geus-Oei and F.H.P. van Velden

Received: 29 March 2022
Accepted: 3 May 2022
Published: 7 May 2022

Publisher's Note: MDPI stays neutral with regard to jurisdictional claims in published maps and institutional affiliations.

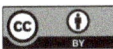

Copyright: © 2022 by the authors. Licensee MDPI, Basel, Switzerland. This article is an open access article distributed under the terms and conditions of the Creative Commons Attribution (CC BY) license (https://creativecommons.org/licenses/by/4.0/).

1. Introduction

In recent years, the role of neuroinflammation has been studied in many neurodegenerative diseases, including Alzheimer's disease (AD) and Parkinson's disease (PD) [1–4]. Noninvasive measurement of regional brain microglial activation with PET imaging has become a popular approach for investigation of neuroinflammation in clinical research [5]. The best established and most often used PET imaging biomarker for microglial activation is the 18 kDa translocator protein (TSPO), a protein abundant in brain microglia, monocytes, and other macrophages. A variety of studies have shown the usefulness of the ^{18}F-DPA-714 in research studies of microglial involvement in neurological disorders [6,7]. Despite the growing usage of ^{18}F-DPA-714 in clinical research, quantification of the ^{18}F-DPA-714 uptake and binding to TPSO remains a challenge for clinical research studies. Conventionally, ^{18}F-DPA-714 binding is quantified through a kinetic modeling analysis, where the compartmental analysis is conducted over the tissue time-activity curves from the dynamic PET studies. However, the main obstacle for such analysis is the invasive nature of the required arterial blood sampling procedure to acquire the arterial input function (AIF). Processing of the arterial blood samples is a time-consuming and complex procedure that affects the feasibility to include AIF measurement in clinical trials.

To avoid the arterial blood sampling procedures, modeling approaches based on reference regions are commonly adopted to quantify cerebral tracer binding for PET imaging. To use a reference region, there is an underlying modeling assumption that the reference region is devoid of specific binding of the PET tracer. However, in the case of ^{18}F-DPA-714, there is a widespread distribution of TSPO in the normal brain, and no region can be regarded as a perfect reference region lacking TSPO binding, especially if microglial activation is widespread. For example, the cerebellum has been a popular reference region of choice in the literature for TSPO binding quantification [8–11]. However, it has been well known that the cerebellum contains a substantial amount of specific binding sites for TSPO tracers [12,13]. Previous reports have suggested that in such cases, reference region methods may lead to a biased measurement of tracer binding [14]. Moreover, the binding capacity in the reference region may be altered under pathological or pharmacological conditions. For example, Gerhard et al. showed that the cerebellum shows elevated TSPO overexpression with the TSPO tracer ^{11}C-(R)PK11195 in subjects with progressive supranuclear palsy [15]. Increased TSPO tracer binding in the cerebellum has also been observed in AD [16,17]. In some conditions, there could even be a global elevation of neuroinflammation and TSPO overexpression throughout the brain [18]. Under such cases, it is nearly impossible to identify a reference region that can properly serve as a true reference region. As a result, quantifying TSPO PET with reference region methods may not be an appropriate choice, especially if a disease or abnormality may cause widespread TSPO overexpression and microglial activation throughout the brain.

To address these limitations, we sought to develop an image-derived input function (IDIF) as a noninvasive surrogate for the AIF measurement. Current methods for extracting IDIF are usually based on image segmentation techniques that focus on extracting large arterial structures such as carotid arteries [19,20] or the left ventricle [21]. Due to the relatively low spatial resolution of PET, such methods need to address the activity spillover and partial volume effects that lead to a mixture of the true blood activity and activity from surrounding tissue [19,22] or use a few blood samples to correct for the activity cross-contamination [20]. An IDIF extraction method for mouse TSPO PET imaging has been developed based on factor analysis by Wimberley et al. [23], but it requires a whole body scan and may be difficult for human brain PET studies without specialized scanners. Currently there does not seem to be a satisfactory IDIF solution for human TSPO PET imaging.

In this work, we developed a new IDIF method by using a model-based matrix factorization (MBMF) to separate the arterial blood and brain tissue radioactivity. We also developed a unique optimization procedure to scale the extracted IDIF from a normalized and dimensionless form into the activity concentration of the arterial blood signal. The developed method was validated through two approaches. First, we validated our method in a small cohort (n = 5) in which we conducted arterial blood sampling and measured AIF directly. The calculated IDIF was compared with the measured AIF through a Logan graphical analysis that measures the volume of distribution (V_T). Second, we applied the IDIF method to a group of healthy controls (n = 28), which had been genotyped for the polymorphism (rs6971) that determines affinity for ^{18}F-DPA-714 for TSPO [24]. Subjects predicted to be high-affinity binders (HAB; rs6971 C/C) and mixed-affinity binders (MAB; rs6971 C/T) were included in the cohort, while low-affinity binders (LAB, rs6971 T/T) were not included in the imaging study. Previous investigations have shown a 20–50% higher V_T for ^{18}F-DPA-714 in HAB subjects compared to MAB subjects [12,25]. We evaluated whether V_T measured with IDIF was able to detect these expected differences in binding in our cohort of healthy controls. Standard uptake values (SUVs) from the 40th to the 60th minutes post injection were also taken as an alternative reference of comparison between the HAB and MAB groups.

2. Materials and Methods

2.1. Standard Protocol Approvals, Registrations, and Patient Consents

Two separate cohorts of human subjects were recruited for this study. For cohort 1, all subjects were recruited under a small pilot study to examine the utility of ^{18}F-DPA-714 imaging for studying neuroinflammation in PD (ClinicalTrials.gov Identifier: NCT03457493). For cohort 2, human subjects were recruited as part of the larger longitudinal NINDS-funded Alabama Udall Center observational study examining the role of inflammation in early PD. Participants were enrolled between March 2018 and May 2021 through the Movement Disorder Clinic at the University of Alabama at Birmingham. The study was approved by institutional review board at UAB, and full written consent was obtained on each participant.

2.2. Participants

For cohort 1, denoted as the blood-sampling cohort in this work, eligible participants were age ≥ 30 years and were healthy controls or subjects diagnosed with PD. Control subjects had no current diagnosis of PD or other neurodegenerative disorder, had no history of PD in first-degrees blood relatives, and had ≤ 3 positive response on the PD Screening Questionnaire [26]. Subjects with PD were diagnosed according to the United Kingdom Brain Bank criteria by a movement disorder specialist. These criteria require bradykinesia and at least one of the following: 4–6 Hz resting tremor, rigidity, or postural instability. There was no restriction to stage of PD for enrollment.

For cohort 2, denoted as the nonblood-sampling cohort, imaging data from MAB and HAB control subjects enrolled as part of the larger longitudinal NINDS-funded Alabama Udall Center study prior to May 2021 were used for the analysis. Eligible participants were age ≥ 40 years. Control subjects had no current diagnosis of PD or other neurodegenerative disorder, had no history of PD in first-degrees blood relatives, and had ≤ 3 positive response on the PD Screening Questionnaire [26]. Subjects were excluded if they had a history of significant autoimmune/inflammatory disorder, current treatment with immunosuppressant therapy, or serious comorbidity that would interfere with study participation.

All participants underwent genetic testing for the rs6971 SNP associated with TSPO binding and were classified into low-, mixed-, or high-affinity binders. Low-affinity binders were not imaged.

2.3. Data Acquisition for the Cohort with Arterial Blood Sampling Procedures

In the blood-sampling cohort, five subjects underwent arterial blood sampling procedures during their ^{18}F-DPA-714 PET scans. These five subjects included two healthy controls and three PD patients. The TSPO genotype was determined by measuring the rs6971 polymorphism of the TSPO gene with single-nucleotide polymorphism (SNP)-based tests. Three of them were HAB, and two were MAB. Arterial blood samples were collected through the radial artery catheter under the following sampling settings: one sample per six seconds for the first minute, one sample per ten seconds for one minute, one sample per minute for three minutes, and one sample every five minutes for the rest of the scan, yielding a total of thirty samples for each study. Both the whole-blood and plasma activity concentrations of ^{18}F-DPA-714 were measured from each arterial blood sample. The blood samples at the 5th, 15th, 30th, and 60th minutes post injection were analyzed with high-performance liquid chromatography (HPLC) to measure the parent fraction for unmetabolized ^{18}F-DPA-714 for four subjects of the study. Decay correction was performed for all blood samples. All subjects underwent dynamic ^{18}F-DPA-714 PET/MR scans. Injection dose for ^{18}F-DPA-714 was 5 mCi (185 MBq). The ^{18}F-DPA-714 PET scan with a GE Signa PET/MR scanner lasted for 60 min for each subject immediately after tracer injection. Images were reconstructed with OSEM using 4 iterations and 16 subsets into a total of 36 frames, with the frame setting of 12 ten-second, 9 20-second, 5 one-minute, and 10 five-minute frames. Attenuation correction was involved in the reconstruction process with MR-based attenuation maps acquired with zero echo time (ZTE) MRI [27]. Time-of-flight information and point spread functions were incorporated in the PET reconstruction. The image volume was 256 × 256 × 89 with the pixel size of 1.17 mm and a slice thickness of 2.78 mm. Decay correction was also performed during the PET reconstruction.

2.4. Data Acquisition for the Cohort without Arterial Blood Sampling

The nonblood-sampling cohort included only healthy controls who underwent PET scans but did not undergo arterial blood sampling during the PET acquisition. Fifteen subjects out of the 28 healthy controls were HAB, and thirteen subjects were MAB. All subjects underwent the same PET dynamic acquisition as described previously.

2.5. Image Post-Processing

The reconstructed dynamic PET data underwent two additional image correction processes. First, we conducted a frame-by-frame 3D PET image registration to minimize the between-frame misalignment due to the involuntary patient motion during the PET acquisition. The last frame was used as the reference for the frame-by-frame registration. Second, partial volume correction was performed for all PET datasets with the geometric transfer matrix method [28] provided by the PETPVC toolbox [29]. The anatomical maps were derived from the segmentation results using Freesurfer, which performs subcortical region segmentation over the T1-weighted scans [30]. All image processing methods were implemented in MATLAB (version 2020a, Mathworks, Inc., Natick, MA, USA) The Freesurfer-derived segmentation maps of the prior step were also applied to the PET dynamic data and used to extract the tissue time-activity curves of the regions of interest. We chose the following nine regions as target regions of evaluation: putamen, caudate, thalamus, hippocampus, frontal cortex, temporal cortex, occipital cortex, parietal cortex, and cerebellum.

2.6. IDIF Extraction Procedure

The IDIF extraction procedure involved three steps: an image segmentation process to extract arterial voxels, a factorization process to separate the blood signal from the tissue signal, and a scaling process to set the separated blood signal back to the accurate activity concentration units. In the first step, we aimed to segment the voxels that are most likely to be within the carotid arteries. For each subject, we first took the Freesurfer-derived segmentation maps to determine the lowest slice of the cerebellum and only segment between this slice and the overall lowest slice in the field of view. For each of those axial slices, we took the first minute of dynamic frames and searched on the left side for the voxel with the highest intensity over these six frames. Assuming an approximated diameter of 6 mm for the carotid arteries [31], this voxel was then dilated with a five-by-five diamond-shaped structural element to form a segmented mask. The same operation was repeated for the right side of the same image slice to complete the carotid segmentation for this slice. All the selected slices underwent the same segmentation procedure to complete the segmentation for carotid arterial blood voxels. With the partial volume effect, the intensity of the segmented voxels that resemble the arterial blood activities is in fact a mixture of the arterial blood activities and the surrounding tissues.

To extract the arterial blood activities, it is assumed that all the surrounding tissue of the selected voxels can be approximated as a single tissue type and shares the same tracer uptake kinetics. Accordingly, the activity concentration of a specific voxel i can be expressed as:

$$C_{i,PET}(t) = \alpha_i C_{AIF}(t) + (1 - \alpha_i) C_{TISSUE}(t) \tag{1}$$

where C_{PET} represents the PET-measured activity, C_{AIF} represents the arterial blood activity, and C_{TISSUE} represents the surrounding tissue activity. α_i is the voxel-dependent mixing fraction of the arterial blood for the specific voxel.

Assuming there is a total of n segmented voxels and m PET image frames for the dynamic study, an n-by-m matrix A can be formed by combining $C_{i,PET}$ from all the m frames and n segmented voxels. With the goal to extract the underlying arterial input function C_{AIF} and tissue activity C_{TISSUE}, we developed a novel method that decomposes the matrix A into a 2-by-m matrix H that contains the two components of C_{AIF} and C_{TISSUE} and an n-by-2 weighting matrix W so that the difference between A and W*H can be minimized. Unlike other blind matrix factorization methods, our matrix factorization method is based on physiological models and shares similar concepts with guided matrix factorization [32] and knowledge-driven matrix factorization [33] by incorporating the prior knowledge of underlying factors during the matrix factorization process. During this model-based matrix factorization (MBMF), it is assumed that C_{AIF} and C_{TISSUE} can both be modeled and parameterized. Accordingly, the factorization process becomes an optimization problem that estimates the underlying parameters for C_{AIF} and C_{TISSUE}, instead of a blind and direct search for the time activity curves of C_{AIF} and C_{TISSUE}. In this study, we used the 7-parameter input function model developed by Feng et al. [22,34] as:

$$C_{AIF}(t) = (A_1(t-\tau) - A_2 - A_3)e^{-\lambda_1(t-\tau)} + A_2 e^{-\lambda_2(t-\tau)} + A_3 e^{-\lambda_3(t-\tau)} \tag{2}$$

And the tissue time-activity function C_{TISSUE} was modeled as a two-tissue compartment model output as [35]:

$$C_{TISSUE}(t) = C_{AIF}(t) \otimes \frac{K_1}{(B_2 - B_1)}\left[(k_3 + k_4 - B_1)e^{-B_1 t} + (B_2 - k_3 - k_4)e^{-B_2 t}\right] \tag{3}$$

where

$$B_{1,2} = \frac{1}{2}[(k_2 + k_3 + k_4) \mp \sqrt{(k_2 + k_3 + k_4)^2 - 4k_2 k_4}] \tag{4}$$

We used the trust-region-reflective optimization algorithm within MATLAB's 'fmincon' function to perform the numerical optimization for the $C_{AIF}(t)$ and $C_{TISSUE}(t)$. In each iteration of the parameter optimization, the parameter set of $\emptyset = \{\tau, A_1, A_2, A_3, \lambda_1, \lambda_2, \lambda_3, K_1, k_2, k_3, k_4\}$ at the current iteration was applied to Equations (2) and (3) and then used to form matrix H. The weighting matrix W at this iteration was derived from MATLAB's linear system solver that minimizes the least-square errors. The optimization then searched for the optimal solution for the parameter set $\emptyset$ by minimizing:

$$\hat{\emptyset} = \mathrm{argmin}_{(\emptyset)} ||WH - A||^2 \tag{5}$$

After the convergence of MBMF, optimal $\emptyset$ was used to determine the extracted and normalized functions $C_{Norm,AIF}$ and $C_{Norm,TISSUE}$ that represented the decomposed arterial blood and tissue components, respectively. Those functions were denoted with 'Norm' because they were in a normalized form after the MBMF extraction, where $\sum_{j=1}^{m} C_{Norm,AIF,j}$ equaled to one (j is the frame index). The last step was to scale the extracted $C_{Norm,AIF}$ from an arbitrary unit to the correct physical magnitude of activity units as C_{AIF}. To scale $C_{Norm,AIF}$ to the correct units of activity concentration, we related $C_{Norm,AIF}$ to the true AIF C_{AIF} by a scaling factor s_{AIF} as:

$$C_{AIF}(t) = s_{AIF} C_{Norm,AIF}(t) \tag{6}$$

Similarly, $C_{Norm,TISSUE}$ was related to the true C_{TISSUE} by a scaling factor s_{TISSUE}. The individual activity of a specific voxel i was estimated by the MBMF extraction as:

$$\tilde{C}_{i,PET}(t) = w_{i,AIF}C_{Norm,AIF}(t) + w_{i,TISSUE}C_{Norm,TISSUE}(t) \tag{7}$$

$w_{i,AIF}$ and $w_{i,TISSUE}$ were the MBMF-estimated mixing fractions for the $C_{Norm,AIF}$ and $C_{Norm,TISSUE}$, respectively. Note $\tilde{C}_{i,PET}$ is not identical to $C_{i,PET}$ since it is a weighted summation of the extracted and estimated functions $C_{Norm,AIF}$ and $C_{Norm,TISSUE}$.

We further derived:

$$\tilde{C}_{i,PET}(t) = \frac{w_{i,AIF}}{s_{AIF}} \cdot C_{AIF}(t) + \frac{w_{i,TISSUE}}{s_{TISSUE}} \cdot C_{TISSUE}(t) \tag{8}$$

From Equation (1), it was assumed that the mixing fractions of the AIF and tissue activity should sum up to one under ideal situation. Therefore, the optimal values of s_{AIF} and s_{TISSUE} were optimized by minimizing:

$$\hat{s}_{AIF}, \hat{s}_{TISSUE} = \operatorname{argmin}_{(s_{AIF}, s_{TISSUE})} \sum_{i=1}^{n} \left(\frac{w_{i,AIF}}{s_{AIF}} + \frac{w_{i,TISSUE}}{s_{TISSUE}} - 1 \right)^2 \tag{9}$$

where $\hat{s}_{AIF}$ and $\hat{s}_{TISSUE}$ denoted the optimized scaling factors for extracted AIF and tissue activity, respectively. n denoted the total number of segmented voxels. We used the trust-region-reflective optimization algorithm with MATLAB's 'fmincon' function to perform the numerical optimization for minimizing Equation (5). The estimated $\hat{s}_{AIF}$ was then plugged into Equation (6) to scale the IDIF into the correct physical units.

2.7. Metabolite Correction

Since the IDIF method extracts the whole-blood activity and cannot separate the metabolite signal from the unmetabolized tracer, we used a population-based approach to convert the extracted IDIF to a metabolite-corrected plasma time-activity curve [36,37]. With the metabolite data and plasma time-activity curves measured in the blood-sampling cohort, the individual parent fraction was multiplied to the plasma-to-whole blood activity fraction. The individual composite fraction was averaged for each time point at the 5th, 15th, 30th, and 60th minutes and then fitted to a single exponential function with constant [37,38]. As a result, the corrected IDIF is expressed as:

$$C_{IDIF,MCPC}(t) = \hat{s}_{AIF} C_{N,AIF}(t)(1 - 0.29(1 - e^{-0.03t})) \tag{10}$$

where t is in the unit of minutes, and MCPC denotes metabolite-corrected plasma concentration of activity.

2.8. ^{18}F-DPA-714 Quantification

Quantification of ^{18}F-DPA-714 binding was estimated through the Logan plot, where the distribution volume (V_T) was approximated by the graphical analysis [39,40]. Logan plot analysis was based on the 30th to the 60th minutes of data [41]. For the blood-sampling cohort, the distribution volume V_T was calculated from the metabolite-corrected AIF, denoted as $V_{T,AIF}$. The distribution volume was also calculated from the metabolite-corrected IDIF, denoted as $V_{T,IDIF}$ and compared to $V_{T,AIF}$. For each subject, nine target regions were chosen from the Freesurfer segmentation and calculated for $V_{T,AIF}$ and $V_{T,IDIF}$. For the nonblood-sampling cohort, $V_{T,IDIF}$ was calculated with the same steps described. The distribution volume with respect to the reference region, denoted as $V_{T,REF}$, was also computed with the cerebellum time-activity curves using the Logan graphical analysis.

2.9. Statistical Analysis

In the blood-sampling cohort, $V_{T,IDIF}$ was compared against the reference $V_{T,AIF}$ with data presented as mean ± SD. Error percentage, presented as mean ± SD, was calculated for $V_{T,IDIF}$ using $V_{T,AIF}$ as the gold standard value. Linear mixed-effect model was used to examine the correlation between $V_{T,IDIF}$ and $V_{T,AIF}$, treating the subject as a random effect with or without the region as a fixed effect.

In the nonblood-sampling cohort, the subjects were divided into the HAB and MAB groups based on the individual genotypes of TSPO binding. The $V_{T,IDIF}$ of the HAB group was compared to that of the MAB group through an unpaired two-sample t-test. Significance was set as $p < 0.05$. The same analysis was also performed for the SUV as well as $V_{T,REF}$ to evaluate their differences between the HAB and MAB groups. Linear mixed effect model was used to evaluate whether there was a significant difference between the HAB and MAB under SUV, $V_{T,IDIF}$, and $V_{T,REF}$, respectively, adjusting for the effects of region with subject as a random effect.

3. Results

3.1. IDIF Predicts AIF

In the first cohort of five subjects, arterial blood sampling was performed to measure the AIF. We then compared the distribution volume calculated with the AIF ($V_{T,AIF}$) and IDIF ($V_{T,IDIF}$) to determine whether IDIF is an appropriate surrogate for measurement of ^{18}F-DPA-714 quantification. The extraction process of the IDIF in one subject of the blood-sampling cohort is demonstrated in Figure 1 for the three steps: segmentation, signal decomposition, and scale optimization. Figure 1a shows the summed PET image over the first 60 s post tracer injection as a maximum intensity projection. Figure 1b,c show one axial slice within the neck area and the segmented contour for the carotid arteries. The extracted tissue and blood components are shown in Figure 1d, and the IDIF after the scale adjustment is plotted in Figure 1e with the measured arterial input function (AIF). The IDIF curve demonstrated a satisfactory agreement with the AIF curve. $\frac{\omega_{i,AIF}}{s_{AIF}}$ averaged 0.28 ± 0.30, and $\frac{\omega_{i,TISSUE}}{s_{TISSUE}}$ averaged 0.55 ± 0.36 across the five subjects. The comparison of IDIF and AIF for the other four subjects in the blood-sampling cohort is shown in Figure S1.

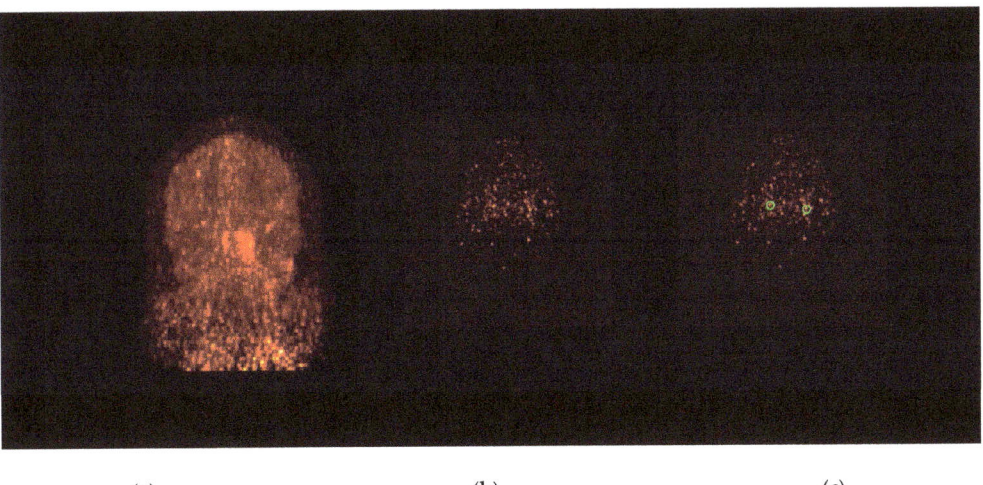

(a)　　　　　　　　　　　(b)　　　　　　　　　　　(c)

Figure 1. *Cont.*

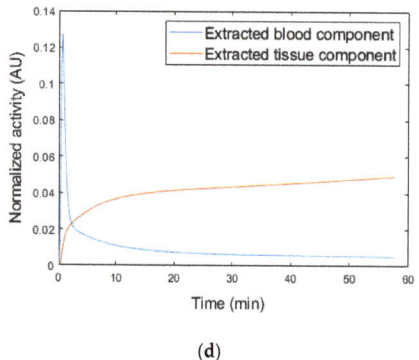
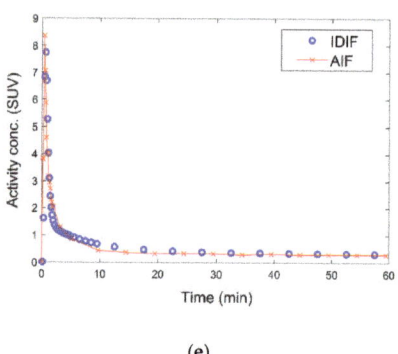

(d)   (e)

Figure 1. Demonstration of the IDIF extraction. (**a**) The coronal maximum intensity projection (MIP) of the summed early frames of the DPA-714 scan of one subject. (**b**) One axial slice of the neck area at the early frame. (**c**) The segmented regions (green contour) for carotid artery over the same slice. (**d**) The MBMF-extracted time-activity curves for the blood and tissue components. Note both curves are in the normalized and dimensionless form. (**e**) The resultant IDIF (blue circle) after the magnitude is re-scaled by the proposed method. The activities measured with arterial blood sampling are plotted as red stars, showing a satisfactory agreement between AIF and IDIF.

Table 1 summarizes the V_T derived from the AIF and IDIF for the nine target regions in the blood-sampling cohort. The overall error for $V_{T,IDIF}$ was $-5.8 \pm 7.8\%$ against the reference $V_{T,AIF}$. In all regions, the mean error of V_T was less than 10% across all subjects. The amount of error for V_T in the healthy controls is similar in the PD patients. Figure 2 shows the scatter plot and the Bland–Altman plot for $V_{T,IDIF}$ and $V_{T,AIF}$ of all the target regions and demonstrates a satisfactory agreement between them. In the linear mixed effect model analysis, the overall $V_{T,IDIF}$ and $V_{T,AIF}$ were highly correlated with each other ($p < 0.001$), adjusting for the effect of regions.

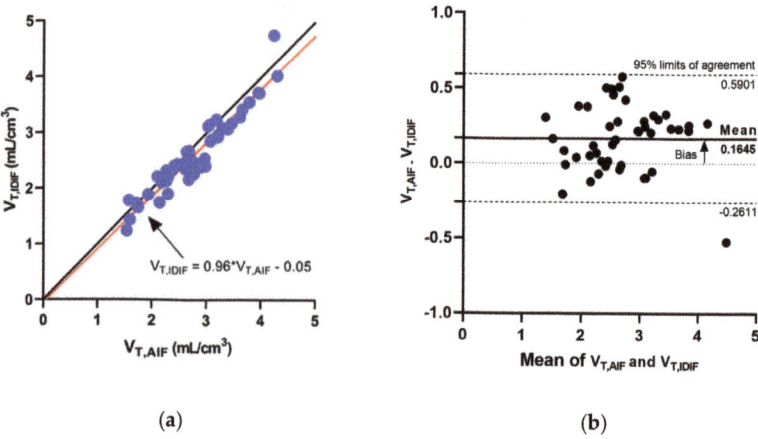

(a)   (b)

Figure 2. (**a**) The scatter plot for $V_{T,IDIF}$ plotted against $V_{T,AIF}$. The dashed line is the unity line. The red line is the fitted regression trend line. The scatter plot shows a strong correlation between $V_{T,IDIF}$ plotted against $V_{T,AIF}$. The statistical test also showed a strong correlation through the mixed effect model analysis. (**b**) The Bland–Altman plot for $V_{T,IDIF}$ and $V_{T,AIF}$.

Table 1. Comparison between the $V_{T,AIF}$ and $V_{T,IDIF}$ in the blood-sampling cohort. Overall error is $-5.8 \pm 7.8\%$ for $V_{T,IDIF}$ when compared to $V_{T,AIF}$. The error does not appear to be dependent on the target region.

	All (n = 5)			PD (n = 3)			HC (n = 2)		
	$V_{T,AIF}$	$V_{T,IDIF}$	Error %	$V_{T,AIF}$	$V_{T,IDIF}$	Error %	$V_{T,AIF}$	$V_{T,IDIF}$	Error %
Putamen	2.44 ± 0.52	2.30 ± 0.52	−5.7 ± 7.7	2.61 ± 0.47	2.43 ± 0.59	−7.7 ± 9.7	2.19 ± 0.95	2.12 ± 0.79	−2.7 ± 5.4
Caudate	1.91 ± 0.48	1.81 ± 0.50	−5.4 ± 11.9	1.91 ± 0.60	1.83 ± 0.61	−3.8 ± 16.4	1.93 ± 0.70	1.79 ± 0.73	−7.6 ± 3.8
Thalamus	2.97 ± 0.63	2.77 ± 0.61	−6.7 ± 7.0	3.12 ± 0.71	2.89 ± 0.75	−7.6 ± 9.4	2.75 ± 1.17	2.59 ± 1.06	−5.3 ± 1.8
Hippocampus	2.61 ± 0.58	2.42 ± 0.44	−6.3 ± 9.3	2.79 ± 0.62	2.57 ± 0.45	−6.6 ± 12.6	2.34 ± 0.96	2.19 ± 0.84	−6.0 ± 3.0
Frontal	2.70 ± 0.49	2.55 ± 0.48	−5.1 ± 7.5	2.79 ± 0.46	2.65 ± 0.54	−5.2 ± 9.5	2.56 ± 0.88	2.41 ± 0.77	−5.0 ± 3.2
Temporal	3.45 ± 0.86	3.34 ± 1.08	−4.5 ± 11.5	3.73 ± 0.92	3.65 ± 1.33	−4.2 ± 15.7	3.03 ± 1.29	2.86 ± 1.12	−4.8 ± 2.8
Occipital	2.96 ± 0.55	2.78 ± 0.55	−6.1 ± 7.3	3.15 ± 0.45	2.95 ± 0.57	−6.5 ± 9.9	2.69 ± 1.05	2.52 ± 0.92	−5.5 ± 4.8
Parietal	3.13 ± 0.52	2.97 ± 0.47	−5.0 ± 7.0	3.26 ± 0.45	3.08 ± 0.51	−5.7 ± 8.7	2.93 ± 0.97	2.79 ± 0.80	−3.9 ± 4.1
Cerebellum	3.16 ± 0.60	2.95 ± 0.58	−6.4 ± 7.1	3.35 ± 0.55	3.11 ± 0.67	−7.4 ± 9.7	2.87 ± 1.14	2.70 ± 0.97	−5.0 ± 1.5

3.2. IDIF Method Distinguishes High-Affinity Binders from Mixed-Affinity Binders

To validate our IDIF quantification methodology, we next tested whether IDIF could distinguish control subjects who were MAB from those who were HAB as determined by TSPO SNP genotyping. In the SUV measurements, all nine brain regions showed significantly higher uptake of ^{18}F-DPA-714 in the HAB group than in the MAB group ($p < 0.05$). The HAB uptake averaged $31 \pm 3\%$ higher than the MAB in SUV (Figure 3). The distribution volume as determined by IDIF also showed significantly higher uptake in HAB vs. MAB overall ($p < 0.05$). Region-wise, mean $V_{T,IDIF}$ was statistically higher in the HAB group in all nine brain regions (Figure 4). $V_{T,IDIF}$ was $37 \pm 3\%$ higher in the HAB group overall. On the other hand, the distribution volume determined by using the cerebellum as a reference region showed only a mildly increased $V_{T,REF}$ of $3 \pm 3\%$ in the HAB group compared to the MAB group (Figure 5). Only one out of the nine brain regions revealed a statistically significant increase in $V_{T,REF}$ in HAB vs. MAB subjects with the reference region approach. The mixed effect model showed a significant difference in the SUV ($p = 0.010$) and $V_{T,IDIF}$ ($p = 0.010$) but not in the $V_{T,REF}$ ($p = 0.069$) after adjusting for the effects of regions.

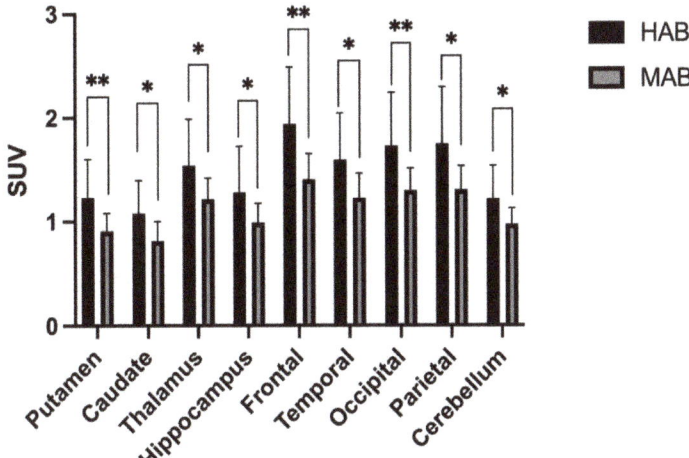

Figure 3. The box plot of the SUV measured for target brain regions for high- and mixed-affinity binders in the nonblood-sampling cohort. * denotes significant differences under two-sample t-test ($p < 0.05$), while ** denotes $p < 0.01$. All nine target regions showed significant differences between the HAB and MAB subjects. SUV is $31 \pm 3\%$ higher in HAB than in MAB.

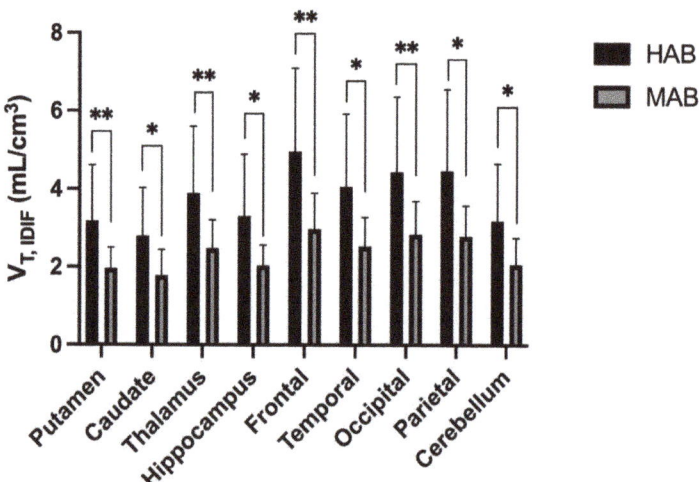

Figure 4. The box plot of the $V_{T,IDIF}$. $V_{T,IDIF}$ is 37 ± 3% higher in HAB than in MAB. All nine regions were found with significant difference (*: $p < 0.05$, **: $p < 0.01$) between the HAB and MAB subjects. The overall increase pattern in the HAB is similar as the SUV pattern of increase.

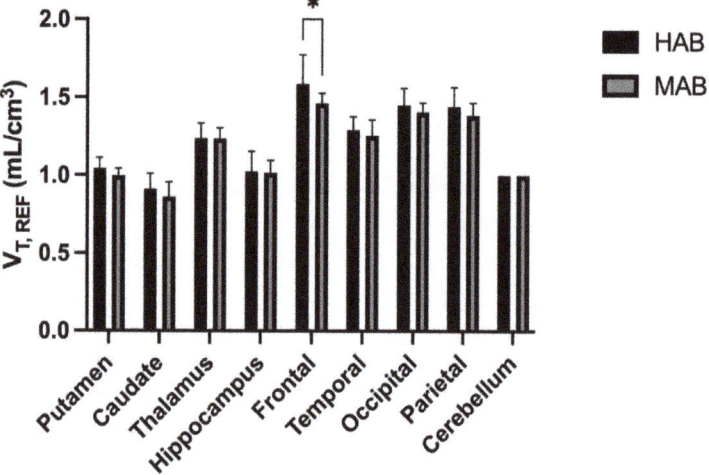

Figure 5. The box plot of the $V^{T,REF}$ using the cerebellum as the reference region. The difference between HAB and MAB is 3 ± 3% and only reaches significance (*: $p < 0.05$) in just one of nine regions.

4. Discussion

Evidence is growing for the central role of neuroinflammation in many neurodegenerative diseases, and accordingly neuroinflammation is both a potential marker for diagnosis and a therapeutic target. As a tool of noninvasive measurement of neuroinflammation, TSPO PET has gained much interest in recent year but poses unique challenges in quantification. Interested readers are referred to a comprehensive review of TSPO PET quantification by Wimberley et al. [42]. One challenge that has been recognized for ^{18}F-DPA-714 imaging is how to achieve an accurate quantification of the tracer binding through kinetic modeling analysis. Since microglial cells are widely distributed in all brain tissues and neuroinflammation can potentially occur throughout the brain, the underlying assumption for reference region-based analysis may be violated when a certain disease affects the reference region and increases the microglial activation similarly to the target region of interest. Although the cerebellum has been used as the reference region by several reports, it is also well known that the cerebellum demonstrates non-negligible ^{18}F-DPA-714-specific binding even in the healthy subjects [12,13]. Therefore, it is not surprising that prior reports have shown that the cerebellar TSPO binding can be elevated in certain diseases that make the cerebellum further deviate from the modeling assumptions for the reference regions [15–17]. Studies have suggested that several neurological disorders can cause globally elevated neuroinflammation including the cerebellum [18,43,44]. For example, Terada et al. have shown that there may be a global pattern of microglial activation in the whole brain for PD patients [45]. Under such a scenario, the reference region-based method may fail to properly measure the ^{18}F-DPA-714 binding differences between the study groups. Accordingly, an accurate and non-invasive method for DPA-714 quantification is significant for TSPO PET in measuring neuroinflammation.

Here, we have shown that our developed IDIF method is a potential alternative for arterial blood sampling methods. This method incorporates image segmentation, signal separation, and a novel approach to scale the extracted TACs to the accurate magnitude. Based on a relatively small validation cohort, our current results show a satisfactory extraction of IDIF that was very similar to the AIF calculated from arterial blood sampling. We found that the V_T measured with AIF and IDIF is highly correlated ($p < 0.001$), and the difference between these two measurements is small with less than 10% overall bias. The data from this cohort show that the IDIF-measured V_T decently resembles the AIF-measured V_T and may be a useful alternative to replace the V_T measured through invasive arterial blood sampling. The proposed method is fully automatic and may eliminate the potential interoperator variabilities. The fact that it does not require any blood sampling or sample processing makes this approach easy to apply to retrospective data analysis and to use in clinical trials. Further studies with larger validation cohorts would be crucial for a more comprehensive validation and performance evaluation for this method.

We further validated the IDIF method by testing whether IDIF can distinguish HAB vs. MAB healthy control subjects. TSPO genotypes, specifically a single nucleotide polymorphism at rs6971, critically affect the ^{18}F-DPA-714 signal. Prior reports have shown that the TSPO ligand binding in HAB subjects is 20–50% higher than that of MAB subjects, depending on the quantification approaches and study settings [12,25]. In our dataset, a simple measurement of SUV shows significantly higher ^{18}F-DPA-714 uptake in the HAB group that matched the expected magnitude of increase as described in the literature. When IDIF-based kinetic modeling analysis was applied, similar results were obtained as the degree of $V_{T,IDIF}$ increase was similar to the SUV increase. All of the nine tested regions showed significant differences through $V_{T,IDIF}$ as expected. On the other hand, the V_T measured using reference region-based analysis with the cerebellum as the reference region showed only a minimal increase in the HAB group of less than five percent. Only one out of nine brain regions showed significant differences between the HAB and MAB subjects using reference region-based analysis. This lack of difference is likely an artifact of the reference region method, arising from the fact that TSPO binding is increased in both the target and reference regions for the HAB group compared to the MAB group. Similar results have been presented in a study conducted by Hameline et al. in which the cerebellum was chosen as the reference region. In this study, the ^{18}F-DPA-714 SUVr obtained from the HAB and MAB subjects was very similar using the reference region-based analysis, supporting our observation that the cerebellum may not serve as an ideal reference region for TSPO imaging as it may cancel out or diminish the effects of TSPO overexpression caused by certain physiological or pathological conditions [46]. Our data suggest that the developed IDIF method may be more suitable for quantifying the TSPO binding than reference region methods.

Other efforts have been developed to noninvasively extract the input function or reference region activities for kinetic modeling analysis. An approach similar to IDIF is the population-based input function (PBIF) method [37]. This method assumes an identical curve shape for arterial input functions across the population. A PBIF can be obtained by averaging the AIF for a cohort with the individual scale determined through one or few blood samples. Compared with the PBIF method, the IDIF method developed in this work estimates the individual curve shape for AIF and scales the estimated AIF with the imaging data. No blood sampling or population AIF data are required in our approach, and therefore it may be easier to apply the IDIF over dynamic PET scans. The supervised clustering algorithm (SVCA), on the other hand, extracts the voxels that most closely follow the tracer kinetics of a low-binding, time-activity curve that is predefined from previously collected cohort datasets [47]. SVCA methods are fully automatic and have been applied in the image quantification of several disease models [48]. However, the challenge for SVCA is that a predefined set of kinetic curves must be present and known for both the healthy controls and subjects with the specific brain disorder that is being studied. In addition, such predefined kinetic curves must be scanner- and protocol-specific, and such requirements may limit its applicability for analyzing the data acquired through clinical trials where the patient sample sizes are often limited [42]. Moreover, some reports have also suggested that the SVCA-extracted reference region time-activity curves may still contain a non-negligible amount of specific binding that may lead to bias in quantifying the TSPO binding [49,50]. It requires further studies to objectively compare the performances of the proposed IDIF method with SVCA and PBIF methods to determine which may provide the most reliable quantification of TSPO binding, and it may likely be dependent on the disease model being investigated.

This study has its limitations, and the proposed method can be further improved. First, our blood-sampling cohort contained only five subjects due to the difficulties of performing arterial blood sampling procedures, particularly under the influences of the global SARS-CoV-2 pandemic during the subject recruitment. A larger cohort with blood sampling may help further verify the accuracy and reliability of the developed IDIF method. Second, since our method is based on matrix factorization to extract the IDIF, the accuracy of the extracted IDIF will depend on the segmented voxels that ideally shall be those possessing high fractions of the arterial blood. Our current segmentation method is a simple method that searches for voxels that are likely to be within the carotid artery. Although it has the benefit that it does not require data from modalities other than PET, the carotid segmentation can certainly be improved with more advanced methods or with the assistance of MR- or CT-based angiography. For example, some of the IDIF methods make use of time-of-flight MR angiography (TOF-MRA) through a simultaneous PET/MR to delineate the carotid arteries [51]. The enhanced segmentation of arterial structures may provide the MBMF with a better source data for matrix factorization and therefore improve the accuracy of IDIF extraction. Third, our experimental design included a 60 min PET dynamic acquisition to reduce the discomfort for the recruited patients, whereas a 90 min acquisition has been more common in the current literature. Although prior reports have shown that a 60 min scan may properly suffice for an accurate measurement of V_T [12,41], a longer scan would be beneficial to increase the parameter sensitivity toward the estimation of binding potential and microrate constants through compartment modeling analysis. Although our proposed IDIF method is not strictly dependent on the scan protocol, how our method would perform under a longer scan requires future studies to evaluate. Fourth, since the IDIF can only extract whole-blood AIF, individual metabolite and plasma activity correction will not be feasible without additional blood sampling procedures. Accordingly, a population-based approach for metabolite correction was taken in this work. Whether the error of V_T measurement is introduced by such a population-based method requires further investigation. Lastly, signal separation of the IDIF and tissue tracer uptake could possibly be improved in our method with other signal separation methods, such as those based on machine learning techniques [52].

5. Conclusions

A novel image-derived input function method for quantifying the TSPO binding with ^{18}F-DPA-714 was developed in this work. We used two separate cohorts as an initial validation for this method and showed that it may serve as a promising alternative for an automatic and noninvasive way to extract the IDIF.

Supplementary Materials: The following supporting information can be downloaded at: https://www.mdpi.com/article/10.3390/diagnostics12051161/s1, Figure S1: The comparison between AIF and IDIF for the other four subjects in the blood-sampling cohort.

Author Contributions: Conceptualization, Y.-H.D.F. and J.E.M.; Data curation, T.A.Y.; Formal analysis, Y.-H.D.F., Y.Z. and R.E.K.; Funding acquisition, D.G.S.; Investigation, Y.-H.D.F., J.E.M. and D.G.S.; Methodology, Y.-H.D.F.; Project administration, T.A.Y.; Software, Y.-H.D.F.; Supervision, D.G.S.; Writing–original draft, Y.-H.D.F.; Writing–review & editing, J.E.M., T.A.Y., Y.Z., R.E.K. and D.G.S. All authors have read and agreed to the published version of the manuscript.

Funding: This study was supported by the Alabama Morris K. Udall Center of Excellence in Parkinson's Research (NS108675) and the Parkinson Association of Central Alabama.

Institutional Review Board Statement: The study was conducted according to the guidelines of the Declaration of Helsinki and approved by the Institutional Review Board of the University of Alabama at Birmingham (protocol code IRB-300001025 approved on 16 October 2017).

Informed Consent Statement: Informed consent was obtained from all subjects involved in the study.

Data Availability Statement: The data presented in this study are available on request from the corresponding author. The data are not publicly available due to the privacy of the enrolled subjects.

Acknowledgments: We thank all study participants and Jennifer Bartels, Allan Joop, and Lauren Ruffrage for research support.

Conflicts of Interest: This study was supported by the Alabama Morris K. Udall Center of Excellence in Parkinson's Research (NS108675) and the Parkinson Association of Central Alabama. Jonathan McConathy is an investigator in studies funded by NIH, Eli Lilly/Avid, Blue Earth Diagnostics, Cytosite Biopharma, and ImaginAb. He is a consultant for Eli Lilly/Avid, GE Healthcare, Blue Earth Diagnostics, ImaginAb, and Canon Medical. Talene Yacoubian has active grants from the American Parkinson Disease Association, Travere Therapeutics, and the NIH. She has received honoraria for presentations from the Movement Disorder Society and for grant reviews from the NIH and the Michael J. Fox Foundation. David Standaert is an investigator in studies funded by AbbVie Inc., the American Parkinson Disease Association, the Michael J. Fox Foundation for Parkinson Research, Alabama Department of Commerce, the Department of Defense, and the NIH. He has served as a consultant for or received honoraria from AbbVie Inc., the Parkinson Study Group, Curium Pharma, the International Parkinson Disease and Movement Disorder Society, Theravance, McGraw Hill, Gray Matter Technologies, and Sanofi-Aventis. No potential conflict of interest relevant to this article exist.

References

1. Heneka, M.T.; Carson, M.J.; El Khoury, J.; Landreth, G.E.; Brosseron, F.; Feinstein, D.L.; Jacobs, A.H.; Wyss-Coray, T.; Vitorica, J.; Ranasoho, R.M.; et al. Neuroinflammation in Alzheimer's disease. *Lancet Neurol.* **2015**, *14*, 388–405. [CrossRef]
2. Latta, C.H.; Brothers, H.M.; Wilcock, D.M. Neuroinflammation in Alzheimer's disease; A source of heterogeneity and target for personalized therapy. *Neuroscience* **2015**, *302*, 103–111. [CrossRef] [PubMed]
3. Hirsch, E.C.; Hunot, S. Neuroinflammation in Parkinson's disease: A target for neuroprotection? *Lancet Neurol.* **2009**, *8*, 382–397. [CrossRef]
4. Hirsch, E.C.; Standaert, D.G. Ten Unsolved Questions about Neuroinflammation in Parkinson's Disease. *Mov. Disord.* **2021**, *36*, 16–24. [CrossRef] [PubMed]
5. Jain, P.; Chaney, A.M.; Carlson, M.L.; Jackson, I.M.; Rao, A.; James, M.L. Neuroinflammation PET Imaging: Current Opinion and Future Directions. *J. Nucl. Med.* **2020**, *61*, 1107–1112. [CrossRef]
6. Werry, E.L.; Bright, F.M.; Piguet, O.; Ittner, L.M.; Halliday, G.M.; Hodges, J.R.; Kiernan, M.C.; Loy, C.T.; Kril, J.J.; Kassiou, M. Recent Developments in TSPO PET Imaging as a Biomarker of Neuroinflammation in Neurodegenerative Disorders. *Int. J. Mol. Sci.* **2019**, *20*, 3161. [CrossRef] [PubMed]

7. De Picker, L.J.; Haarman, B.C.M. Applicability, potential and limitations of TSPO PET imaging as a clinical immunopsychiatry biomarker. *Eur. J. Nucl. Med. Mol. Imaging* **2021**, *49*, 164–173. [CrossRef]
8. Arlicot, N.; Vercouillie, J.; Ribeiro, M.-J.; Tauber, C.; Venel, Y.; Baulieu, J.-L.; Maia, S.; Corcia, P.; Stabin, M.G.; Reynolds, A.; et al. Initial evaluation in healthy humans of [18F]DPA-714, a potential PET biomarker for neuroinflammation. *Nucl. Med. Biol.* **2012**, *39*, 570–578. [CrossRef]
9. Corcia, P.; Tauber, C.; Vercouillie, J.; Arlicot, N.; Prunier, C.; Praline, J.; Nicolas, G.; Venel, Y.; Hommet, C.; Baulieu, J.-L.; et al. Molecular imaging of microglial activation in amyotrophic lateral sclerosis. *PLoS ONE* **2012**, *7*, e52941. [CrossRef]
10. Kropholler, M.A.; Boellaard, R.; Schuitemaker, A.; Folkersma, H.; van Berckel, B.N.; Lammertsma, A.A. Evaluation of reference tissue models for the analysis of [11C](R)-PK11195 studies. *J. Cereb. Blood Flow Metab.* **2006**, *26*, 1431–1441. [CrossRef]
11. Lyoo, C.H.; Ikawa, M.; Liow, J.-S.; Zoghbi, S.S.; Morse, C.L.; Pike, V.W.; Fujita, M.; Innis, R.B.; Kreisl, W.C. Cerebellum Can Serve As a Pseudo-Reference Region in Alzheimer Disease to Detect Neuroinflammation Measured with PET Radioligand Binding to Translocator Protein. *J. Nucl. Med.* **2015**, *56*, 701–706. [CrossRef] [PubMed]
12. Lavisse, S.; García-Lorenzo, D.; Peyronneau, M.-A.; Bodini, B.; Thiriez, C.; Kuhnast, B.; Comtat, C.; Remy, P.; Stankoff, B.; Bottlaender, M. Optimized Quantification of Translocator Protein Radioligand (1)(8)F-DPA-714 Uptake in the Brain of Genotyped Healthy Volunteers. *J. Nucl. Med.* **2015**, *56*, 1048–1054. [CrossRef] [PubMed]
13. Owen, D.; Guo, Q.; Kalk, N.; Colasanti, A.; Kalogiannopoulou, D.; Dimber, R.; Lewis, Y.L.; Libri, V.; Barletta, J.; Ramada-Magalhaes, J.; et al. Determination of [(11)C]PBR28 binding potential in vivo: A first human TSPO blocking study. *J. Cereb. Blood Flow Metab.* **2014**, *34*, 989–994. [CrossRef] [PubMed]
14. Salinas, C.A.; Searle, G.E.; Gunn, R.N. The simplified reference tissue model: Model assumption violations and their impact on binding potential. *J. Cereb. Blood Flow Metab.* **2015**, *35*, 304–311. [CrossRef]
15. Gerhard, A.; Trender-Gerhard, I.; Turkheimer, F.; Quinn, N.P.; Bhatia, K.P.; Brooks, D.J. In Vivo imaging of microglial activation with [11C](R)-PK11195 PET in progressive supranuclear palsy. *Mov. Disord.* **2006**, *21*, 89–93. [CrossRef]
16. Edison, P.; Archer, H.A.; Gerhard, A.; Hinz, R.; Pavese, N.; Turkheimer, F.E.; Hammers, A.; Tai, Y.F.; Fox, N.; Kennedy, A.; et al. Microglia, amyloid, and cognition in Alzheimer's disease: An [11C](R)PK11195-PET and [11C]PIB-PET study. *Neurobiol. Dis.* **2008**, *32*, 412–419. [CrossRef]
17. Varrone, A.; Oikonen, V.; Forsberg, A.; Joutsa, J.; Takano, A.; Solin, O.; Haaparanta-Solin, M.; Nag, S.; Nakao, R.; Al-Tawil, N.; et al. Positron emission tomography imaging of the 18-kDa translocator protein (TSPO) with [18F]FEMPA in Alzheimer's disease patients and control subjects. *Eur. J. Nucl. Med. Mol. Imaging* **2015**, *42*, 438–446. [CrossRef]
18. Hillmer, A.T.; Sandiego, C.M.; Hannestad, J.; Angarita, G.; Kumar, A.; McGovern, E.M.; Huang, Y.; O'Connor, K.C.; Carson, R.; O'Malley, S.S.; et al. In Vivo imaging of translocator protein, a marker of activated microglia, in alcohol dependence. *Mol. Psychiatry* **2017**, *22*, 1759–1766. [CrossRef]
19. Mabrouk, R.; Rusjan, P.; Mizrahi, R.; Jacobs, M.F.; Koshimori, Y.; Houle, S.; Ko, J.H.; Strafella, A.P. Image derived input function for [18F]-FEPPA: Application to quantify translocator protein (18 kDa) in the human brain. *PLoS ONE* **2014**, *9*, e115768. [CrossRef]
20. Zanotti-Fregonara, P.; Liow, J.-S.; Fujita, M.; Dusch, E.; Zoghbi, S.S.; Luong, E.; Boellaard, R.; Pike, V.W.; Comtat, C.; Innis, R.B. Image-derived input function for human brain using high resolution PET imaging with [C](R)-rolipram and [C]PBR28. *PLoS ONE* **2011**, *6*, e17056. [CrossRef]
21. Macaskill, M.G.; Walton, T.; Williams, L.; Morgan, T.E.F.; Alcaide-Corral, C.J.; Dweck, M.R.; Gray, G.A.; Newby, D.E.; Lucatelli, C.; Sutherland, A.; et al. Kinetic modelling and quantification bias in small animal PET studies with [18F]AB5186, a novel 18 kDa translocator protein radiotracer. *PLoS ONE* **2019**, *14*, e0217515. [CrossRef] [PubMed]
22. Fang, Y.H.; Muzic, R.F., Jr. Spillover and partial-volume correction for image-derived input functions for small-animal 18F-FDG PET studies. *J. Nucl. Med.* **2008**, *49*, 606–614. [CrossRef] [PubMed]
23. Wimberley, C.; Nguyen, D.L.; Truillet, C.; Peyronneau, M.-A.; Gulhan, Z.; Tonietto, M.; Boumezbeur, F.; Boisgard, R.; Chalon, S.; Bouilleret, V.; et al. Longitudinal mouse-PET imaging: A reliable method for estimating binding parameters without a reference region or blood sampling. *Eur. J. Nucl. Med. Mol. Imaging* **2020**, *47*, 2589–2601. [CrossRef] [PubMed]
24. Owen, D.R.; Yeo, A.J.; Gunn, R.N.; Song, K.; Wadsworth, G.; Lewis, A.; Rhodes, C.; Pulford, D.J.; Bennacef, I.; Parker, C.A.; et al. An 18-kDa translocator protein (TSPO) polymorphism explains differences in binding affinity of the PET radioligand PBR28. *J. Cereb. Blood Flow Metab.* **2012**, *32*, 1–5. [CrossRef]
25. Lavisse, S.; Goutal, S.; Wimberley, C.; Tonietto, M.; Bottlaender, M.; Gervais, P.; Kuhnast, B.; Peyronneau, M.-A.; Barret, O.; Lagarde, J.; et al. Increased microglial activation in patients with Parkinson disease using [(18)F]-DPA714 TSPO PET imaging. *Parkinsonism Relat. Disord.* **2021**, *82*, 29–36. [CrossRef]
26. Tanner, C.; Gilley, D.; Goetz, C. A brief screening questionnaire for parkinsonism. *Ann. Neurol.* **1990**, *28*, 267–268.
27. Sekine, T.; ter Voert, E.E.; Warnock, G.; Buck, A.; Huellner, M.W.; Veit-Haibach, P.; Delso, G. Clinical Evaluation of Zero-Echo-Time Attenuation Correction for Brain ^{18}F-FDG PET/MRI: Comparison with Atlas Attenuation Correction. *J. Nucl. Med.* **2016**, *57*, 1927–1932. [CrossRef]
28. Rousset, O.G.; Ma, Y.; Evans, A.C. Correction for partial volume effects in PET: Principle and validation. *J. Nucl. Med.* **1998**, *39*, 904–911.
29. Thomas, B.; Cuplov, V.; Bousse, A.; Mendes, A.; Thielemans, K.; Hutton, B.F.; Erlandsson, K. PETPVC: A toolbox for performing partial volume correction techniques in positron emission tomography. *Phys. Med. Biol.* **2016**, *61*, 7975–7993. [CrossRef]
30. Fischl, B. FreeSurfer. *Neuroimage* **2012**, *62*, 774–781. [CrossRef]

31. Krejza, J.; Arkuszewski, M.; Kasner, S.E.; Weigele, J.; Ustymowicz, A.; Hurst, R.W.; Cucchiara, B.L.; Messe, S.R. Carotid artery diameter in men and women and the relation to body and neck size. *Stroke* **2006**, *37*, 1103–1105. [CrossRef] [PubMed]
32. Vendrow, J.; Haddock, J.; Rebrova, E.; Needell, D. On a guided nonnegative matrix factorization. In Proceedings of the ICASSP 2021—2021 IEEE International Conference on Acoustics, Speech and Signal Processing (ICASSP), Toronto, ON, Canada, 6–11 June 2021.
33. Zhou, Y.; Li, Z.; Yang, X.; Zhang, L.; Srivastava, S.; Jin, R.; Chan, C. Using Knowledge Driven Matrix Factorization to Reconstruct Modular Gene Regulatory Network. In Proceedings of the Twenty-Third AAAI Conference on Artificial Intelligence, AAAI 2008, Chicago, IL, USA, 13–17 July 2008.
34. Feng, D.; Wong, K.-P.; Wu, C.-M.; Siu, W.-C. A technique for extracting physiological parameters and the required input function simultaneously from PET image measurements: Theory and simulation study. *IEEE Trans. Inf. Technol. Biomed.* **1997**, *1*, 243–254. [CrossRef] [PubMed]
35. Huang, S.-C.; Phelps, M.E.; Hoffman, E.J.; Sideris, K.; Selin, C.J.; Kuhl, D.E. Noninvasive determination of local cerebral metabolic rate of glucose in man. *Am. J. Physiol.-Endocrinol. Metab.* **1980**, *238*, E69–E82. [CrossRef] [PubMed]
36. Wu, J.; Lin, S.F.; Gallezot, J.D.; Chan, C.; Prasad, R.; Thorn, S.L.; Stacy, M.R.; Huang, Y.; Zonouz, T.H.; Liu, Y.-H.; et al. Quantitative Analysis of Dynamic 123I-mIBG SPECT Imaging Data in Healthy Humans with a Population-Based Metabolite Correction Method. *J. Nucl. Med.* **2016**, *57*, 1226–1232. [CrossRef] [PubMed]
37. Buchert, R.; Dirks, M.; Schütze, C.; Wilke, F.; Mamach, M.; Wirries, A.-K.; Pflugrad, H.; Hamann, L.; Langer, L.B.; Wetzel, C.; et al. Reliable quantification of (18)F-GE-180 PET neuroinflammation studies using an individually scaled population-based input function or late tissue-to-blood ratio. *Eur. J. Nucl. Med. Mol. Imaging* **2020**, *47*, 2887–2900. [CrossRef]
38. Feeney, C.; Scott, G.; Raffel, J.; Roberts, S.; Coello, C.; Jolly, A.; Searle, G.; Goldstone, A.; Brooks, D.; Nicholas, R.S.; et al. Kinetic analysis of the translocator protein positron emission tomography ligand [18F] GE-180 in the human brain. *Eur. J. Nucl. Med. Mol. Imaging* **2016**, *43*, 2201–2210. [CrossRef]
39. Logan, J.; Fowler, J.S.; Volkow, N.D.; Wolf, A.P.; Dewey, S.L.; Schlyer, D.J.; MacGregor, R.R.; Hitzemann, R.; Bendriem, B.; Gatley, S.J.; et al. Graphical analysis of reversible radioligand binding from time-activity measurements applied to [N-11C-methyl]-(-)-cocaine PET studies in human subjects. *J. Cereb. Blood Flow Metab.* **1990**, *10*, 740–747. [CrossRef]
40. Logan, J. Graphical analysis of PET data applied to reversible and irreversible tracers. *Nucl. Med. Biol.* **2000**, *27*, 661–670. [CrossRef]
41. Golla, S.S.; Boellaard, R.; Oikonen, V.; Hoffmann, A.; van Berckel, B.N.; Windhorst, A.D.; Virta, J.; Haaparanta-Solin, M.; Luoto, P.; Savisto, N.; et al. Quantification of [18F]DPA-714 binding in the human brain: Initial studies in healthy controls and Alzheimer's disease patients. *J. Cereb. Blood Flow Metab.* **2015**, *35*, 766–772. [CrossRef]
42. Wimberley, C.; Lavisse, S.; Hillmer, A.; Hinz, R.; Turkheimer, F.; Zanotti-Fregonara, P. Kinetic modeling and parameter estimation of TSPO PET imaging in the human brain. *Eur. J. Nucl. Med. Mol. Imaging* **2021**, *49*, 246–256. [CrossRef]
43. Vera, J.H.; Guo, Q.; Cole, J.H.; Boasso, A.; Greathead, L.; Kelleher, P.; Rabiner, E.A.; Kalk, N.; Bishop, C.; Gunn, R.N.; et al. Neuroinflammation in treated HIV-positive individuals: A PET study. *Neurology* **2016**, *86*, 1425–1432. [CrossRef] [PubMed]
44. Dimber, R.; Guo, Q.; Bishop, C.; Adonis, A.; Buckley, A.; Kocsis, A.; Owen, D.; Kalk, N.; Newbould, R.; Gunn, R.N.; et al. Evidence of Brain Inflammation in Patients with Human T-Lymphotropic Virus Type 1-Associated Myelopathy (HAM): A Pilot, Multimodal Imaging Study Using 11C-PBR28 PET, MR T1-Weighted, and Diffusion-Weighted Imaging. *J. Nucl. Med.* **2016**, *57*, 1905–1912. [CrossRef] [PubMed]
45. Terada, T.; Yokokura, M.; Yoshikawa, E.; Futatsubashi, M.; Kono, S.; Konishi, T.; Miyajima, H.; Hashizume, T.; Ouchi, Y. Extrastriatal spreading of microglial activation in Parkinson's disease: A positron emission tomography study. *Ann. Nucl. Med.* **2016**, *30*, 579–587. [CrossRef] [PubMed]
46. Matheson, G.J.; Plaven-Sigray, P.; Forsberg, A.; Varrone, A.; Farde, L.; Cervenka, S. Assessment of simplified ratio-based approaches for quantification of PET [(11)C]PBR28 data. *EJNMMI Res.* **2017**, *7*, 58. [CrossRef] [PubMed]
47. García-Lorenzo, D.; Lavisse, S.; Leroy, C.; Wimberley, C.; Bodini, B.; Remy, P.; Veronese, M.; Turkheimer, F.; Stankoff, B.; Bottlaender, M. Validation of an automatic reference region extraction for the quantification of [(18)F]DPA-714 in dynamic brain PET studies. *J. Cereb. Blood Flow Metab.* **2018**, *38*, 333–346. [CrossRef]
48. Schubert, J.; Tonietto, M.; Turkheimer, F.; Zanotti-Fregonara, P.; Veronese, M. Supervised clustering for TSPO PET imaging. *Eur. J. Nucl. Med. Mol. Imaging* **2021**, *49*, 257–268. [CrossRef]
49. Zanotti-Fregonara, P.; Kreisl, W.C.; Innis, R.B.; Lyoo, C.H. Automatic Extraction of a Reference Region for the Noninvasive Quantification of Translocator Protein in Brain Using (11)C-PBR28. *J. Nucl. Med.* **2019**, *60*, 978–984. [CrossRef]
50. Plaven-Sigray, P.; Matheson, G.J.; Cselenyi, Z.; Jucaite, A.; Farde, L.; Cervenka, S. Test-retest reliability and convergent validity of (R)-[(11)C]PK11195 outcome measures without arterial input function. *EJNMMI Res.* **2018**, *8*, 102. [CrossRef]
51. Su, Y.; Blazey, T.M.; Snyder, A.Z.; Raichle, M.E.; Hornbeck, R.C.; Aldea, P.; Morris, J.C.; Benzinger, T.L.S. Quantitative amyloid imaging using image-derived arterial input function. *PLoS ONE* **2015**, *10*, e0122920. [CrossRef]
52. Kuttner, S.; Wickstrøm, K.K.; Lubberink, M.; Tolf, A.; Burman, J.; Sundset, R.; Jenssen, R.; Appel, L.; Axelsson, J. Cerebral blood flow measurements with (15)O-water PET using a non-invasive machine-learning-derived arterial input function. *J. Cereb. Blood Flow Metab.* **2021**, *41*, 2229–2241. [CrossRef]

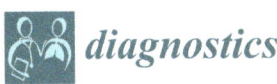

Communication

Cerebral [^{18}F]-FDOPA Uptake in Autism Spectrum Disorder and Its Association with Autistic Traits

Rik Schalbroeck [1,2,3,*], Lioe-Fee de Geus-Oei [3,4], Jean-Paul Selten [1,2], Maqsood Yaqub [5], Anouk Schrantee [6], Therese van Amelsvoort [1], Jan Booij [6] and Floris H. P. van Velden [3]

1. School for Mental Health and Neuroscience, Maastricht University, 6229 ER Maastricht, The Netherlands; j.selten@rivierduinen.nl (J.-P.S.); t.vanamelsvoort@maastrichtuniversity.nl (T.v.A.)
2. Rivierduinen Institute for Mental Healthcare, 2333 ZZ Leiden, The Netherlands
3. Section of Nuclear Medicine, Department of Radiology, Leiden University Medical Center, 2333 ZA Leiden, The Netherlands; l.f.de_geus-oei@lumc.nl (L.-F.d.G.-O.); f.h.p.van_velden@lumc.nl (F.H.P.v.V.)
4. Biomedical Photonic Imaging Group, University of Twente, 7522 NB Enschede, The Netherlands
5. Department of Radiology and Nuclear Medicine, Amsterdam University Medical Centers, Location VU Medical Center, 1081 HV Amsterdam, The Netherlands; maqsood.yaqub@amsterdamumc.nl
6. Department of Radiology and Nuclear Medicine, Amsterdam University Medical Centers, Location Academic Medical Center, 1105 AZ Amsterdam, The Netherlands; a.g.schrantee@amsterdamumc.nl (A.S.); j.booij@amsterdamumc.nl (J.B.)

* Correspondence: rschalbroeck@gmail.com

Abstract: Dopaminergic signaling is believed to be related to autistic traits. We conducted an exploratory 3,4-dihydroxy-6-[^{18}F]-fluoro-L-phenylalanine positron emission tomography/computed tomography ([^{18}F]-FDOPA PET/CT) study, to examine cerebral [^{18}F]-FDOPA influx constant (k_i^{cer} min^{-1}), reflecting predominantly striatal dopamine synthesis capacity and a mixed monoaminergic innervation in extrastriatal neurons, in 44 adults diagnosed with autism spectrum disorder (ASD) and 22 controls, aged 18 to 30 years. Autistic traits were assessed with the Autism Spectrum Quotient (AQ). Region-of-interest and voxel-based analyses showed no statistically significant differences in k_i^{cer} between autistic adults and controls. In autistic adults, striatal k_i^{cer} was significantly, negatively associated with AQ attention to detail subscale scores, although Bayesian analyses did not support this finding. In conclusion, among autistic adults, specific autistic traits can be associated with reduced striatal dopamine synthesis capacity. However, replication of this finding is necessary.

Keywords: autism spectrum disorder; autistic traits; [^{18}F]-FDOPA; positron emission tomography; dopamine; monoamine

1. Introduction

The atypical functioning of dopaminergic and other monoaminergic systems has long been hypothesized to contribute to autistic traits [1]. For instance, according to the dopamine hypothesis of autism spectrum disorder (ASD) [2,3], alterations in the midbrain dopaminergic system are associated with clinical and sub-clinical autistic traits, including difficulties in social interaction and communication, and stereotyped behaviors. However, there is a lack of studies assessing in vivo monoamine functioning in autistic adults [4].

Positron emission tomography/computed tomography (PET/CT) studies have used 3,4-dihydroxy-6-[^{18}F]-fluoro-L-phenylalanine ([^{18}F]-FDOPA) to assess the presynaptic dopamine synthesis capacity in ASD. One study reported that [^{18}F]-FDOPA uptake was decreased in the anterior medial prefrontal cortex in (mostly sedated) autistic children (n = 14), relative to typically developing controls (n = 10) [5]. Another study found that [^{18}F]-FDOPA uptake was increased in the frontal and striatal regions in adults with Asperger syndrome (n = 8) relative to controls (n = 5) [6]. However, in both studies, sample sizes were small, and the associations with measures of autistic traits were not examined.

The social defeat hypothesis of schizophrenia posits that a subordinate or outsider position leads to an increased baseline activity or sensitization of the mesolimbic dopamine system and, thereby, to an increased risk of schizophrenia [7]. Since ASD is a risk factor for schizophrenia [8], we recently conducted a large [^{18}F]-FDOPA PET/CT study to test the pre-registered hypothesis of increased striatal dopamine synthesis capacity in non-psychotic individuals with ASD [9]. Contrary to our hypothesis, the results indicated no differences in striatal [^{18}F]-FDOPA uptake between individuals with ASD ($n = 44$) and controls ($n = 22$), and no association between this uptake and social defeat.

Here, we extend our previous study with exploratory region of interest (ROI) and voxel-based analyses, in which we compare striatal as well as extrastriatal [^{18}F]-FDOPA uptake between adults with ASD and controls, and examine their associations with self-reported autistic traits.

2. Materials and Methods

2.1. Participants and Procedures

The full procedures are described in our previous publication [9]. We recruited Dutch participants aged 18 to 30 years, who were abstinent from current or recent psychotropic medication use (see Supplementary Methods S1 for details). Those with ASD, had received their diagnosis from a registered mental health clinician, and this diagnosis was confirmed by the first author using the Autism Diagnostic Observation Schedule-2 (ADOS-2) module 4 [10,11]. We included 44 autistic participants and 22 controls (frequency-matched on age, sex, and smoking status). All the participants provided informed consent. The study was approved by the medical ethics committee of the Leiden University Medical Center (reference NL54244.058.15).

2.2. Autism Spectrum Quotient

The Autism Spectrum Quotient (AQ) is a 50 item self-report questionnaire that assesses the presence of autistic traits [12]. Items are scored between 1 (definitely agree) and 4 (definitely disagree). After reverse-scoring, the higher total scores reflect the presence of more autistic traits. Additionally, in line with the original validation of the Dutch AQ [13], we calculated scores on the "social interaction" and "attention to detail" subscales. Higher scores on these subscales indicate greater difficulties in social interactions, and a greater attention to, and interests in, patterns and details, respectively. The AQ was completed by both samples.

2.3. MRI and PET/CT Acquisition and Processing

Details of magnetic resonance imaging (MRI) and PET/CT acquisitions and processing steps have been previously described [9]. In short, a structural T1-weighted MRI scan was obtained on a 3T Ingenia (Philips Healthcare, Best, The Netherlands). A 90 min dynamic PET scan was obtained on a Biograph Horizon with TrueV option (Siemens Healthineers, Erlangen, Germany) or Vereos (Philips Healthcare, Best, The Netherlands), directly after the administration of approximately 150 MBq [^{18}F]-FDOPA. A low dose CT scan (110/120 kVp, 35 mAs) was acquired for attenuation–correction purposes. Participants consumed 150 mg of carbidopa and 400 mg entacapone, 1 hour before starting the PET/CT scan.

We used [^{18}F]-FDOPA uptake in gray matter (GM) cerebellum as a reference to calculate the influx constant (k_i^{cer} min^{-1}; hereon labeled as k_i^{cer}) throughout the brain using reference Patlak graphical analysis [14]. The ROIs were automatically identified from the co-registered MRI scan using PVElab (v2.3; Neurobiology Research Unit, Copenhagen, Denmark; [15,16]), using a maximum probability atlas [17]. The ROIs included the GM of the whole striatum and three striatal anatomical sub-regions (putamen, nucleus accumbens, and caudate nucleus), which were selected on the basis of their putative role in ASD [2,3], and their reliability in terms of imaging [^{18}F]-FDOPA uptake [18].

In addition to the ROI analysis, the parametric image of each participant was transformed to standard space to facilitate voxel-based comparisons. To do so, we first normalized the participant's co-registered MRI scan using SPM12 (Institute of Neurology, London, UK). The resulting transformation matrix was applied to the parametric image, which was then smoothed using an 8 mm full width at half maximum (FWHM) Gaussian filter [18].

2.4. Statistical Analysis

With reference to the ROI method, data were analyzed using JASP version 0.16 [19]. We used multiple linear regression analysis to compare the regional k_i^{cer} values between ASD and controls and to assess the associations of k_i^{cer} with the AQ total and subscale scores. We adjusted for four confounders: age, sex, smoker status (yes/no), and scanner type (Vereos/Biograph Horizon). A two-tailed p-value of 0.05 was used to evaluate the statistical significance. In addition, Bayesian analyses were conducted (see Supplementary Methods S2). Voxel-based comparisons were made in SPM12. An independent samples t-test was used to examine group differences in k_i^{cer}, and multiple linear regression analysis was used to examine associations between k_i^{cer} and AQ scores. Confounders included age, sex, smoker status, and scanner type. A family-wise error (FWE) rate of $\alpha = 0.05$ was used to evaluate the statistical significance. We conducted several additional control analyses to assess the robustness of the findings. First, we repeated our analyses restricting ourselves to voxels with k_i^{cer} values above 0.001 and 0.005, effectively excluding voxels showing little specific [^{18}F]-FDOPA uptake. Second, we repeated our analyses with unsmoothed data and after smoothing with a 4 mm FWHM Gaussian filter (i.e., instead of the 8 mm FWHM Gaussian filter that we used for the main analysis). Third, we conducted the analyses for the two PET/CT scanners separately.

3. Results

3.1. Sample Characteristics

Sample characteristics are reported in Table 1. Participants with ASD had significantly higher AQ total scores ($t_{64} = 8.74$, $p < 0.001$), as well as social interaction ($t_{64} = 8.34$, $p < 0.001$) and attention to detail ($t_{64} = 5.55$, $p < 0.001$) subscale scores. With regard to self-reported lifetime diagnosed mental health conditions, in the control group, participants reported having ever been diagnosed with a depressive disorder ($n = 1$) and anxiety disorder ($n = 1$). In the ASD sample, participants reported having ever been diagnosed with a depressive disorder ($n = 9$), attention deficit/hyperactivity disorder ($n = 4$), anxiety disorder ($n = 2$), and post-traumatic stress disorder ($n = 2$). None of the participants had currently or recently used any medication for these conditions.

Table 1. Sample characteristics of adults with autism spectrum disorder (ASD) and controls.

Variable	ASD ($n = 44$)	Controls ($n = 22$)
Male, no. (%)	28 (64%)	14 (64%)
Age in years, mean (SD)	23.74 (2.64)	23.47 (2.48)
IQ, mean (SD)	103.75 (5.19)	105.05 (4.90)
Smoker, no. (%)	2 (5%)	1 (5%)
Scanned on Vereos PET/CT scanner, no. (%)	31 (70%)	13 (59%)
Approximate injected [^{18}F]-FDOPA dose in MBq, mean (SD)	161.55 (7.26)	157.24 (8.57)
AQ total score, mean (SD)	132.41 (20.05)	91.73 (12.01)
AQ social interaction subscale, mean (SD)	105.25 (17.65)	71.27 (10.22)
AQ attention to detail subscale, mean (SD)	27.16 (4.94)	20.45 (4.19)

SD, standard deviation; IQ, intelligence quotient; MBq, megabecquerel; and AQ, autism spectrum quotient.

3.2. ROI Analyses

Table 2 shows the k_i^{cer} values in striatal ROIs and their associations with the AQ total and subscale scores. We found no significant differences in the striatal k_i^{cer} values between ASD and controls. Moreover, within the control sample, and within the combined ASD and control sample, we found no significant associations between the AQ scores and striatal k_i^{cer} values. In contrast, in the ASD sample, k_i^{cer} values in the whole striatum, putamen, and nucleus accumbens were significantly negatively associated with AQ attention to detail subscale scores. These associations remained negative when we examined the results without adjusting for confounders or for the two PET/CT scanners separately, although they became statistically non-significant. No other statistically significant associations were observed.

Table 2. Striatal [^{18}F]-FDOPA uptake (k_i^{cer} min^{-1}) in ASD adults and controls, and its association with self-reported autistic traits.

	k_i^{cer}, Mean (SD)			Association Between k_i^{cer} Value and AQ Scores								
				ASD			Controls			Combined Sample		
ROI	ASD	Controls	p-value	Total	Social	Detail	Total	Social	Detail	Total	Social	Detail
Whole striatum	0.0145 (0.0023)[a]	0.0143 (0.0024)[a]	0.87[a]	β = −0.04, p = 0.81	β = 0.04, p = 0.80	β = −0.35, p = 0.04	β = 0.08, p = 0.74	β = 0.08, p = 0.74	β = 0.03, p = 0.90	β = 0.02, p = 0.87	β = 0.06, p = 0.65	β = −0.14, p = 0.28
Putamen	0.0157 (0.0025)	0.0153 (0.0026)	0.61	β = 0.03, p = 0.86	β = 0.12, p = 0.46	β = −0.36, p = 0.04	β = 0.10, p = 0.67	β = 0.06, p = 0.80	β = 0.13, p = 0.56	β = 0.10, p = 0.43	β = 0.14, p = 0.28	β = −0.08, p = 0.52
Nucleus accumbens	0.0114 (0.0024)	0.0108 (0.0024)	0.38	β = −0.09, p = 0.58	β = 0.00, p = 0.99	β = −0.43, p = 0.01	β = 0.13, p = 0.59	β = 0.14, p = 0.57	β = 0.04, p = 0.85	β = 0.09, p = 0.49	β = 0.12, p = 0.33	β = −0.10, p = 0.45
Caudate nucleus	0.0135 (0.0022)	0.0137 (0.0025)	0.69	β = −0.12, p = 0.48	β = −0.06, p = 0.72	β = −0.29, p = 0.09	β = 0.05, p = 0.84	β = 0.10, p = 0.69	β = −0.09, p = 0.72	β = −0.09, p = 0.48	β = −0.05, p = 0.66	β = −0.19, p = 0.12

ASD, autism spectrum disorder; AQ, autism spectrum quotient; SD, standard deviation; ROI, region of interest; total, AQ total scores; social, AQ social interaction subscale scores; and detail, AQ attention to detail subscale scores. Analyses adjusted for age, sex, smoking status, and PET/CT scanner type. [a], as reported in [9].

Bayesian analyses supported the observed null findings over the alternative hypotheses (Supplementary Method S2 and Supplementary Table S1). Notably, these analyses also did not provide support for a relationship between AQ attention to detail subscale scores and k_i^{cer} values.

3.3. Voxel-Based Comparisons

Figure 1 (panels A and B) shows the average k_i^{cer} for ASD and control participants in voxels throughout the brain. In striatal as well as extrastriatal regions, we found no statistically significant differences in the k_i^{cer} values between ASD and controls, and in neither sample did we observe significant associations between the k_i^{cer} values and the AQ total or social interaction subscale scores. These results were similar, regardless of whether we adjusted for confounders, applied varying k_i^{cer} thresholds, used unsmoothed data or data smoothed with a 4 FWHM Gaussian filter, or examined the results for the two PET/CT scanners separately. We did observe, in accordance with the ROI analysis, that k_i^{cer} values in a small cluster of voxels in the left nucleus accumbens, significantly negatively correlated with the AQ attention to detail subscale in the ASD sample (and not in controls) (Figure 1C). At more lenient p-value thresholds, this association extended to larger parts of the striatum bilaterally.

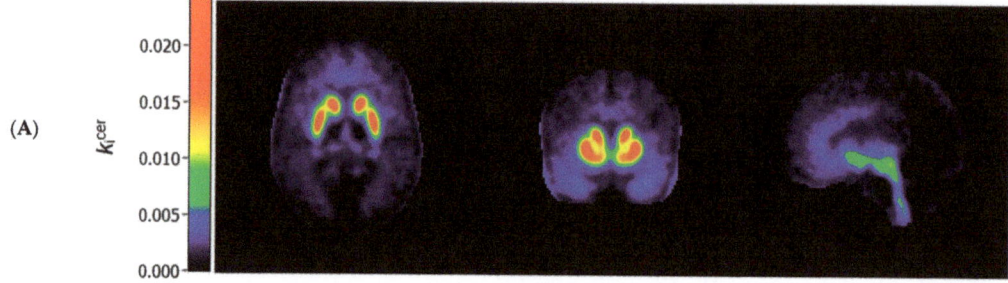

Figure 1. Cont.

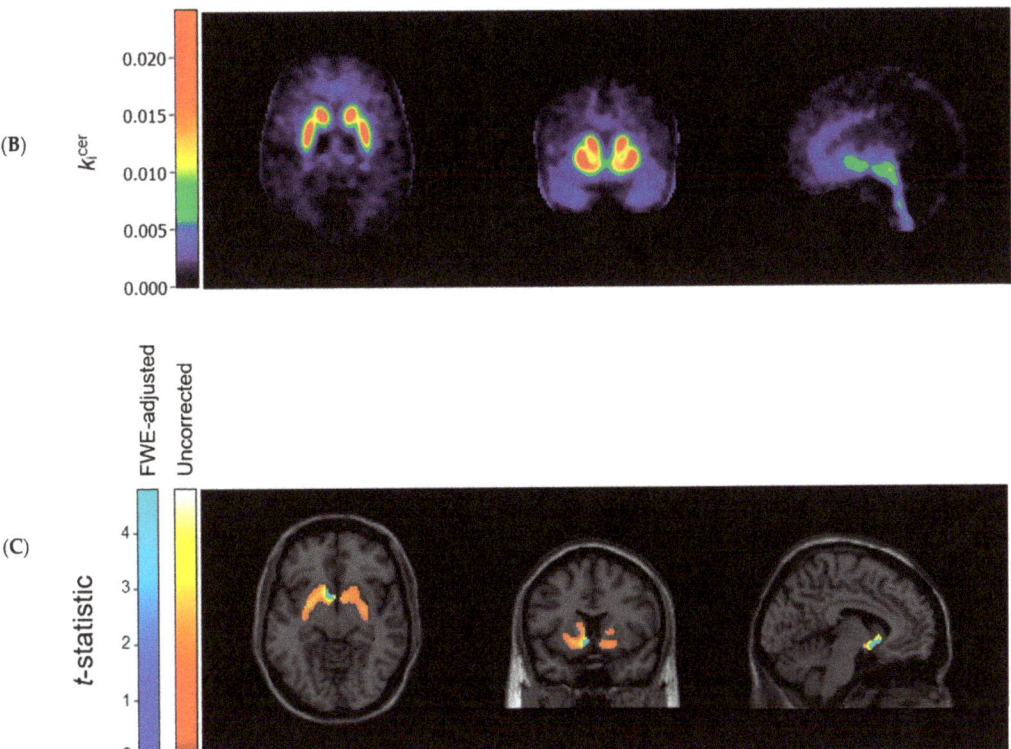

Figure 1. Axial (left), coronal (middle), and sagittal (right) view of the mean cerebral [^{18}F]-FDOPA uptake (k_i^{cer} min^{-1}; unadjusted and unsmoothed) in (**A**) adults with autism spectrum disorder ($n = 44$) and (**B**) controls ($n = 22$). Panel (**C**) shows statistically significant negative associations between scores on the autism spectrum quotient attention to detail subscale and k_i^{cer} values in autistic adults, overlaid on a single subject T1-weighted MRI scan, when family-wise error (FWE) rate-adjusted or unadjusted p-values of 0.05 are used (8 mm smoothing, threshold of $k_i^{cer} \geq 0.005$).

4. Discussion

In this exploratory study, we found no significant differences in the striatal and extrastriatal [^{18}F]-FDOPA uptake between unmedicated autistic adults and controls. In the ASD sample, but not in the control or combined samples, the AQ attention to detail subscale scores were significantly and negatively correlated with dopamine synthesis capacity in the whole striatum, the putamen, and particularly the nucleus accumbens, although these findings were not supported by Bayesian analyses.

The results of our exploratory analyses confirm our previous ROI analysis, in which we found no differences in [^{18}F]-FDOPA uptake in the striatum and its functional sub-regions (i.e., associative, limbic, and sensorimotor striatum) between ASD and controls [9]. We extend these findings by showing that [^{18}F]-FDOPA uptake does not differ in anatomical sub-regions of the striatum (i.e., putamen, nucleus accumbens, and caudate nucleus) nor in extrastriatal brain regions. In the striatum, [^{18}F]-FDOPA is decarboxylated to fluorodopamine through amino acid decarboxylase (AADC) and stored in vesicles within presynaptic terminals [20]. Although it is well-established that striatal [^{18}F]-FDOPA uptake represents dopamine synthesis capacity, the radiotracer is taken up and stored by all AADC-containing, monoaminergic neurons [21]. On the one hand, this can be considered a limitation of the method, since to some extent it remains unknown what [^{18}F]-FDOPA uptake in extrastriatal regions reflects. On the other hand, since we observed no significant difference in uptake in the whole brain, this can indicate that, for instance, also serotonergic functioning in the raphe nuclei is unaltered in ASD [22].

Our findings partially differ from the study by Ernst et al. [5], who reported a decreased [^{18}F]-FDOPA uptake in the anterior medial prefrontal cortex in autistic children ($n = 14$), and from the study by Nieminen von Wendt et al. [6], who found an increased [^{18}F]-FDOPA uptake in the striatal and frontal regions in adults with Asperger syndrome ($n = 8$). Future studies can assess whether the differences between samples in factors, such as age, ASD diagnosis, and symptom severity, can have contributed to these partially discrepant findings.

Although we found no group differences in [^{18}F]-FDOPA uptake, we did find significant negative associations between AQ attention to detail subscale scores and dopamine synthesis capacity in striatal ROIs among ASD adults. These findings should be interpreted with caution since multiple tests were performed, and Bayesian analyses were inconsistent with these observations. Nevertheless, it is of interest that a recent study also showed that in individuals with ASD ($n = 18$), but not in controls ($n = 20$), striatal dopamine D_1 receptor binding was negatively associated with the same AQ attention to detail subscale [23]. This finding can be accounted for by either increased endogenous dopamine or by the expression of fewer D_1 receptors. This latter explanation seems more plausible, since the authors note that the assessment of D_1 receptor binding is unlikely to be strongly influenced by the availability of endogenous dopamine. Our findings of no increased striatal dopamine synthesis capacity in ASD, and a recent report of a decreased striatal dopamine release in response to monetary reward in adults with ASD ($n = 10$) compared to controls ($n = 12$) [24], support this interpretation, as these suggest that endogenous synaptic dopamine is not higher in ASD. Together, these findings can then be interpreted as indicating that a reduction in striatal dopamine signaling is associated with attentional processes relevant to ASD, which accords with previous theoretical and empirical work on the role of striatal dopamine in ASD [1–3,25].

If striatal dopamine is indeed related to attentional processing in ASD, and we emphasize that this finding requires replication in an independent cohort, then it can do so in different ways. For example, striatal dopamine can be involved in the direction of attention to salient information [25–27], which would fit with our finding that associations were strongest in the nucleus accumbens, a region known to play a role in these cognitive processes [28]. It is also possible that our findings reflect alterations secondary to the perturbations in other neurotransmitter systems. Future studies, combining molecular imaging methods with objective assessments of cognitive functioning would be useful in this respect. Of note, there has been a relative scarcity of molecular imaging studies in ASD [4], and future (preferably longitudinal) assessments of different aspects of the dopamine and other neurotransmitter systems would help elucidate the role of these systems in ASD. Such assessments can also increase our knowledge on the reasons why certain medications might (not) work in autistic individuals. Given their high prescription rates [29], this seems useful and necessary.

The strengths of the present study are its large sample size and the completion of additional analyses to ensure the robustness of our findings. Note that, as reported previously [9], the mean cerebellar standardized uptake values were comparable for ASD and controls and, therefore, possible differences in non-specific uptake of [^{18}F]-FDOPA can be excluded. A first limitation of the study is the exclusion of participants who used medication or had been diagnosed with a low IQ or a psychotic disorder, as we do not know how our findings generalize to those populations. Second, autistic traits were assessed by self-report only. Third, since the study was exploratory, we did not conduct a priori sample size calculations for the present study purposes. Fourth, data were collected on two PET/CT systems. However, reconstruction parameters for the two scanners were harmonized using published guidelines [30], and scanner type was added as a covariate to the analyses. Fifth, we chose to use [^{18}F]-FDOPA analyses methods based on previous literature (e.g., [18]) and conducted additional sensitivity analyses (e.g., with varying k_i^{cer}

thresholds); however, future studies should explore the added value of more sophisticated analysis methods. For example, the role of partial volume correction should be further investigated, as some studies have indicated GM/WM differences between autistic individuals and healthy controls [31,32].

In conclusion, our exploratory findings indicate that [^{18}F]-FDOPA uptake in the brain does not significantly differ between autistic adults and controls. The striatal dopamine synthesis capacity can be negatively associated with scores on the AQ attention to detail subscale in autistic adults, but replication of this finding is necessary.

Supplementary Materials: The following are available online at https://www.mdpi.com/2075-4418/11/12/2404/s1. Table S1: Bayes factors (BF$_{10}$) for the analyses examining striatal [^{18}F]-FDOPA uptake (k_i^{cer} min^{-1}) in autistic adults and controls, and its association with self-reported autistic traits.

Author Contributions: Conceptualization, R.S., L.-F.d.G.-O., J.-P.S., T.v.A., J.B. and F.H.P.v.V.; Methodology, R.S., L.-F.d.G.-O., J.-P.S., M.Y., A.S., T.v.A., J.B. and F.H.P.v.V.; Software, R.S., F.H.P.v.V., A.S. and M.Y.; Validation, R.S., F.H.P.v.V., A.S. and M.Y.; Formal Analysis, R.S. and F.H.P.v.V.; Investigation, R.S., L.-F.d.G.-O. and F.H.P.v.V.; Resources, L.-F.d.G.-O., J.-P.S., M.Y., A.S., T.v.A., J.B. and F.H.P.v.V.; Data Curation, R.S., L.-F.d.G.-O., J.-P.S. and F.H.P.v.V.; Writing—Original Draft Preparation, R.S.; Writing—Review and Editing, L.-F.d.G.-O., J.-P.S., M.Y., A.S., T.v.A., J.B. and F.H.P.v.V.; Visualization, R.S., F.H.P.v.V., A.S. and M.Y.; Supervision, L.-F.d.G.-O., J.-P.S., J.B. and F.H.P.v.V.; Project Administration, R.S., L.-F.d.G.-O., J.-P.S. and F.H.P.v.V.; Funding Acquisition, L.-F.d.G.-O., J.-P.S. and F.H.P.v.V. All authors have read and agreed to the published version of the manuscript.

Funding: The study was funded in part by Stichting J.M.C. Kapteinfonds.

Institutional Review Board Statement: The study was conducted according to the guidelines of the Declaration of Helsinki, and approved by the Medical Ethical Committee of Leiden University Medical Center (reference NL54244.058.15; date of approval: 5 July 2016).

Informed Consent Statement: Informed consent was obtained from all subjects involved in the study.

Data Availability Statement: The datasets generated during and/or analyzed during the current study are available from the corresponding author upon reasonable request.

Acknowledgments: We would like to thank Jacqueline Aanholt-Bijlemeer, Ina Boot, Neanke Bouwman, Robert Bovenkerk, Johan van Brecht, Michael Bruijns, Paul de Bruin, Mark van Buchem, Petra Dibbets-Schneider, Demi Jansen, Jordi Vonk-van Oosten, and Patrick van der Zwet for facilitating the MRI and PET/CT scans. Furthermore, we would like to express our gratitude to Daniëlle Bos, Carlijn Clemens, Truda Driesen, Debora Op 't Eijnde, Erik Giltay, Jori Henke, and Jessie Kosterman for their assistance with conducting this study. We would also like to thank Ronald Boellaard, Patricia Cambraia Lopes, Elsmarieke van de Giessen, Sandeep Golla, Claus Svarer, and Charlotte van der Vos for their support with PET/CT data processing, and Fabian Termorshuizen for his support with the statistical analyses. Finally, we would like to thank JADOS (in particular Elles van Woerkum and Paul Stoffer), Anna Souverijn, Marcel Melchers, Els van der Ven, Villa Abel, PAS Nederland, Leviaan, aspergersyndroom.nl, autsider.net, RIAN Autismenetwerk, and the Dutch Association for Autism (Nederlandse Vereniging voor Autisme) for their help with recruiting study participants.

Conflicts of Interest: The authors declare no conflict of interest.

References

1. Baron-Cohen, S.; Wheelwright, S.; Skinner, R.; Martin, J.; Clubley, E. The autism-spectrum quotient (AQ): Evidence from asperger syndrome/high-functioning autism, males and females, scientists and mathematicians. *J. Autism Dev. Disord.* **2001**, *31*, 5–17. [CrossRef] [PubMed]
2. Brown, W.D.; Taylor, M.; Roberts, A.D.; Oakes, T.R.; Schueller, M.; Holden, J.E.; Malischke, L.; DeJesus, O.T.; Nickles, R.J. FluoroDOPA PET shows the nondopaminergic as well as dopaminergic destinations of levodopa. *Neurology* **1999**, *53*, 1212–1218. [CrossRef] [PubMed]
3. Cauda, F.; Geda, E.; Sacco, K.; D'Agata, F.; Duca, S.; Geminiani, G.; Keller, R. Grey matter abnormality in autism spectrum disorder: An activation likelihood estimation meta-analysis study. *J. Neurol. Neurosurg. Psychiatry* **2011**, *82*, 1304–1313. [CrossRef] [PubMed]

4. Cools, R.; D'Esposito, M. Inverted-U-shaped dopamine actions on human working memory and cognitive control. *Biol. Psychiatry* **2011**, *69*, e113–e125. [CrossRef] [PubMed]
5. Damasio, A.R.; Maurer, R.G. A neurological model for childhood autism. *Arch. Neurol.* **1978**, *35*, 777–786. [CrossRef] [PubMed]
6. Egerton, A.; Demjaha, A.; McGuire, P.; Mehta, M.A.; Howes, O.D. The test–retest reliability of 18F-DOPA PET in assessing striatal and extrastriatal presynaptic dopaminergic function. *Neuroimage* **2010**, *50*, 524–531. [CrossRef]
7. Ernst, M.; Zametkin, A.; Matochik, J.; Pascualvaca, D.; Cohen, R. Low medial prefrontal dopaminergic activity in autistic children. *Lancet* **1997**, *350*, 638. [CrossRef]
8. Fuccillo, M.V. Striatal circuits as a common node for autism pathophysiology. *Front. Neurosci.* **2016**, *10*, 27. [CrossRef]
9. Hammers, A.; Allom, R.; Koepp, M.J.; Free, S.L.; Myers, R.; Lemieux, L.; Mitchell, T.N.; Brooks, D.J.; Duncan, J.S. Three-dimensional maximum probability atlas of the human brain, with particular reference to the temporal lobe. *Hum. Brain Mapp.* **2003**, *19*, 224–247. [CrossRef]
10. Hoekstra, R.A.; Bartels, M.; Cath, D.C.; Boomsma, D.I. Factor structure, reliability and criterion validity of the Autism-Spectrum Quotient (AQ): A study in Dutch population and patient groups. *J. Autism Dev. Disord.* **2008**, *38*, 1555–1566. [CrossRef]
11. Hus, V.; Lord, C. The autism diagnostic observation schedule, module 4: Revised algorithm and standardized severity scores. *J. Autism Dev. Disord.* **2014**, *44*, 1996–2012. [CrossRef] [PubMed]
12. JASP Team. *JASP (Version 0.16)*; University of Amsterdam: Amsterdam, The Netherlands, 2021.
13. Kapur, S.; Mizrahi, R.; Li, M. From dopamine to salience to psychosis—Linking biology, pharmacology and phenomenology of psychosis. *Schizophr. Res.* **2005**, *79*, 59–68. [CrossRef]
14. Kubota, M.; Fujino, J.; Tei, S.; Takahata, K.; Matsuoka, K.; Tagai, K.; Sano, Y.; Yamamoto, Y.; Shimada, H.; Takado, Y. Binding of Dopamine D_1 receptor and noradrenaline transporter in individuals with autism spectrum disorder: A PET study. *Cereb. Cortex* **2020**, *30*, 6458–6468. [CrossRef] [PubMed]
15. Lai, M.-C.; Kassee, C.; Besney, R.; Bonato, S.; Hull, L.; Mandy, W.; Szatmari, P.; Ameis, S.H. Prevalence of co-occurring mental health diagnoses in the autism population: A systematic review and meta-analysis. *Lancet Psychiatry* **2019**, *6*, 819–829. [CrossRef]
16. Lord, C.; Petkova, E.; Hus, V.; Gan, W.; Lu, F.; Martin, D.M.; Ousley, O.; Guy, L.; Bernier, R.; Gerdts, J. A multisite study of the clinical diagnosis of different autism spectrum disorders. *Arch. Gen. Psychiatry* **2012**, *69*, 306–313. [CrossRef]
17. Moore, R.Y.; Whone, A.L.; McGowan, S.; Brooks, D.J. Monoamine neuron innervation of the normal human brain: An ^{18}F-DOPA PET study. *Brain Res.* **2003**, *982*, 137–145. [CrossRef]
18. Nieminen-von Wendt, T.S.; Metsähonkala, L.; Kulomäki, T.A.; Aalto, S.; Autti, T.H.; Vanhala, R.; Eskola, O.; Bergman, J.; Hietala, J.A.; von Wendt, L.O. Increased presynaptic dopamine function in Asperger syndrome. *Neuroreport* **2004**, *15*, 757–760. [CrossRef]
19. Patlak, C.S.; Blasberg, R.G. Graphical evaluation of blood-to-brain transfer constants from multiple-time uptake data. Generalizations. *J. Cereb. Blood Flow Metab.* **1985**, *5*, 584–590. [CrossRef] [PubMed]
20. Pavăl, D. A dopamine hypothesis of autism spectrum disorder. *Dev. Neurosci.* **2017**, *39*, 355–360. [CrossRef]
21. Pavăl, D.; Micluția, I.V. The dopamine hypothesis of autism spectrum disorder revisited: Current status and future prospects. *Dev. Neurosci.* **2021**, *43*, 73–83. [CrossRef]
22. Pavese, N.; Simpson, B.; Metta, V.; Ramlackhansingh, A.; Chaudhuri, K.R.; Brooks, D.J. [^{18}F]FDOPA uptake in the raphe nuclei complex reflects serotonin transporter availability. A combined [^{18}F]FDOPA and [^{11}C]DASB PET study in Parkinson's disease. *Neuroimage* **2012**, *59*, 1080–1084. [CrossRef]
23. Quarantelli, M.; Berkouk, K.; Prinster, A.; Landeau, B.; Svarer, C.; Balkay, L.; Alfano, B.; Brunetti, A.; Baron, J.-C.; Salvatore, M. Integrated software for the analysis of brain PET/SPECT studies with partial-volume-effect correction. *J. Nucl. Med.* **2004**, *45*, 192–201.
24. Radua, J.; Via, E.; Catani, M.; Mataix-Cols, D. Voxel-based meta-analysis of regional white-matter volume differences in autism spectrum disorder versus healthy controls. *Psychol. Med.* **2011**, *41*, 1539–1550. [CrossRef] [PubMed]
25. Salgado, S.; Kaplitt, M.G. The nucleus accumbens: A comprehensive review. *Stereotact. Funct. Neurosurg.* **2015**, *93*, 75–93. [CrossRef]
26. Schalbroeck, R.; van Velden, F.H.P.; de Geus-Oei, L.-F.; Yaqub, M.; van Amelsvoort, T.; Booij, J.; Selten, J.-P. Striatal dopamine synthesis capacity in autism spectrum disorder and its relation with social defeat: An [^{18}F]-FDOPA PET/CT study. *Transl. Psychiatry* **2021**, *11*, 47. [CrossRef]
27. Selten, J.-P.; Booij, J.; Buwalda, B.; Meyer-Lindenberg, A. Biological mechanisms whereby social exclusion may contribute to the etiology of psychosis: A narrative review. *Schizophr. Bull.* **2017**, *43*, 287–292. [CrossRef]
28. Svarer, C.; Madsen, K.; Hasselbalch, S.G.; Pinborg, L.H.; Haugbøl, S.; Frøkjær, V.G.; Holm, S.; Paulson, O.B.; Knudsen, G.M. MR-based automatic delineation of volumes of interest in human brain PET images using probability maps. *Neuroimage* **2005**, *24*, 969–979. [CrossRef] [PubMed]
29. Verwer, E.E.; Golla, S.; Kaalep, A.; Lubberink, M.; van Velden, F.; Bettinardi, V.; Yaqub, M.; Sera, T.; Rijnsdorp, S.; Lammertsma, A.A.; et al. Harmonisation of PET/CT contrast recovery performance for brain studies. *Eur. J. Nucl. Med. Mol. Imaging* **2021**, *48*, 2856–2870. [CrossRef]
30. Wong, A.Y.; Hsia, Y.; Chan, E.W.; Murphy, D.G.; Simonoff, E.; Buitelaar, J.K.; Wong, I.C. The variation of psychopharmacological prescription rates for people with autism spectrum disorder (ASD) in 30 countries. *Autism Res.* **2014**, *7*, 543–554. [CrossRef] [PubMed]

31. Zürcher, N.R.; Bhanot, A.; McDougle, C.J.; Hooker, J.M. A systematic review of molecular imaging (PET and SPECT) in autism spectrum disorder: Current state and future research opportunities. *Neurosci. Biobehav. Rev.* **2015**, *52*, 56–73. [CrossRef]
32. Zürcher, N.R.; Walsh, E.C.; Phillips, R.D.; Cernasov, P.M.; Tseng, C.-E.J.; Dharanikota, A.; Smith, E.; Li, Z.; Kinard, J.L.; Bizzell, J.C. A simultaneous [^{11}C]raclopride positron emission tomography and functional magnetic resonance imaging investigation of striatal dopamine binding in autism. *Transl. Psychiatry* **2021**, *11*, 33. [CrossRef] [PubMed]

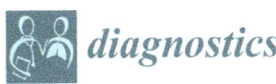

Case Report

Quantitative, Dynamic ^{18}F-FDG PET/CT in Monitoring of Smoldering Myeloma: A Case Report

Christos Sachpekidis *, Matthias Türk and Antonia Dimitrakopoulou-Strauss

Clinical Cooperation Unit Nuclear Medicine, German Cancer Research Center, Heidelberg 69120, Germany; matthias.tuerk@gmx.de (M.T.); a.dimitrakopoulou-strauss@dkfz.de (A.D.-S.)
* Correspondence: c.sachpekidis@dkfz-heidelberg.de or christos_saxpe@yahoo.gr; Tel.: +49-6221-42-2478; Fax: +49-6221-42-2476

Abstract: We report on a 52-year-old patient with an initial diagnosis of smoldering myeloma (SMM), who was monitored by means of dynamic and static positron emission tomography/computed tomography (PET/CT) with the radiotracer ^{18}F-fluorodeoxyglucose (^{18}F-FDG). Baseline PET/CT revealed no pathological signs. Six months later, a transition to symptomatic, multiple myeloma (MM) was diagnosed. The transition was not accompanied by focal, hypermetabolic lesions on PET/CT. However, a diffusely increased ^{18}F-FDG uptake in the bone marrow, accompanied by a marked increase of semi-quantitative (standardized uptake value, SUV) and quantitative, pharmacokinetic ^{18}F-FDG parameters, was demonstrated. After successful treatment, including tandem autologous transplantation, the diffuse uptake in the bone marrow as well as the semi-quantitative and quantitative parameters showed a marked remission. This response was also confirmed by the clinical follow-up of the patient. These findings suggest that in MM a diffuse ^{18}F-FDG uptake in the bone marrow may indeed reflect an actual bone marrow infiltration by plasma cells. Moreover, SUV values and kinetic parameters, not only from myeloma lesions but also from random bone marrow samples, may be used for MM monitoring. This could be particularly helpful in the follow-up of myeloma patients negative for ^{18}F-FDG-avid focal lesions.

Keywords: smoldering myeloma; multiple myeloma; quantitative; dynamic ^{18}F-FDG PET/CT; autologous stem cell transplantation

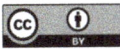

1. Introduction

Multiple myeloma (MM) is a neoplastic plasma cell disorder, characterized by the uncontrolled, clonal proliferation of plasma cells in the bone marrow. It is the second most common hematologic malignancy after non-Hodgkin lymphoma and accounts for approximately 1% of neoplastic diseases [1]. MM is almost always preceded by a premalignant precursor condition (monoclonal gammopathy of undetermined significance, MGUS), which then develops into asymptomatic or smoldering myeloma (SMM) and, finally, into symptomatic disease [2,3]. SMM represents a highly heterogeneous entity with a progression risk to MM of 10% per year during the first five years after diagnosis [4]. Different risk stratification models for progression of SMM to MM have been developed, the most popular being the Mayo Clinic model, which utilizes M-protein, bone marrow plasma cell infiltration and the ratio of serum free light chain, and the Spanish model, which uses flow-cytometry to define the proportion of aberrant plasma cells in the marrow and the presence of immunoparesis [5,6]. The identification of those SMM patients who have a high risk of progression to active, symptomatic disease is of utmost clinical importance, since these patients would benefit from early treatment commencement [7,8]. In this context, in 2014, the definition of MM was revised by the International Myeloma Working group (IMWG), including the subset of SMM patients with an 80% two-year risk of progression to symptomatic MM, based on findings from bone marrow biopsy, serum free light chain and magnetic resonance imaging (MRI) [9].

The role of positron emission tomography/computed tomography (PET/CT) with the radiotracer ^{18}F-fluorodeoxyglucose (^{18}F-FDG) in multiple myeloma (MM) has been markedly upgraded in recent years. A steadily increasing amount of literature has highlighted the value of the imaging modality in diagnosis, prognosis and treatment response evaluation of the disease [10–15]. Proof of the established role of PET/CT in MM management, is its inclusion in the latest updated criteria for the diagnosis of the disease by IMWG. In particular, the detection of one or more osteolytic lesions on CT or PET/CT fulfills the criteria of bone disease and, therefore, of symptomatic MM requiring treatment [10]. Although still limited, the first results of the application of ^{18}F-FDG PET/CT in asymptomatic SMM have been promising, reflecting the potential role of the modality in predicting the risk of progression to symptomatic disease [16,17].

On the other hand, in myeloma—more than in other malignancies—issues on the evaluation of ^{18}F-FDG PET/CT exist. This is mainly attributed to the different patterns of bone marrow involvement in the disease, which results in poor inter-observer reproducibility in scan interpretation [18]. In an attempt to standardize the interpretation of ^{18}F-FDG PET/CT scans in MM, several efforts have been undertaken, making use of visual [18,19] as well as semi-quantitative and quantitative approaches [20–24]. However, none of these methods have been yet extensively applied in clinical practice.

We herein report on a patient with an initial diagnosis of SMM who was monitored throughout the physical history of the disease by means of quantitative, dynamic ^{18}F-FDG PET/CT.

2. Case Report

A 52-year-old male patient with a diagnosis of SMM of IgG-lambda type (initial bone marrow plasma cell infiltration rate 10%) was referred to the nuclear medicine department for staging purposes. The patient underwent both dynamic and static PET/CT (Biograph mCT, S128, Siemens Co., Erlangen, Germany) with ^{18}F-FDG. In particular, after an intravenous bolus administration of ^{18}F-FDG, dynamic PET/CT was performed over the lower abdomen and pelvis for 60 min using a 24-frame protocol (10 frames of 30 s, 5 frames of 60 s, 5 frames of 120 s and 4 frames of 600 s). After the end of the dynamic acquisition, whole body, static imaging from the head to the feet was performed with an image duration of 2 min per bed position for the emission scans. Data analysis of PET/CT consisted of the conventional visual (qualitative) and semi-quantitative (standardized uptake value, SUV) evaluation, as well as the quantitative analysis of the dynamic ^{18}F-FDG PET/CT data, which was based on two-tissue compartment modeling (Figure 1) [25–28] and fractal analysis [29].

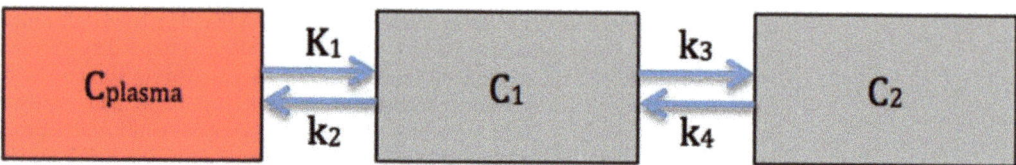

Figure 1. Schematic representation of the two-tissue compartment model applied for ^{18}F-FDG. K_1, k_2, k_3 and k_4 are rate constants (1/min) and describe the directional exchanges between the three compartments. C_{plasma} represents the vascular compartment, C_1 represents the free and non-specifically bound tracer in tissue (non-displaceable compartment) and C_2 represents the specifically bound (phosphorylated) tracer in tissue. K_1 reflects the carrier-mediated transport of ^{18}F-FDG from plasma to tissue and k_2 reflects the transport of the radiopharmaceutical back from tissue to plasma, while k_3 represents the phosphorylation rate and k_4 the dephosphorylation rate of the glucose analogue.

Baseline PET/CT at SMM diagnosis revealed no pathological findings suggestive of myeloma. Merely, a discretely increased, diffuse tracer uptake in the bone marrow was noticed, which was, however, not higher than liver uptake (Figure 2A). Six months later, a transition from asymptomatic SMM to symptomatic MM was diagnosed, after a pathological fracture of the right humerus—treated with surgery and radiotherapy—accompanied by respective increases of the M-protein (from 3.1 g/dL to 6.1 g/dL), and the lambda light chains in serum (from 135 mg/L to 306 mg/L) and urine (from unmeasurable levels to 20.6 mg/24 h). The patient was re-assessed with dynamic and static PET/CT, which demonstrated no focal hypermetabolic lesions. However, a new, intense, diffuse ^{18}F-FDG uptake in the bone marrow of the axial skeleton was now delineated (Figure 2B). With regard to the semi-quantitative PET/CT parameters, SUV_{mean} and SUV_{max} of the iliac bone increased by 82% and 91%, respectively, in comparison to the baseline scan. Similar changes were observed in the pharmacokinetic parameters derived from dynamic PET/CT: the regional blood volume (V_B) increased by 150%, the tracer influx (K_i) increased by 200%, and fractal dimension (FD) also increased by 16% (Table 1; Figure 3). The patient was treated with bortezomib-based induction therapy, followed by tandem high-dose chemotherapy (HDT) and autologous stem cell transplantation (ASCT). Two months after therapy, a third PET/CT demonstrated a pronounced remission of the diffuse bone marrow uptake (Figure 2C), accompanied by a marked decrease of the respective semi-quantitative and quantitative parameters to levels similar to or even lower than those of baseline PET/CT (Table 1; Figure 3). These findings were in line with respective changes of the M-protein (decrease to 1.1 g/dL), and the lambda light chains in serum (decrease to 24 mg/L) and urine (decrease to unmeasurable levels). The patient, furthermore, received maintenance therapy with lenalidomide. At last contact, he had not shown any disease progression, having reached a progression-free survival (PFS) of 74 months.

Table 1. Semi-quantitative and quantitative parameters of the bone marrow (iliac bone) derived from dynamic PET/CT at the three time points of scanning. The units of parameters fractional blood volume (V_B), K_1, k_3 and influx (K_i) are 1/min. SUV_{mean}, SUV_{max} and fractal dimension (FD) have no unit.

Parameter	Baseline PET/CT (SMM)	First Follow-Up PET/CT (MM Transition)	Second Follow-Up PET/CT (MM after ASCT)
SUV_{mean}	2.2	4.0	1.4
SUV_{max}	3.3	6.3	1.6
V_B	0.02	0.05	0.001
K_1	0.31	0.39	0.18
k_3	0.03	0.09	0.04
Influx (K_i)	0.01	0.03	0.01
FD	1.09	1.26	1.05

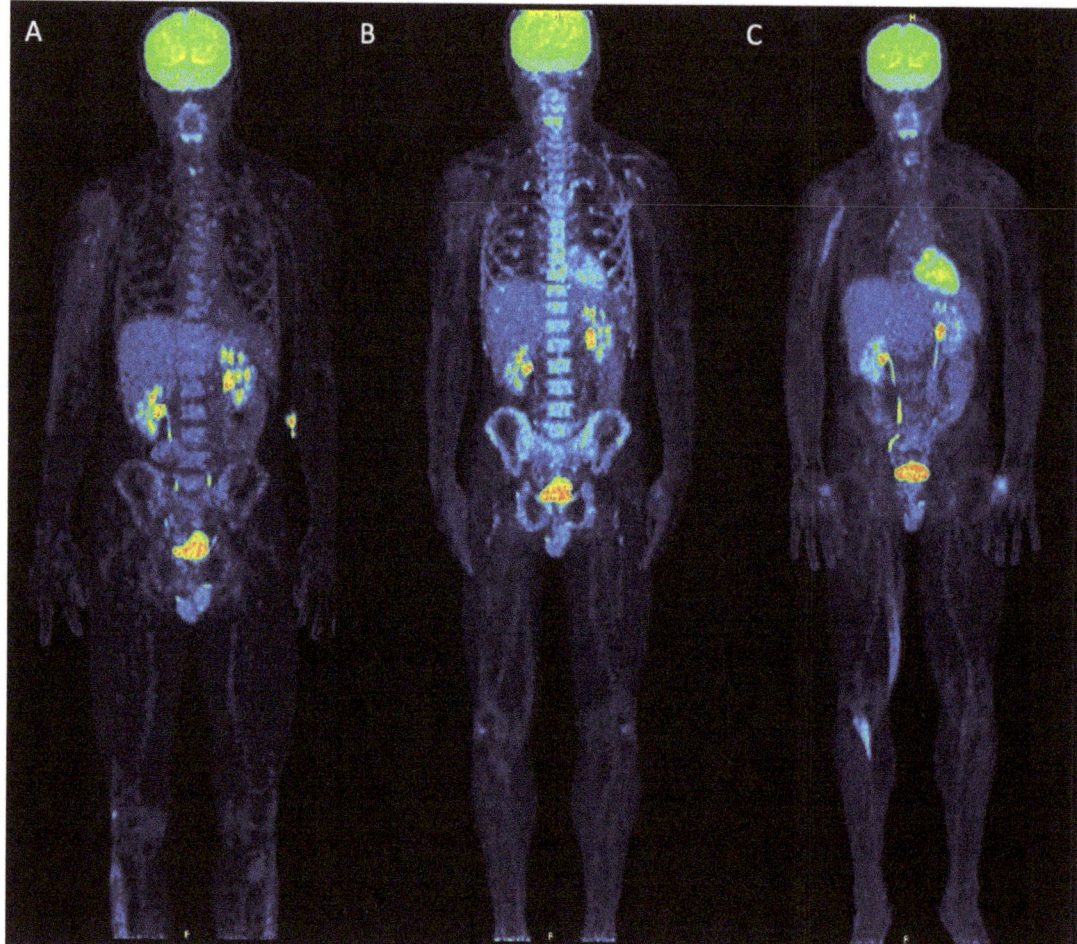

Figure 2. Maximum intensity projection (MIP) ^{18}F-FDG PET/CT images upon SMM diagnosis (**A**), at transition to symptomatic MM (**B**) and after therapeutic intervention (**C**). Baseline PET/CT upon asymptomatic SMM showed no pathological findings. A discretely increased, diffuse tracer uptake in the bone marrow ($\leq$liver uptake) is observed. The foci of increased ^{18}F-FDG uptake in the lower abdomen/pelvis correspond to physiological urinary tracer activity in the ureters, while the focal ^{18}F-FDG accumulation in the right knee joint most likely represents an inflammatory process. Semi-quantitative calculations revealed a SUV_{mean} of the iliac bone of 2.2 (SUV_{max} 3.3). According to the quantitative, pharmacokinetic analysis, the influx of ^{18}F-FDG in the bone marrow was 0.01 (1/min) (**A**). The first follow-up PET/CT scan at the time of symptomatic myeloma transition (6 months later) revealed an intense, diffuse ^{18}F-FDG uptake in the bone marrow of the axial skeleton without any focal lesions. SUV_{mean} of the iliac bone increased to 4.0 (SUV_{max} 6.3), while the tracer influx increased to 0.03 (1/min) (**B**). Two months after successful treatment, which involved tandem HDT and ASCT, the patient underwent a second follow-up PET/CT scan. This demonstrated a pronounced remission of the diffuse bone marrow uptake and a reduction of the respective SUV values (SUV_{mean} 1.4, SUV_{max} 1.6) and influx (0.01 (1/min)) of ^{18}F-FDG. The elongated uptake in the right arm, right thigh and lower leg correspond to muscular activity. Physiological urinary tracer activity is observed in the ureters (**C**).

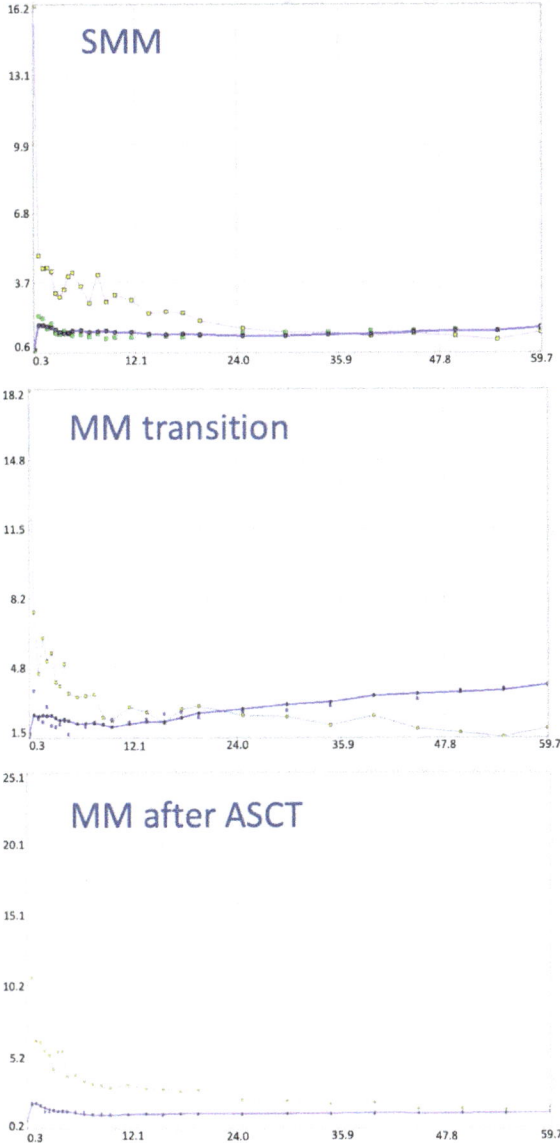

Figure 3. Time activity curves (TACs) depicting ^{18}F-FDG concentration during the 60 min of dynamic PET acquisition upon SMM diagnosis (upper row), at transition to symptomatic myeloma (middle row) and after therapy with tandem HDT and ASCT (lower row). The curves are derived from the bone marrow of the iliac bone (thick blue curve with green dots) and from the common iliac artery (thin blue curve with golden dots). The TAC at baseline imaging shows a relatively stable tracer concentration over time. The transition from asymptomatic SMM to symptomatic MM is accompanied by a change in the respective TAC of the radiotracer, showing a steadily increasing accumulation in the bone marrow compared to the definitely lower tracer concentration upon SMM. After the therapeutic intervention, we notice a decrease of the ^{18}F-FDG concentration in the bone marrow, which is also reflected in the slope of the curve.

3. Discussion

^{18}F-FDG PET/CT is regarded as a reliable outcome predictor and an elective imaging technique for treatment response evaluation of MM due to its ability in differentiating active from inactive sites of the disease [30]. Three independent, easily attainable with routine PET/CT parameters have been recognized to adversely affect both PFS and overall survival (OS). In particular, the presence of more than three focal ^{18}F-FDG-avid lesions, a $SUV_{max} > 4.2$ of the lesions and the presence of extramedullary disease (EMD) are associated with an adverse outcome [12,31]. Moreover, the complete remission of the ^{18}F-FDG-avid lesions after therapy has been shown to confer superior PFS and OS; contrarily, the persistence of pathologic findings on PET/CT after treatment is associated with a worse prognosis [12–14,31,32].

Thus far, the vast majority of PET/CT studies in MM were restricted either to descriptive analyses, mainly through the identification of focal, hypermetabolic lesions, and/or semi-quantitative analyses of parameters derived from static imaging of focal lesions. Little light, however, has been shed on the interpretation and prognostic value of the diffuse bone marrow involvement—irrespective of the presence of focal lesions—on PET/CT. Moreover, the quantitative aspect of PET, which is feasible only after performance of dynamic scanning, has only been scarcely utilized, due to the routine application of conventional, static protocols.

In the present case, we monitored by means of dynamic and static PET/CT a patient with an initially asymptomatic SMM, who demonstrated a transition to symptomatic myeloma, and was subsequently successfully treated. The patient did not show any typical signs of myeloma involvement on PET/CT, i.e., focal, hypermetabolic lesions, at any phase during the course of the disease. However, at transition from SMM to symptomatic MM, a diffusely increased ^{18}F-FDG uptake in the bone marrow was observed; this was accompanied by a marked increase of both the semi-quantitative (SUV values) and the quantitative, pharmacokinetic parameters, derived from bone marrow of the iliac crest. Importantly, after the successful therapeutic intervention, the diffuse uptake in the bone marrow as well as the semi-quantitative and quantitative parameters showed a pronounced remission. This response was also confirmed by the long-term, clinical follow-up of the patient.

Our findings suggest, firstly, that in untreated MM, a diffuse ^{18}F-FDG uptake in the bone marrow may reflect an actual bone marrow infiltration by plasma cells. Particularly in patients suffering from SMM, the appearance of a diffuse hypermetabolic bone marrow pattern—regardless of the concurrent emergence of focal lesions—during the course of the entity may reflect transition to symptomatic disease and should, therefore, lead to further investigation. We are, indeed, aware of the several causes leading to a false-positive, diffuse, homogeneous, bone marrow ^{18}F-FDG uptake on PET/CT, such as severe anemia, previous administration of granulocyte colony-stimulating factor (G-CSF), chemotherapy or erythropoietin [33]. However, in the present case, all potential causes of a false-positive bone marrow ^{18}F-FDG uptake could be excluded from the patient's history.

Secondly, SUV values not only from myeloma lesions—as consistently highlighted by previous studies—but also from random bone marrow samples, may be used to monitor disease transition and response to treatment. This could be particularly helpful in the follow-up of myeloma patients negative for ^{18}F-FDG-avid focal lesions. The metabolic state of the bone marrow as evaluated by SUV calculations and/or in comparison to reference organs has recently been put into focus of MM research, rendering promising results as a potentially prognostic factor [22,34]. The present findings are in support of this direction.

Finally, the information acquired after the application of full dynamic PET/CT was in line with the respective qualitative (visual) and semi-quantitative (SUV) findings during the different phases of the disease. The dynamic ^{18}F-FDG PET/CT protocol offers the unique advantages to investigate the tracer accumulation over time through generation of the respective time activity curves (TACs) as well as to extract pharmacokinetic indices that reflect dedicated parameters of the tracer's metabolism, such as perfusion, transport or phosphorylation. This quantitative aspect is a major advantage of PET/CT, which is neglected when using conventional, static, whole-body protocols (usually 60 min post-injection) and descriptive analysis as the only diagnostic tool. In the present case, quantitative, dynamic PET/CT showed that the transition of asymptomatic SMM to symptomatic disease was accompanied by a marked increase of ^{18}F-FDG accumulation in the bone marrow over time, compared to baseline PET/CT. Moreover, several quantitative ^{18}F-FDG parameters, including the regional blood volume (V_B), the tracer influx rate (K_i), the carrier-mediated transport of the tracer from plasma to bone marrow (K_1), the phosphorylation rate of ^{18}F-FDG in the bone marrow (k_3) as well as the degree of tracer heterogeneity—reflected by the parameter fractal dimension (FD)—showed a distinct increase. Contrarily, a pronounced decrease of the respective TAC and pharmacokinetic parameters were observed after the successful therapeutic intervention. These results are in line with previous findings of our group regarding the potential role of dynamic PET in MM prognosis and treatment response evaluation [22,35–37]. By complementing the information offered by conventional imaging with the multiparametric, pharmacokinetic data extracted by dynamic PET/CT, the diagnostic certainty of the reading physician could be enhanced, particularly in patients with ambiguous findings. Moreover, our understanding of the pathophysiology of the disease and its response to treatment can be improved.

Although these findings could suggest the wider usage of dynamic PET/CT in MM, more data, preferably derived from large prospective studies, are warranted to prove the potential benefit of the modality. Moreover, we note some practical considerations related to the possible implementation of dynamic PET/CT in clinical routine: firstly, it is more time-consuming than conventional PET/CT, since it requires in most cases a 60-min acquisition, followed by the conventional, static, whole-body PET/CT acquisition. This may lead to patient discomfort as well as to logistical issues in a nuclear medicine department. Furthermore, data interpretation is challenging, based on sophisticated software tools and application of the—rather complex—compartment modeling and fractal analysis. According to the previous, for the time being, qualitative and semi-quantitative analysis will remain the main evaluation tools of PET/CT in MM. However, dynamic PET/CT could be applied in selected cases, for example in the context of clinical trials in MM, adding significant quantitative information and reducing inter-observer variability. Moreover, the recent advent of new PET/CT scanners, which allow dynamic studies over several bed positions by using a continuous bed movement, will facilitate the use of dynamic PET protocols and reduce the whole acquisition time, making dynamic PET/CT an attractive and cost-effective approach in oncological imaging [38].

4. Conclusions

A patient with an initial diagnosis of asymptomatic SMM was monitored by means of dynamic and static ^{18}F-FDG PET/CT during the course of the disease. Upon SMM diagnosis, the patient had no pathological signs on PET/CT. The transition from SMM to symptomatic MM was not accompanied by the typical signs of myeloma involvement on PET/CT, i.e., focal, hypermetabolic lesions. However, a diffusely increased ^{18}F-FDG uptake in the bone marrow was observed, while at the same time, a marked increase of both semi-quantitative (SUV values) and quantitative, pharmacokinetic parameters was demonstrated. Following treatment, the diffuse uptake in the bone marrow as well as the semi-quantitative and quantitative parameters showed a pronounced remission. This response was also confirmed by the long-term, clinical follow-up of the patient. Altogether, the here-presented findings suggest, firstly, that in MM a diffuse ^{18}F-FDG uptake in the bone marrow may reflect an actual bone marrow infiltration by plasma cells. Secondly, SUV values not only from myeloma lesions—as highlighted by previous studies—but also from random bone marrow samples, may be used for MM monitoring; this could be particularly helpful in the follow-up of myeloma patients negative for ^{18}F-FDG-avid focal lesions. Finally, several pharmacokinetic parameters, derived from dynamic PET/CT, can be used to increase the diagnostic certainty and provide valuable information on dedicated parameters of the tracer's metabolism.

Author Contributions: C.S. performed the PET/CT studies and evaluations, analyzed the data and drafted the manuscript; M.T. analyzed the data and revised the manuscript; A.D.-S. designed the study, performed the PET/CT evaluations and revised the manuscript. All authors have read and agreed to the published version of the manuscript.

Funding: The study was part of a special research area project (SFB TRR 79) funded by the German Research Foundation and the Dietmar-Hopp-Foundation.

Institutional Review Board Statement: The present case report is part of a study, which was conducted according to the guidelines of the Declaration of Helsinki, and was approved (10.05.2010) by the ethical committee of the University of Heidelberg (S-076/2010) and the Federal Agency of Radiation Protection in Germany ("Bundesamt für Strahlenschutz").

Informed Consent Statement: Written informed consent, including consent for publication, was obtained from the patient.

Data Availability Statement: The authors confirm that the data supporting the findings of this case report are available within the article.

Conflicts of Interest: The authors declare no conflict of interest. The funders had no role in the design of the study; in the collection, analyses, or interpretation of data; in the writing of the manuscript, or in the decision to publish the results.

References

1. Palumbo, A.; Anderson, K. Multiple myeloma. *N. Engl. J. Med.* **2011**, *364*, 1046–1060. [CrossRef]
2. Kyle, R.A.; Greipp, P.R. Smoldering multiple myeloma. *N. Engl. J. Med.* **1980**, *302*, 1347–1349. [CrossRef] [PubMed]
3. Landgren, O.; Kyle, R.A.; Rajkumar, S.V. From myeloma precursor disease to multiple myeloma: New diagnostic concepts and opportunities for early intervention. *Clin. Cancer. Res.* **2011**, *17*, 1243–1252. [CrossRef]
4. Mateos, M.V.; Kumar, S.; Dimopoulos, M.A.; González-Calle, V.; Kastritis, E.; Hajek, R.; De Larrea, C.F.; Morgan, G.J.; Merlini, G.; Goldschmidt, H.; et al. International Myeloma Working Group risk stratification model for smoldering multiple myeloma (SMM). *Blood Cancer J.* **2020**, *10*, 102. [CrossRef] [PubMed]
5. Dispenzieri, A.; Kyle, R.A.; Katzmann, J.A.; Therneau, T.M.; Larson, D.; Benson, J.; Clark, R.J.; Melton, L.J., 3rd; Gertz, M.A.; Kumar, S.K.; et al. Immunoglobulin free light chain ratio is an independent risk factor for progression of smoldering (asymptomatic) multiple myeloma. *Blood* **2008**, *111*, 785–789. [CrossRef]
6. Pérez-Persona, E.; Vidriales, M.B.; Mateo, G.; García-Sanz, R.; Mateos, M.V.; de Coca, A.G.; Galende, J.; Martín-Nuñez, G.; Alonso, J.M.; de Las Heras, N.; et al. New criteria to identify risk of progression in monoclonal gammopathy of uncertain significance and smoldering multiple myeloma based on multiparameter flow cytometry analysis of bone marrow plasma cells. *Blood* **2007**, *110*, 2586–2592. [CrossRef] [PubMed]
7. Mateos, M.V.; Hernández, M.T.; Giraldo, P.; de la Rubia, J.; de Arriba, F.; López Corral, L.; Rosiñol, L.; Paiva, B.; Palomera, L.; Bargay, J.; et al. Lenalidomide plus dexamethasone for high-risk smoldering multiple myeloma. *N. Engl. J. Med.* **2013**, *369*, 438–447. [CrossRef]
8. Lonial, S.; Jacobus, S.; Fonseca, R.; Weiss, M.; Kumar, S.; Orlowski, R.Z.; Kaufman, J.L.; Yacoub, A.M.; Buadi, F.K.; O Brien, T.; et al. Randomized Trial of Lenalidomide Versus Observation in Smoldering Multiple Myeloma. *J. Clin. Oncol.* **2020**, *38*, 1126–1137. [CrossRef] [PubMed]
9. Rajkumar, S.V.; Dimopoulos, M.A.; Palumbo, A.; Blade, J.; Merlini, G.; Mateos, M.V.; Kumar, S.; Hillengass, J.; Kastritis, E.; Richardson, P.; et al. International Myeloma Working Group updated criteria for the diagnosis of multiple myeloma. *Lancet Oncol.* **2014**, *15*, e538–e548. [CrossRef]
10. Cavo, M.; Terpos, E.; Nanni, C.; Moreau, P.; Lentzsch, S.; Zweegman, S.; Hillengass, J.; Engelhardt, M.; Usmani, S.Z.; Vesole, D.H.; et al. Role of 18F-FDG PET/CT in the diagnosis and management of multiple myeloma and other plasma cell disorders: a consensus statement by the International Myeloma Working Group. *Lancet Oncol.* **2017**, *18*, e206–e217. [CrossRef]
11. Zamagni, E.; Nanni, C.; Patriarca, F.; Englaro, E.; Castellucci, P.; Geatti, O.; Tosi, P.; Tacchetti, P.; Cangini, D.; Perrone, G.; et al. A prospective comparison of 18F-fluorodeoxyglucose positron emission tomography-computed tomography, magnetic resonance imaging and whole-body planar radiographs in the assessment of bone disease in newly diagnosed multiple myeloma. *Haematologica.* **2007**, *92*, 50–55. [CrossRef] [PubMed]
12. Bartel, T.B.; Haessler, J.; Brown, T.L.; Shaughnessy, J.D., Jr.; van Rhee, F.; Anaissie, E.; Alpe, T.; Angtuaco, E.; Walker, R.; Epstein, J.; et al. F18-fluorodeoxyglucose positron emission tomography in the context of other imaging techniques and prognostic factors in multiple myeloma. *Blood* **2009**, *114*, 2068–2076. [CrossRef] [PubMed]

13. Usmani, S.Z.; Mitchell, A.; Waheed, S.; Crowley, J.; Hoering, A.; Petty, N.; Brown, T.; Bartel, T.; Anaissie, E.; van Rhee, F.; et al. Prognostic implications of serial 18-fluoro-deoxyglucose emission tomography in multiple myeloma treated with total therapy 3. *Blood* 2013, *121*, 1819–1823. [CrossRef] [PubMed]
14. Zamagni, E.; Nanni, C.; Mancuso, K.; Tacchetti, P.; Pezzi, A.; Pantani, L.; Zannetti, B.; Rambaldi, I.; Brioli, A.; Rocchi, S.; et al. PET/CT improves the definition of complete response and allows to detect otherwise unidentifiable skeletal progression in multiple Myeloma. *Clin. Cancer. Res.* 2015, *21*, 4384–4390. [CrossRef] [PubMed]
15. Moreau, P.; Attal, M.; Caillot, D.; Macro, M.; Karlin, L.; Garderet, L.; Facon, T.; Benboubker, L.; Escoffre-Barbe, M.; Stoppa, A.M.; et al. Prospective evaluation of magnetic resonance imaging and [18F]fluorodeoxyglucose positron emission tomography-computed tomography at diagnosis and before maintenance therapy in symptomatic patients with multiple myeloma included in the IFM/DFCI 2009 Trial: Results of the IMAJEM study. *J. Clin. Oncol.* 2017, *35*, 2911–2918. [CrossRef] [PubMed]
16. Siontis, B.; Kumar, S.; Dispenzieri, A.; Drake, M.T.; Lacy, M.Q.; Buadi, F.; Dingli, D.; Kapoor, P.; Gonsalves, W.; Gertz, M.A.; et al. Positron emission tomography-computed tomography in the diagnostic evaluation of smoldering multiple myeloma: Identification of patients needing therapy. *Blood Cancer J.* 2015, *5*, e364. [CrossRef]
17. Zamagni, E.; Nanni, C.; Gay, F.; Pezzi, A.; Patriarca, F.; Bellò, M.; Rambaldi, I.; Tacchetti, P.; Hillengass, J.; Gamberi, B.; et al. 18F-FDG PET/CT focal, but not osteolytic, lesions predict the progression of smoldering myeloma to active disease. *Leukemia* 2016, *30*, 417–422. [CrossRef] [PubMed]
18. Nanni, C.; Zamagni, E.; Versari, A.; Chauvie, S.; Bianchi, A.; Rensi, M.; Bellò, M.; Rambaldi, I.; Gallamini, A.; Patriarca, F.; et al. Image interpretation criteria for FDG PET/CT in multiple myeloma: A new proposal from an Italian expert panel. IMPeTUs (Italian Myeloma criteria for PET USe). *Eur. J. Nucl. Med. Mol. Imaging* 2016, *43*, 414–421. [CrossRef] [PubMed]
19. Nanni, C.; Versari, A.; Chauvie, S.; Bertone, E.; Bianchi, A.; Rensi, M.; Bellò, M.; Gallamini, A.; Patriarca, F.; Gay, F.; et al. Interpretation criteria for FDG PET/CT in multiple myeloma (IMPeTUs): Final results. IMPeTUs (Italian myeloma criteria for PET USe). *Eur. J. Nucl. Med. Mol. Imaging* 2018, *45*, 712–719. [CrossRef]
20. Fonti, R.; Larobina, M.; Del Vecchio, S.; De Luca, S.; Fabbricini, R.; Catalano, L.; Pane, F.; Salvatore, M.; Pace, L. Metabolic tumor volume assessed by 18F-FDG PET/CT for the prediction of outcome in patients with multiple myeloma. *J. Nucl. Med.* 2012, *53*, 1829–1835. [CrossRef]
21. McDonald, J.E.; Kessler, M.M.; Gardner, M.W.; Buros, A.F.; Ntambi, J.A.; Waheed, S.; van Rhee, F.; Zangari, M.; Heuck, C.J.; Petty, N.; et al. Assessment of Total lesion glycolysis by (18)F FDG PET/CT significantly improves prognostic value of GEP and ISS in myeloma. *Clin. Cancer. Res.* 2017, *23*, 1981–1987. [CrossRef] [PubMed]
22. Sachpekidis, C.; Merz, M.; Kopp-Schneider, A.; Jauch, A.; Raab, M.S.; Sauer, S.; Hillengass, J.; Goldschmidt, H.; Dimitrakopoulou-Strauss, A. Quantitative dynamic 18F-fluorodeoxyglucose positron emission tomography/computed tomography before autologous stem cell transplantation predicts survival in multiple myeloma. *Haematologica* 2019, *104*, e420–e423. [CrossRef]
23. Takahashi, M.E.S.; Mosci, C.; Souza, E.M.; Brunetto, S.Q.; Etchebehere, E.; Santos, A.O.; Camacho, M.R.; Miranda, E.; Lima, M.C.L.; Amorim, B.J.; et al. Proposal for a Quantitative 18F-FDG PET/CT Metabolic Parameter to Assess the Intensity of Bone Involvement in Multiple Myeloma. *Sci. Rep.* 2019, *9*, 16429. [CrossRef] [PubMed]
24. Terao, T.; Machida, Y.; Tsushima, T.; Kitadate, A.; Miura, D.; Narita, K.; Takeuchi, M.; Matsue, K. Prognostic Implications of Metabolic Total Volume and Total Lesion Glycolysis Assessed By PET/CT Combined with High Levels of Bone Marrow Plasma Cells Percentages As a Potential Risk Model in Patients with Newly Diagnosed Multiple Myeloma. *Blood* 2019, *134* (Suppl. 1). [CrossRef]
25. Sokoloff, L.; Smith, C.B. Basic principles underlying radioisotopic methods for assay of biochemical processes in vivo. In *The Metabolism of the Human Brain Studied with Positron Emission Tomography*; Greitz, T., Ingvar, D.H., Widén, L., Eds.; Raven Press: New York, NY, USA, 1983; pp. 123–148.
26. Miyazawa, H.; Osmont, A.; Petit-Taboué, M.C.; Tillet, I.; Travère, J.M.; Young, A.R.; Barré, L.; MacKenzie, E.T.; Baron, J.C. Determination of 18F-fluoro-2-deoxy-D-glucose rate constants in the anesthetized baboon brain with dynamic positron tomography. *J. Neurosci. Methods* 1993, *50*, 263–272. [CrossRef]
27. Pan, L.; Cheng, C.; Haberkorn, U.; Dimitrakopoulou-Strauss, A. Machine learning-based kinetic modeling: A robust and reproducible solution for quantitative analysis of dynamic PET data. *Phys. Med. Biol.* 2017, *62*, 3566–3581. [CrossRef]
28. Dimitrakopoulou-Strauss, A.; Pan, L.; Sachpekidis, C. Kinetic modeling and parametric imaging with dynamic PET for oncological applications: General considerations, current clinical applications, and future perspectives. *Eur. J. Nucl. Med. Mol. Imaging* 2020. [CrossRef]
29. Dimitrakopoulou-Strauss, A.; Strauss, L.G.; Burger, C.; Mikolajczyk, K.; Lehnert, T.; Bernd, L.; Ewerbeck, V. On the fractal nature of positron emission tomography (PET) studies. *World J. Nucl. Med.* 2003, *4*, 306–313.
30. Sachpekidis, C.; Goldschmidt, H.; Dimitrakopoulou-Strauss, A. Positron Emission Tomography (PET) Radiopharmaceuticals in Multiple Myeloma. *Molecules* 2019, *25*, 134. [CrossRef] [PubMed]
31. Zamagni, E.; Patriarca, F.; Nanni, C.; Zannetti, B.; Englaro, E.; Pezzi, A.; Tacchetti, P.; Buttignol, S.; Perrone, G.; Brioli, A.; et al. Prognostic relevance of 18-F FDG PET/CT in newly diagnosed multiple myeloma patients treated with up-front autologous transplantation. *Blood* 2011, *118*, 5989–5995. [CrossRef] [PubMed]
32. Davies, F.E.; Rosenthal, A.; Rasche, L.; Petty, N.M.; McDonald, J.E.; Ntambi, J.A.; Steward, D.M.; Panozzo, S.B.; van Rhee, F.; Zangari, M.; et al. Treatment to suppression of focal lesions on positron emission tomography-computed tomography is a therapeutic goal in newly diagnosed multiple myeloma. *Haematologica* 2018, *103*, 1047–1053. [CrossRef] [PubMed]

33. Lin, E.C.; Alavi, A. Normal variants and benign findings. In *PET and PET/CT: A Clinical Guide*, 2nd ed.; Lin, E.C., Alavi, A., Eds.; Thieme: New York, NY, USA; Stuttgart, Germany, 2005.
34. Zamagni, E.; Nanni, C.; Dozza, L.; Carlier, T.; Bailly, C.; Tacchetti, P.; Versari, A.; Chauvie, S.; Gallamini, A.; Gamberi, B.; et al. Standardization of 18F-FDG-PET/CT According to Deauville Criteria for Metabolic Complete Response Definition in Newly Diagnosed Multiple Myeloma. *J. Clin. Oncol.* **2020**, *39*, 116–125. [CrossRef] [PubMed]
35. Dimitrakopoulou-Strauss, A.; Hoffmann, M.; Bergner, R.; Uppenkamp, M.; Haberkorn, U.; Strauss, L.G. Prediction of progression-free survival in patients with multiple myeloma following anthracycline-based chemotherapy based on dynamic FDG-PET. *Clin. Nucl. Med.* **2009**, *34*, 576–584. [CrossRef] [PubMed]
36. Sachpekidis, C.; Mai, E.K.; Goldschmidt, H.; Hillengass, J.; Hose, D.; Pan, L.; Haberkorn, U.; Dimitrakopoulou-Strauss, A. (18)F-FDG dynamic PET/CT in patients with multiple myeloma: Patterns of tracer uptake and correlation with bone marrow plasma cell infiltration rate. *Clin. Nucl. Med.* **2015**, *40*, e300-7. [CrossRef] [PubMed]
37. Sachpekidis, C.; Hillengass, J.; Goldschmidt, H.; Wagner, B.; Haberkorn, U.; Kopka, K.; Dimitrakopoulou-Strauss, A. Treatment response evaluation with 18F-FDG PET/CT and 18F-NaF PET/CT in multiple myeloma patients undergoing high-dose chemotherapy and autologous stem cell transplantation. *Eur. J. Nucl. Med. Mol. Imaging* **2017**, *44*, 50–62. [CrossRef] [PubMed]
38. Zhang, X.; Xie, Z.; Berg, E.; Judenhofer, M.S.; Liu, W.; Xu, T.; Ding, Y.; Lv, Y.; Dong, Y.; Deng, Z.; et al. Total-Body Dynamic Reconstruction and Parametric Imaging on the uEXPLORER. *J. Nucl. Med.* **2020**, *61*, 285–291. [CrossRef]

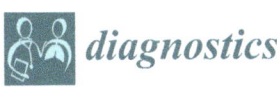

Correction

Correction: Rijnsdorp et al. Impact of the Noise Penalty Factor on Quantification in Bayesian Penalized Likelihood (Q.Clear) Reconstructions of ^{68}Ga-PSMA PET/CT Scans. *Diagnostics* 2021, *11*, 847

Sjoerd Rijnsdorp [1,*], Mark J. Roef [2] and Albert J. Arends [1]

[1] Department of Medical Physics, Catharina Hospital Eindhoven, Michelangelolaan 2, 5623 EJ Eindhoven, The Netherlands; bertjan.arends@catharinaziekenhuis.nl
[2] Department of Nuclear Medicine, Catharina Hospital Eindhoven, Michelangelolaan 2, 5623 EJ Eindhoven, The Netherlands; mark.roef@catharinaziekenhuis.nl
* Correspondence: srijnsdorp@outlook.com

In the original article [1], there was a mistake in Figure 3 as published. Due to a mistake in the publication process, Figure 2 and Figure 3 were the same. The corrected Figure 3 appears below. The authors apologize for any inconvenience caused and state that the scientific conclusions are unaffected. The original article has been updated.

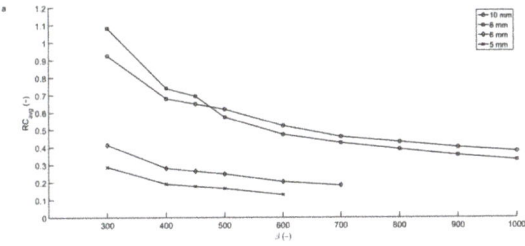

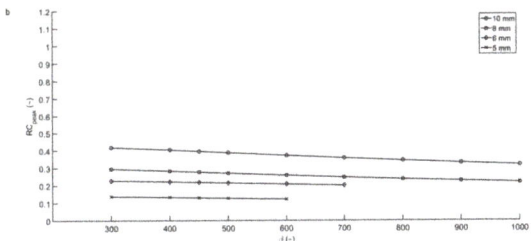

Figure 3. Average and peak recovery coefficients from the Micro Hollow Sphere phantom. For an acquisition time of two minutes per bed position, the apparent RC_{avg} (**a**) of the 8 mm sphere measured with T/B ratio 10:1 exceeds that of the bigger spheres for low β, as the center of this sphere happened to coincide with the center of a voxel. Taking RC_{peak} as a measure for the recovery coefficient (**b**), the recovery coefficients are lower, but more robust.

Conflicts of Interest: The authors declare no conflict of interest.

Reference

1. Rijnsdorp, S.; Roef, M.J.; Arends, A.J. Impact of the Noise Penalty Factor on Quantification in Bayesian Penalized Likelihood (Q.Clear) Reconstructions of ^{68}Ga-PSMA PET/CT Scans. *Diagnostics* **2021**, *11*, 847. [CrossRef] [PubMed]

MDPI
St. Alban-Anlage 66
4052 Basel
Switzerland
Tel. +41 61 683 77 34
Fax +41 61 302 89 18
www.mdpi.com

Diagnostics Editorial Office
E-mail: diagnostics@mdpi.com
www.mdpi.com/journal/diagnostics

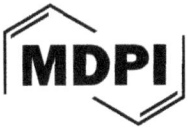

www.ingramcontent.com/pod-product-compliance
Lightning Source LLC
LaVergne TN
LVHW070743100526
838202LV00013B/1291